Perioperative Nursing Data Set

The Perioperative Nursing Vocabulary

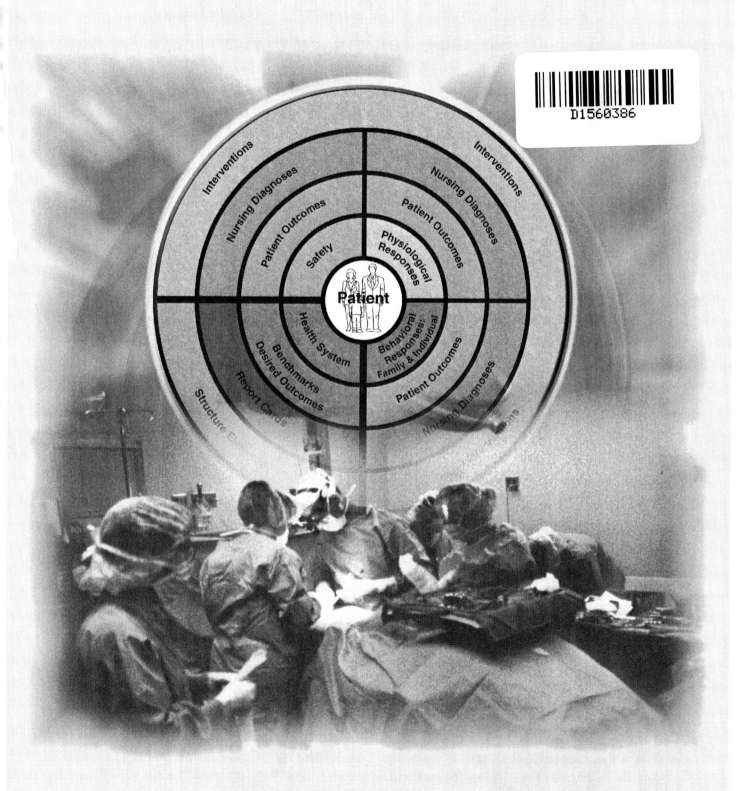

Revised Second Edition

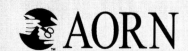

AORN

PERIOPERATIVE NURSING DATA SET©
The Perioperative Nursing Vocabulary
Revised Second Edition

Edited by
Carol Petersen, RN, BSN, MAOM, CNOR
Manager, Perioperative Nursing Data Set
AORN Center for Nursing Practice

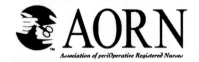

2170 South Parker Road, Suite 300
Denver, Colorado 80231
303-755-6300
www.aorn.org

NOTICE
No responsibility is assumed by AORN, Inc, for any injury and/or damage to persons or property as a matter of products liability, negligence, or otherwise, or from any use or operation of any standards, recommended practices, methods, products, instructions, or ideas contained in the material herein. Because of rapid advances in the health care sciences in particular, independent verification of diagnoses, medication dosages, and individualized care and treatment should be made. The material contained herein is not intended to be a substitute for the exercise of professional medical or nursing judgment.

Table of Contents

PART III: Applications of the PNDS

PART IV: Appendices

Index to Supplementary Materials

Foreword to the Revised Second Edition

Since the Perioperative Nursing Data Set (PNDS) was recognized in 1999 by the American Nurses Association (ANA), ongoing efforts have focused primarily on disseminating information about the PNDS and helping nurses use it in all types of clinical, education, management, and research applications. The results of these efforts include the following:

- Our vendor partners have licensed the vocabulary and embedded it in documentation software.
- Documentation is moving toward a standardization process using the data set.
- The PNDS is being used to educate new nurses, document competencies, and evaluate nursing staff.

This move toward standardization supports perioperative nurses in their efforts to provide evidence-based practice and to co-manage costs and quality. Equally important, perioperative nurses are documenting patient care that demonstrates the professional aspects of their role. This data will answer the question of why facilities need a registered nurse in the OR as well as in other perioperative settings.

Although the PNDS can be used in both paper and electronic documentation, the real advantage comes when it is implemented in the electronic health record (EHR). The manner in which data is documented, captured, and mined is a critical factor for improving health care. The PNDS is particularly suited for the EHR. It contains the framework of uniquely coded clinical terms and knowledge that describe patient care provided during a surgical or invasive procedure regardless of the setting.

Using standardized nomenclature such as the PNDS in electronic documentation provides the vehicle for gathering and aggregating data for analysis. The impact of using and mining the PNDS data is significant on several levels:

- The immediate impact is for enhanced communication and the linkage to clinical support for the perioperative nurse.
- Health care organizations benefit from effective standardized outcome reporting and quality improvement activities.

- The PNDS provides reliable and valid clinical data that can be used by researchers to uncover new clinical relationships.

Recently, AORN has undertaken a three-year project to create an integrated electronic content repository with a database-driven authoring system and PNDS electronic representation for integration in the EHR. The AORN recommended practices and the PNDS are the focus of this project because, together, these resources provide the tools necessary to guide and document perioperative nursing practice across the continuum of care. When the project is complete, the coded nursing interventions contained in both the PNDS and the recommended practices will be linked, and the terminology used to describe these interventions will be consistent. This linkage will facilitate standardized documentation of the nursing interventions in the electronic system.

Using this powerful combination of resources will provide data that nursing researchers need to evaluate perioperative nursing care. As researchers complete studies on nursing care delivered to perioperative patients, more evidence will become available to use in the creation of the content that informs nursing practice.

Although this edition has been reorganized and given a new look, **the data set itself has not changed.** Chapter 6, which is new, introduces the Perioperative Dashboard, a Web-based management tool and national database allowing members to benchmark their facility's health system data against averages for similar health facilities. New applications are presented in the exemplars in Part III and the appendices. Only minor corrections and updates have been made to the remaining chapters.

Much of the work on the PNDS should be attributed to the enormous efforts of volunteer AORN members who donated their time and energy to the Association while maintaining a job and home. All those who contributed to the applications section of this book are true representatives of these dedicated professional nurses. Volunteer members, however, could not do the job without AORN resources or staff to support and augment their endeavors. Indeed, the collaborative will of both volunteers and Association staff have successfully generated a truly valued treasure—the PNDS.

Acknowledgments

This publication would not have been possible without the authors, contributors, and reviewers who worked on the first and second editions. The editors gratefully acknowledge the following individuals for their contributions to the development of the PNDS.

Research Consultant: Susan V.M. Kleinbeck, RN, PhD, CNOR

Clinical Consultants: Dorothy M. Fogg, RN, MA; Ramona Conner, RN, MSN; Carol Petersen, RN, MAOM, CNOR

AORN Task Force on Perioperative Data Elements member volunteers: Cynthia A. Abbott, RN, PhD, CNOR, LTC; Jane A. Ensminger, RN, BSN, CNOR; Susan V. M. Kleinbeck, RN, PhD, CNOR; Julia A. Kneedler, RN, EdD; Kimberly E. Lovelace, RN, CNOR; Jeanette Polaschek, RN, MS; Margaret J. Sudduth, RN, MHS, CNOR; Suzanne F. Ward, RN, MA, MN, CNOR; **AORN staff members at the time of development:** Carol Dungan Applegeet, RN, MSN, CNOR, CNAA, FAAN; Linda J. Brazen, RN, CNOR; Margaret A. Camp, RN, MSN; Dorothy M. Fogg, RN, MA; Eileen J. Ullmann, RN, MHS, CNOR; American Nurses Association (ANA) consultant: Kathy Milholland, RN, PhD.

Data Elements Coordinating Committee (DECC): Joy Don Baker, RN, MS, MBA, CNOR; Renae N. Burchiel, RN, MN, CNOR; Jane A. Ensminger, RN, BSN, CNOR, Chair of DECC; Nancy Marie Fortunato, RN, MEd, CNOR, CPSN; Kelly M. Gollar, RN, MSN, CNOR; Aileen R. Killen, RN, PhD, CNOR; Cecil A. King, RN, MSN, CNOR; Susan V. M. Kleinbeck, RN, PhD, CNOR; Julia A. Kneedler, RN, EdD; Kimberly E. Lovelace, RN, CNOR; Anne S. Medlin, RN, BSN, CNOR; Kathy Milholland, RN, PhD, ANA Consultant; Paula J. Morton, RN, MS; Elizabeth C. Parsons, RN, MSN, CNOR; Mark L. Phippen, RN, MN, CNOR; David J. Reyes, RN, BSN, CNOR; Margaret J. Sudduth, RN, MHS, CNOR; Jacklyn Takahashi Schuchardt, RN, MSN, CNOR; Joan M. Spear, RN, MBA, CNOR; Linda A. Tollerud, RN, BA; Joan A. Uebele, RN, MS; Donna S. Watson, RN, MSN, ARNP, FNP, Chair of DECC; **AORN staff members at the time of development:** Mary A. O'Neale, RN, MN, CNOR; Carol Dungan Applegeet, RN, MSN, CNOR, CNAA, FAAN; Dorothy M. Fogg, RN, MA; Suzanne C. Beyea, RN, PhD; Leslie H. Nicoll, RN, MBA, PhD; and Deb Smith, PNDS project coordinator.

The Value of a Clinical Information Infrastructure

A number of crises confront both the nursing profession and the health care system. The nursing shortage, limited data about nursing contributions to patient outcomes, and decreasing resources have all contributed to RN positions being eliminated or remaining vacant. These crises developed in part from the lack of reliable and valid data to determine and quantify the value and cost-effectiveness of RNs. Recent reports support the premise that mortality and morbidity decreases with an increased RN staffing ratio.[1] As a profession, however, nursing lacks valid and reliable sources of data that provide the knowledge required for clinical practice, education, management, and research. Without that information, the nursing profession—specifically perioperative nursing—is threatened.

Florence Nightingale once stated,
In attempting to arrive at the truth, I have applied everywhere for information, but in scarcely an instance have I been able to obtain hospital records fit for any purposes of comparison. If they could be obtained they would enable us to decide many other questions besides the ones alluded to. They would show subscribers how their money was being spent, what amount of good was really being done with it, or whether the money was not doing mischief rather than good.[2]

Does nursing face the same problems that existed then? Most expert health care informaticians would agree that her statement is as true today as it was nearly 150 years ago. This lack of comparable data severely limits the nursing profession's ability to develop a scientific basis for its practice and an evidence-based model of nursing practice.

Solutions to this problem exist. Without a critical mass of nurse clinicians, educators, managers, and researchers demanding a nursing information infra-structure, however, this problem may continue for another 150 years. An information infrastructure consists of a software framework that allows health concepts to be represented and related to other concepts. The architecture of the information infrastructure would

- support interface or end user terminologies,
- provide a common language for the documentation of clinical care, and
- incorporate reference terminologies that are essential for optimal information retrieval, aggregation, and analysis.

These essential characteristics—an infrastructure architecture, common vocabularies, mappings from one language to others, and reference terminologies for data retrieval—ensure the ability to obtain data that is vital to health care decisions and evidence-based practice. An information infrastructure requires health information systems that enable uniform and universal sharing of clinical data. This will ensure reliable data that is retrievable in a manner to support evidence-based health care and outcomes analysis.

Regardless of their role, nurses must value such an information infrastructure and be willing to contribute to its development and implementation. The PNDS is a clinically relevant interface terminology that provides
- uniformity to perioperative nursing documentation and
- the foundation for understanding nursing contributions in surgical settings.

Without reliable and valid sources of clinical data, nurses will never have the information required to provide evidence-based practice and establish their contributions to patient outcomes and the health care system. The same data derived from such an information infrastructure would provide policy makers, legislators, and insurers the crucial nursing data required to understand how nurses contribute to cost-effective, quality care. Data such as these will quantify the value of professional nursing regardless of the clinical setting. The solution to this problem includes the following:
- clinically useful, reliable, and valid interface and reference terminologies (**Table 1-1**);
- wide acceptance and utilization of interface terminologies in online nursing documentation systems;

- industry-wide acceptance and utilization of a reference terminology within all health care information systems;
- a commitment by the nursing profession to integrate interface terminologies in all aspects of practice and education;
- managers and researchers who demand useful data from clinical information systems;
- an aggressive research agenda to obtain the data required for nursing practice and education from nursing information systems; and
- partnerships with software vendors to standardize documentation across systems and integrate recognized interface and reference terminologies.

With this solution, comparable data could be retrieved and analyzed within and across clinical situations and settings.

The potential and capacity for all of this to occur does exist. Within nursing, interface vocabularies have been developed to describe nursing diagnoses, interventions, and outcomes. In addition, a mapping between nursing (interface) terminologies and a reference terminology (Systematized Nomenclature of Medicine [SNOMED RT/CT©]) is under development. This will ultimately support the ability to perform analyses and comparisons across patient populations and care settings, regardless of which clinical interface vocabulary is used for documentation.

The nursing profession is, however, sadly lacking the requisite support by nurse clinicians, educators, managers, and researchers required to create an

information infrastructure. Also missing is a clear understanding and consensus that an infrastructure is a critical requirement for nursing science and the profession. Nursing must take action now to create such an information infrastructure and recognize that any further delays in this agenda will only contribute to nurses' ongoing difficulty to be compensated and recognized for their contributions. Further delays also continue to impede the development of valid and reliable knowledge about nursing practice.

Perioperative nurses have made significant steps toward making an information infrastructure for perioperative nursing practice a reality.
- AORN has developed a clinically useful interface terminology, the PNDS, which has been recognized by the American Nurses Association (ANA).
- SNOMED© and AORN are in a collaborative agreement to develop a mapping between their reference terminology and our interface vocabulary.
- Several software vendors hold signed licensing agreements to integrate the PNDS in their software products.
- AORN has developed draft data fields for a preoperative assessment form and an intra-operative clinical record that incorporates the PNDS; these are now used in both paper and electronic formats.
- Clinicians, educators, and managers also have begun to utilize the PNDS in a variety of clinical applications (see Chapter 5).

Numerous obstacles, however, must be overcome before perioperative nurses can fully benefit from

TABLE 1-1: Definitions		
Term	**Definition**	**Examples**
Nursing Terminology	Data sets that describe nursing practice or management.	The Nursing Management Minimum Nursing Data Set
Interface Terminology	Data sets or vocabularies that are "used in documenting or facilitating care."[1] Includes ANA-recognized nursing terminologies.	The Perioperative Nursing Data Set The Nursing Intervention Classification The Nursing Outcomes Classification
Reference Terminology	"Often represented in a complex knowledge base and is rich with rigorously controlled rules and relationships (used predominantly for data analysis)."[1]	SNOMED© RT/CT

1.   J S Rose et al, "Common medical terminology comes of age, Part One," *Journal of Health Care Information Management* 15 (Fall 2001) 307-318.

such an information infrastructure. First, there must be a commitment by all perioperative nurses, regardless of their role or practice setting, to use the PNDS in clinical, education, management, and research applications. Most importantly, all professional nurses must understand that data derived from a nursing information system plays a crucial role in providing the knowledge required to support clinical practice, education, and management. The linkages between clinical documentation applications and research, education, and management have not been clearly articulated in nursing. Understanding those connections is critical to the success of an information infrastructure in nursing practice.

BENEFITS FOR CLINICIANS

In today's fast-paced clinical environments, many clinicians resist change, asking questions such as, "Will this take more time?" "What's in it for me?" and "How will this help patients?" Many clinicians do not recognize the link between an online documentation system and improving nursing practice. Until recently, the retrieval of valid and reliable data in a usable format was problematic and labor intensive. In other words, important information about nursing care was never effectively categorized, analyzed, interpreted, and provided to the end user—clinical nurses. In addition, few nurses receive formal education in informatics and, as a consequence, have limited understanding of computers. Even fewer clinical nurses have the requisite skills and knowledge to retrieve and analyze clinical data from a database in a nursing information system. Little discussion has explored the potential for nursing science development through use of databases established by clinicians who are recording patient data in an electronic database that is ready for data mining.

This problem may be further complicated by the reliance on free-text narrative notes in both paper and online documentation. This makes it nearly impossible to retrieve comparable data. For example, different nurses might document a stage II decubitus ulcer using various terms including *bedsore, pressure ulcer, skin breakdown,* or *pressure sore*. This individualization of terms and documentation leads to confusion and makes data useless. Nursing does not have a history of using structured vocabulary or standard terms for documentation. So when clinical nurses are asked to use an interface terminology to achieve consistency in documentation, they may not understand the potential benefits and may resist the change.

Bottom line—what is in this for nurses, specifically perioperative nurses? First and foremost, without data that supports having nurses in surgical settings, that role will be constantly threatened. Perioperative nurses need clear-cut answers to the question, "Does nursing make a difference?" Only solid clinical evidence can answer this question definitively. Without large clinical databases that provide information about the relationship to nursing practice and patient outcomes, the value of nursing will always be questioned. Without documented clinical evidence, many payers, administrators, and others will consider replacing the perioperative RN with personnel with fewer qualifications and less education. Threats to the nursing profession exist without data pertinent to nursing care.

So, how do clinicians, managers, and researchers obtain the necessary data to understand nursing contributions in surgical settings? First, perioperative nurses need to implement standardized documentation throughout the surgical experience. This ensures that comparable data is collected in similar clinical settings. For example, if nurses want to benchmark or compare their facility to another, both facilities must collect the same data elements. They must record the data using the same terms or words. For example, if clinical facilities wanted to compare their pain management programs, the data in both facilities should be recorded in a similar manner. This would require using the same pain assessment instruments, measurements of the extent of relief, and descriptions of interventions taken to treat the pain. Using the PNDS, the nurse could record interventions such as "assesses pain control," "implements pain guidelines," and "evaluates response to pain management" and an expected outcome that the patient reports adequate pain control throughout the perioperative period.

This outcome statement and the nursing interventions linked to that outcome are defined in the PNDS and, when used in a consistent manner across facilities, provide data about clinical practice and patient outcomes. This would facilitate the ability to compare the effectiveness of interventions to the level of pain relief. Without consistency in documentation and vocabulary, data simply cannot be analyzed and compared in a meaningful way.

Imagine the difficulty of determining the number of cases of postoperative pneumonia if physicians used different words to describe the complication. Physicians could name it *lung infection, inflammation of the lung, aspiration pneumonia,* or another favorite term. If this diagnosis of postoperative pneumonia was recorded in an inconsistent manner, meaningful information about the incidence of postoperative pneumonia could not be retrieved. Uniformity and consistency is critical to information retrieval and understanding clinical processes. Nurses must embrace this concept or the data sources required to validate nursing practice will never exist. This does not mean that all clinical records must look the same, but that the words used to record practice must be defined and coded in the same manner. In all clinical settings, it is critical that nurses use a nursing process format to document care and avoid charting only the tasks performed.

Valid and reliable nursing data are the foundation for measuring the value of nursing contributions. Patient databases can provide an understanding of the effectiveness of specific nursing activities and interventions. In addition, information systems can provide data that will help nurses identify risk states for complications and risk-reducing strategies. Data analysis also can identify nursing interventions and activities that are futile and based on tradition and myth rather than science. All of this information is crucial to nursing science development, but it begins with use of standardized documentation formats and interface terminologies.

Currently, clinical documentation standards are determined by the clinicians in each specific facility. Few universal standards exist for similar clinical situations or patient populations. In fact, experienced nurses transferring to a new facility in the same specialty practice often report feeling as though "I don't know how to chart." This lack of uniformity leads to uncertainty by nurses about what to chart and how to record it. These factors make it extremely difficult to obtain comparable data for similar clinical situations or events.

In ORs across the United States, it might be anticipated that similar clinical information is obtained and recorded for adult patients undergoing general surgery. This is not the case, however. An analysis of a national sample of more than 150 perioperative records representing both inpatient and ambulatory settings uncovered a disappointing reality about the current status of intraoperative nursing documentation. One major finding included the marginal consistency in the collection of structural data elements (ie, start time, stop time, anesthesia type, wound classification). Also, nursing diagnoses, interventions, and patient outcomes

were documented in fewer than 22% of the records. The professional aspects of intraoperative nursing care were embedded in the care delivered and not accurately or fully represented in the clinical documentation.

To understand the contributions of perioperative nurses to surgical outcomes, the framework for documentation must be structured in a manner that includes nursing diagnoses, interventions, and outcomes. Subsequent to this analysis, AORN's Nursing Practices Committee compiled a list of proposed data fields for both a preoperative and intraoperative record and is currently disseminating information to clinicians and vendors regarding this uniform approach to documentation (see Chapter 4, exemplars 1, 6, and 8.). These data fields were proposed when the committee members recognized that the benefits of structured vocabulary could only be fully realized when national documentation standards are established and implemented within and across practice settings.

Structured or standardized vocabularies provide uniformity to the language used by clinicians to develop care plans and document nursing care. The PNDS provides wording and definitions for nursing diagnoses, interventions, and outcomes, thus furnishing clinicians with the same terms to describe patient care. This consistency of terms supports documentation, but more importantly, using the same terms across clinical situations and settings allows data to be collected in a uniform way and subsequently analyzed. For example, nurses within an institution consistently document "skin remains smooth, intact, non-reddened, non-irritated, and free from bruising other than surgical incision" after surgery. If this statement is recorded in a consistent manner, characteristics can be collected about the patients who acquire a skin injury as well as the percentage of cases and the staff mix for those cases. In addition, if nursing interventions are recorded in a consistent manner, the most effective interventions can be determined. If other institutions document outcomes using the same vocabulary, benchmarking on an outcome is meaningful.

Standardization and uniformity provide nursing with the best knowledgebase possible from which to make clinical decisions. Access to data from large groups of patients in a variety of settings ensures nurses' ability to measure their contributions and confirm, define, and improve the quality of nursing care and establish best practices.

In another example, the nurse might identify the problem of "risk for infection related to surgical procedure." The outcome statement is "the patient is free from signs and symptoms of infection." When the surgeon closes the wound, it is hard to speculate whether an infection will occur during the first 30 postoperative days. So at the completion of surgery, the interim outcome statement might be stated as "the patient has a primarily closed, clean wound." Within the care plan, the nurse may have planned interventions such as implements aseptic technique, classifies surgical wound, assesses susceptibility for infection, performs skin preparation, protects from cross contamination, monitors for signs and symptoms of infection, minimizes length of invasive procedure, administers prescribed prophylactic treatments, initiates traffic control, and administers care to wound sites.

The nurse documenting the actual care provided would include the following in the nursing notes:
- implements aseptic technique;
- initiates traffic control;
- performs skin prep (hair removed by Nurse Smith) with iodophor scrub;
- classifies surgical wound (Clean); dry sterile dressing applied to midline abdominal incision with four 4x4 sponges and paper tape; nasogastric tube to low suction-no drainage noted; and
- cefazolin 1 gram IV at 10 AM.

By documenting aspects of care using a uniform set of terms and descriptors, the PNDS gives clinical nurses a united voice and a way to truly measure and quantify nursing contributions.

In the example above, nurses using a clinical database could obtain information about the occurrence of various wound classes, the timing of preoperative antibiotics, the most common types of surgical preparation, and the relationship between skin preparations and wound infections. In addition to facilitating the analysis of group data, the professional nursing interventions are represented in the clinical record and measurable, thus providing valuable information to patients, providers, and payers about nursing contributions.

BENEFITS FOR MANAGERS

Managers need reliable and valid data to make informed decisions regarding staffing, purchasing, and scheduling. Structured or standardized vocabulary used in clinical situations provides both the terms and definitions required to establish databases that support the evaluation of resource utilization and allow comparisons across clinical situations and institutions, as demonstrated in Chapter 6. Calculating, managing, and reimbursing the costs of clinical and administrative functions in the perioperative environment provides just one example of how comparable data could be utilized by perioperative managers.

Most importantly, databases developed from structured term sets such as the PNDS allow managers to compare clinical data from a large number of patients. Such comparisons permit managers to measure, monitor, and evaluate quality and the effectiveness of care. These data are required to co-manage both costs and quality and assist with effective decision making.

Managers who were monitoring quality of care or addressing risk management issues might use the PNDS to identify concerns and issues. For example, using the example of the "risk of infection" diagnosis, a manager might ask the following questions.
- What is the rate of infection in this surgical department?
- What types of skin preparations are used for patients who develop an infection?
- How many "clean" wounds later develop an infection?
- Have patients who developed infections receive prophylactic antibiotics?
- Did patients who developed infections receive their antibiotics at the appropriate time?
- What was the average skill mix for patients undergoing surgery who later developed a wound infection? Was there an RN in the operating suite?

If nurses have charted using the PNDS vocabulary and format, this information would be retrievable and could be used to identify practice issues and at the same time improve the quality of care.

Managers need solid information to make everyday management decisions as well. Perhaps a surgeon requests two RN circulators for a specific procedure. His request requires others to work extra hours or may result in other cases being postponed or cancelled. His rationale for this request is, "It is better for the patient." A database that explores the relationship of outcomes to staffing patterns would provide the data required to make decisions about this request. In this case, the data could speak and leave little opportunity for making an opinion-based decision.

Managers also can use the PNDS to develop nurse position descriptions, position accountabilities, evaluation forms, and nurse competency statements. Managers want to be certain that nurses have the knowledge, skills, and abilities needed to fulfill the professional role functions of an RN working in the operating room. For example, a typical competency outcome statement would be "Provides pain management for patients." Examples of competency statements using the PNDS are provided in Chapter 5 (exemplar 2) and Appendix B.

Within a competency statement, it would be specified that the nurse would assess pain control and identify cultural and value components related to pain. When caring for a patient with pain, the nurse would implement pain guidelines, provide pain instruction, and implement alternative methods of pain control. The nurse also would evaluate the patient's responses to interventions. Identifying critical behaviors using the PNDS gives clarity to role expectations using a nursing process format. Competency forms developed in this manner could be used for the interviewing process to assess skill and experience levels. They also can serve as a framework for planning orientation programs and clinical learning opportunities and for evaluating progress toward competence in required skills.

This uniformity or commonality supports developing position descriptions and competencies in clear, concise language. An organizing framework might be safety, physiologic response, knowledge, and rights/ethics. By organizing position descriptions in the same framework that care is provided, role expectations are clear and consistent with the provision of nursing care.

Managers also can use the PNDS as a framework for establishing policies and procedures related to clinical skills. The PNDS describes nursing interventions and activities required to achieve clinical outcomes in perioperative settings. Uniformity in language between policies and procedures and documentation supports nurses' ability to provide and document nursing care in a consistent manner.

The PNDS also provides the basis for developing practice guidelines, critical pathways, and best practices. Collecting data in a uniform manner supports analyses related to treatment responses.

Therefore, clinicians can determine and implement the most efficient and effective intervention, thus ensuring high-quality, cost-effective care.

BENEFITS FOR EDUCATORS

A specialty-based standardized vocabulary helps educators identify the essential content for educational and orientation programs. A standardized vocabulary also helps educators teach students and orient new personnel. In Chapter 5, educators provide examples of how they use the PNDS in designing activities to facilitate student learning about the care and management of patients. Other exemplars in Chapter 5 illustrate how to integrate the PNDS into perioperative orientation for novice and experienced nurses in the OR. Sample lesson plans, learning activities, and a program outline are included to effectively demonstrate the benefits of using the PNDS for educational purposes.

BENEFITS FOR RESEARCHERS

The potential benefits of structured vocabulary for researchers has never been fully appreciated or realized. A tremendous potential resource for answering many nursing research questions lies within the majority of nursing information systems. The grim reality, however, is that most of that data is not retrievable in a useful format. Furthermore, the lack of consistent documentation standards and the limited use of structured vocabulary have ensured that data sets cannot be grouped or compared across settings.

The PNDS and other structured vocabularies, when fully implemented, provide the framework to help clinicians and researchers identify which interventions contribute to specific outcomes. If a database contained information about patients' ages, analyses could be performed to determine how care requirements differ for patients of varying age groups. Standardized vocabulary allows for better data collection and the ability to compare data across clinical situations and settings. Most importantly, it supports the ability to create a data repository and aggregate data sources. Use of the PNDS in perioperative settings would provide large populations of surgical patients from which to explore data about physiologic and behavioral responses to surgery as well as understand the characteristics of events leading to medical error.

In this way, the conceptual model of the Perioperative Patient Focused Model (Chapter 2, exhibit 2-A) guides a research agenda for perioperative nursing. This model proposes that care events in surgical settings focus on the patient and family and occur within the structure of the health care system. Within the model, the professional nurse provides care to achieve patient outcomes that are established based on identified needs and problems. Professional perioperative nurses focus on three domains—safety, physiologic responses, and behavioral responses. This model provides a framework for practice and research in perioperative settings and the PNDS.

A structured vocabulary such as the PNDS provides outcomes that are explicit, clearly defined, observable, and measurable. These outcome statements provide the basis for outcome research and analysis. Measuring performance against observable criteria allows researchers and clinicians the opportunity to identify areas for clinical improvement. For example, the PNDS provides the outcome statement "the patient is free from signs and symptoms of electrical injury." It is the goal of any surgical department that this goal is achieved 100% of the time. If data indicate that injuries are occurring and the goal is not being met, the next step is to examine the reasons. When interventions and outcomes are recorded with the same terms, data that will explain such variations in care can be retrieved.

Examples of research using the PNDS include
- determining the frequency of nursing diagnoses, signs and symptoms, physiologic and psychologic needs, observations, procedures, and communication with allied departments;
- exploring the relationship between surgical diagnosis and intensity of nursing care;
- exploring the relationship between patient outcomes and organizational data (eg, staffing, environment, clinical resources);
- understanding the relationship between outcomes and interventions (ie, effectiveness research);
- defining effective nursing actions as they relate to specific medical and nursing diagnoses;
- identifying actions that prevent or enhance specific patient outcomes;
- determining signs and symptoms that result in nursing action;
- determining expected outcomes or patient responses during specific stages of illness or recovery;

- comparing benefits of specific nursing interventions;
- exploring the relationship of specific interventions to patient outcomes;
- measuring quality;
- identifying risk states for skin breakdown or for electrical or laser injury; and
- establishing staffing patterns based on patients' problems, needs, or classification (intensity of care).

In the example related to infection, researchers might ask the following questions.
- Who are the patients at greatest risk for developing an infection?
- What surgeries are most frequently associated with infections?
- Which providers have the highest rates of infection?
- Is there a relationship between skill mix and infection rates?
- Is there a relationship between urgent and emergency surgeries and infection rates?
- On which postoperative day were surgical site infections confirmed in the 10 most commonly performed surgeries?
- What are the costs associated with infection?
- Does the length of time for a surgical site skin preparation influence infection rates for various procedures?
- Do patients who receive follow-up care have infections detected earlier than patients who receive conventional care?

An information infrastructure with data derived from information systems populated with structured nursing vocabularies will provide nurses with the requisite knowledge to make evidence-based clinical decisions. By providing a common means of communication, structured vocabularies facilitate our abilities to manage information in an electronic format and compare clinical outcomes across settings. A standardized vocabulary helps nurses document care while providing a foundation for examining and evaluating the quality and effectiveness of that care. Reliable and valid data also provide a framework for nursing research by helping nurses understand the relationship of nursing interventions to patient outcomes, informing decisions about the relationship of staffing to patient outcomes, and providing data about the contributions of nurses to patient outcomes.

CONCLUSION

Every nurse can make a difference as we move toward an information infrastructure for nursing. First, ask the various software vendors questions about their utilization of nursing structured vocabularies. Next, inform them about AORN's commitment to representing nursing contributions in a structured manner within documentation. These activities help

- increase everyone's awareness of the importance of including nursing in the electronic patient record, and
- recognize the importance of being able to retrieve information related to nurses' contributions.

Two additional steps include sharing information with other nurses about the value of standardized vocabularies and showing others how easy it is to use structured vocabulary in nursing care plans and documentation forms.

The profession of nursing must establish a critical mass of clinicians and informatics nurses who support efforts related to an information legacy for nursing. Nurses can help this process by sharing information about resources such as the AORN web page or by working locally, regionally, or nationally to implement structured vocabularies in nursing. Working together regardless of our clinical setting or specialty will help us build the information infrastructure required to understand nursing practice.

Most importantly, individual nurses need to understand the value of an information infrastructure that contains reliable and valid data comparable across clinical settings, systems, and situations.

Nurses also need to understand that a quality information infrastructure will mean that nursing data that can be retrieved in a meaningful way, thus providing the essential knowledge to ensure an evidence-based practice model. Without evidence, nurses will never know which clinical situations or conditions require a nurse, how to determine cost-effective interventions, and how to accurately establish staffing patterns.

For nurses who want to learn more about structured vocabulary, consider reading the various articles related to standardized language published in nursing journals. Attend classes or continuing education sessions regarding structured vocabulary. Determine whether your hospital has plans to adopt one or more nursing vocabularies. Talk to other nurses about the importance of high quality data to inform clinical decisions. Share with them the importance of using structured vocabulary to describe clinical problems (ie, nursing diagnoses), interventions, and outcomes.

If clinicians ask for an information infrastructure for nursing, it will be developed and supported. As nurses, we recognize the difference we make in patient care and health outcomes. An information infrastructure will provide the evidence others need to acknowledge what nurses have known for centuries—Nursing does make a difference, and every patient deserves a registered nurse.

References
1. J Needleman, P I Buerhaus, *Nurse Staffing and Patient Outcomes in Hospitals* (Boston: Harvard School of Public Health, 2001) 21-60.

2. F Nightingale, *Notes on Hospitals,* third ed (London: Longman, Green, Longman, Roberts, and Green, 1863).

## Chapter Two

What Is the PNDS?

The PNDS provides clear, consistent, and precise terms and definitions for clinical problems (nursing diagnoses), nursing interventions, and patient outcomes. When clinical data is recorded using a structured vocabulary, such as the PNDS, information can be aggregated and analyzed for management, quality improvement, or research purposes.[1] The data set addresses the delivery of nursing care across the surgical continuum and has applications within any perioperative setting.

During the past several years, AORN members, computerized patient record vendors, clinical practitioners, language experts, informatics specialists, and AORN staff consultants have recommended a variety of changes to the data set. Recommendations have been prompted by

- changes in patient needs;
- analysis of PNDS applications in the clinical setting;
- changes in the perioperative environment, technology, and surgical and other invasive procedures; and
- efforts to reflect RN first assistant (RNFA) contributions to patient care.

In an effort to include these recommendations, the PNDS has been reviewed, revised, and edited into a new format.[2]

PNDS Review

The original PNDS provided an essential foundation for the perioperative clinical specialty; however, the complex nature of vocabulary development and the diversity of clinical roles in the perioperative setting require periodic multilevel reviews of content and vocabulary. As the PNDS continues to be applied in perioperative settings, there will be continual growth and refinement in the vocabulary. Each new edition with changes, additions, and deletions will require repeated content validation from numerous experts in clinical practice, vocabulary development, and informatics. Final approval for all revisions comes from the AORN Board of Directors. Participants in the review process of this new edition included

- members of committees that developed the original PNDS,
- perioperative RNs and RNFAs with content expertise in a variety of specialties,
- nationally recognized vocabulary experts,
- nurse informaticians working with clinical applications,
- members of the AORN Nursing Practices Committee,
- staff members in the AORN Center for Nursing Practice and the Research Department, and
- doctorally prepared consultants.[2]

Guidelines for the Revision

Underlying assumptions are prevailing, guiding principles. Assumptions are viewed as self-evident, unquestioned, and a starting point for reasoning. The assumptions that guided the systematic evaluation and change of the PNDS are

- the PNDS is a vocabulary, not a standard of care;
- the definition of perioperative goes beyond intraoperative practice;
- elements of the PNDS have a unique identifier, and no unique identifier may be used more than once;
- the attributes of consistency and standardization are desirable in a vocabulary;
- redundancy or duplication cannot be eliminated completely from the PNDS vocabulary; and
- consistent levels of abstraction facilitate application of the PNDS to the clinical setting.[2]

The first version PNDS comprised 29 outcomes, 127 interventions, and 64 nursing diagnoses. The second edition has 28 outcomes, 133 interventions, and 74 nursing diagnoses. In this revision, the PNDS enhances nurses' ability to specify and evaluate patient outcomes at any point and time across the surgical continuum.

Redundancy or duplication cannot be completely removed. There are occasions during the process of perioperative nursing that an intervention is appropriately repeated. For example, "Verifies allergies" (I123) should be, and is, included in the interventions addressing nurse administation of pharmaceuticals (O9) and nurse/patient discussions about self-administration of medications (O19). Identification of the ideal divide between standardization and acceptable duplication will occur as the PNDS is used and revised over several iterations.

PERIOPERATIVE OUTCOMES

During a surgical experience, a patient may be alert, oriented, and fully able to converse preoperatively; rendered unconscious intraoperatively; or discharged ambulatory from the postanesthesia care unit. During that same episode of care, several nursing diagnoses may be identified, diverse nursing interventions will be provided, and numerous changes in health status may be noted. Ideally, a patient's health status would improve after surgery; however, the patient's condition may preclude overall improvement, or complications may occur during or after surgery. Outcome statements describe those positive or negative changes in a patient's health status attributed to the provided care.[3]

In the PNDS, outcomes are positive statements that reflect goals that patients are expected to achieve by the end of an entire perioperative experience. Nurses, however, provide care in various clinical settings and evaluate interim, expected outcomes for specific time frames during a surgical experience. Measurement of these phases of care was not adequately or specifically addressed in the first edition of the PNDS. To address this, the concept of outcome measurement across the surgical continuum was reconsidered.

Outcome Measurement
The measurement of perioperative outcomes is complex, multifaceted, and influenced by the timing, validity, and reliability of the screening procedure.[4] Some perioperative outcomes can be measured directly through observation of the patient's physical condition (eg, absence of a skin injury, hemodynamic monitoring of cardiac function). Other outcomes must be measured indirectly by surrogate measures (eg, signature on a discharge teaching form to measure knowledge, self-report of patient satisfaction) and depend on the subjective report of patients and their families. Measuring quality with outcome measures is further complicated by

- risk adjusting for severity of illness (eg, a healthy adult compared to a frail elder),
- the feasibility of collecting data (eg, cost and access to the patient), and
- the timing of data collection (eg, immediately following surgery compared to 30 days after surgery).[5]

The ability to directly link a clinical outcome to the process of clinical care depends on the timing of the observation.[6] Direct evaluation should occur at the time nursing care is provided, and it is expected that the patient's progress is monitored and evaluated in an ongoing manner. Outcomes measurements also may occur after a specific interval and before the patient is transferred to a different clinical unit or caregiver. For example, in the perioperative setting, anxiety may be measured before and after surgery by both the admitting nurse and the OR nurse.

As the patient moves through the continuum of care, different outcomes might be expected. For example, it would be expected that a patient undergoing a nerve block of the right arm would have intact circulation, sensation, and motion of that extremity before surgery. Immediately postoperatively, the patient might have intact circulation in that extremity; however, the nurse might not be able to assess sensation or motion due to the effects of the nerve block. If the patient was discharged the same day, it might be difficult to fully assess the patient's extremity for nerve injury. Therefore, a subsequent assessment would be performed at the follow-up visit. These types of measurement issues prompted two changes in the publication of the second edition of the PNDS:
- development of outcome indicators and deletion of the less specific outcome criteria, and
- facilitation of outcomes evaluation across the continuum by providing examples of interim outcome statements.

Outcome Indicators
PNDS outcome indictors provide clinical, adminis-trative, or fiscal measures of performance. Outcome indictors also link nursing interventions to the outcomes of patient care.[7] Outcome indicators are measured by collecting patient assessment data, reviewing the patient record, listening to patient/family self-reports, or examining facility/administrative data. For example, the suggested outcome indicators for the outcome, "The patient participates in decisions affecting his or her perioperative plan of care" (O23) are

- **cognition**—verbalizes understanding of treatment options, describes sequence of planned procedure, repeats provided information correctly, asks questions based on information provided, and participates in plan of care;
- **affective response**—verbalizes concerns about decisions;
- **clinical documentation**—surgical consent for procedure is signed according to facility policy; Self-Determination Act is implemented according to patient wishes;
- **supportive resources**—family member participates in perioperative plan of care according to patient's preference; and
- **patient satisfaction**—expresses satisfaction with level of involvement in plan of care and decision-making process.

In the revised second edition of the PNDS, the categories related to the outcome indicators are noted in **bold** print. For each outcome statement, examples of positively stated clinical findings are presented. Each indicator category and clinical finding comprises an outcome indicator and helps the nurse determine the degree to which the outcome was achieved.

The patient's condition and clinical situation guide the nurse in determining which outcome indicators to measure and evaluate. Measurements must be made for all of the outcome indicators. Certain outcome indicators would be more appropriate for specific time frames and clinical situations. A variety of outcome indicators are presented for each outcome statement, and the lists are not considered exhaustive. The clinical nurse determines the degree of goal achievement based on subjective and objective clinical findings and within context of the clinical situation.

Interim Outcome Statements

A PNDS interim outcome statement represents an interval outcome as the patient progresses toward achieving the desired or overall expected outcome.[8] An interim outcome statement reflects the degree of progress toward the overall goal that has occurred in response to the implemented interventions.[5] The second edition of the PNDS includes examples of interim outcomes that demonstrate how interval measurements can be used during a perioperative experience. Interim outcome statements support the nurse's ability to accurately represent the patient's level of outcome achievement at a specific point and time during the surgical continuum.

CODING THE DATA ELEMENTS: THE UNIQUE CODING SYSTEM

A criterion for recognition of a data set by the ANA is that each data element has a unique code and a machine-readable audit trail. A single unique code number was thus assigned to each discrete concept in the PNDS. The unique identifier will never change after it is assigned. If a concept becomes outdated or is no longer needed or used, the unique identifier will not be deleted, but rather flagged as obsolete. In other words, unique identifiers are never reassigned to another concept. Unique identifiers are used to create a machine-readable audit trail that is useful if the data elements are embedded in an electronic record.

For the PNDS, code numbers or unique identifiers begin with a letter (ie, "D" for domain, "O" for outcomes, "I" for interventions, "X" for nursing diagnoses) followed by a numerical value. The four domains were coded safety (D1), physiologic response (D2), behavioral response (D3), and health system (D4). The remaining nursing data elements were alphabetized and coded: outcomes (eg, O1, O2, O3), nursing diagnoses (eg, X1, X2, X3), and interventions (eg, I1, I2, I3). This coding system allows the inclusion of new outcomes, interventions, diagnoses, and health system data elements.

Clinically, the coding system can be applied to patient care documentation, computer programs, procedure statements, or care plans. Some discrete concepts (terms) in the PNDS are not coded. Those concepts are the activities under each intervention, interim outcomes, outcome indicators, and the elements listed under the health systems domain. Items that are not coded may be edited or rearranged to meet the needs of the individual patient or facility.

For example, the freedom from electrical injury outcome (O4) has three example interim outcome statements:

- The patient's skin, other than incision, remains unchanged between admission and discharge from the OR.
- The patient's vital signs are stable at discharge from the OR.
- The patient reports comfort at the dispersive electrode site on admission to the postoperative unit.

An exhaustive list of interim outcomes for O4 cannot be provided, as a patient could experience any number of interim adverse (ie, negative) or favorable (ie, positive) outcomes. Therefore, the label "example interim outcome statement" is used in the second edition of the PNDS. For example, the nurse may note that the patient's dispersive grounding pad site is reddened at the time of discharge from the OR. The nurse might decide to reassess the site in the postanesthesia care unit after approximately 30 minutes. At the time of reassessment, if the skin is non-reddened and intact, the interim outcome statement might read, "the patient's skin is smooth, continuous, and free from redness or blisters at ground pad site 30 minutes following the removal of the pad." When determining an interim outcome, the nurse identifies

- who (the subject) is achieving the outcome,
- what the clinical findings or observations are, and
- the time frame when the measurement of the outcome occurs.

Interim outcome statements also address the clinical reality that certain outcomes cannot be assessed until a condition has had a chance to develop (eg, an intraoperative ulceration in the skin is not always evident at discharge from the OR, the first signs of a wound infection are not present the day of surgery).[4] To state that the patient has met the outcome of "freedom from electrical injury" at the time the wound is closed could be justifiably challenged. The nurse can report, however, that the intervention to take preventive measures to prevent injury due to electrical sources (I72) resulted in the patient's skin, other than incision, remaining unchanged from admission to discharge from the OR.

Nursing Diagnoses

Perioperative nursing care focuses on preventive practice, rather than on identification of problems. Simply by undergoing surgery, patients are immediately at risk for several problems. That is, most patients who undergo an operative or invasive procedure procedure will

- experience a planned break in skin integrity, and thus have an increased risk of infection;
- risk acquiring a physical injury from perioperative positioning, extraneous objects, chemicals, electricity, or a fall during transfer or transportation; and
- experience changes in cardiac, pulmonary, and fluid and electrolyte status.

For these reasons, the perioperative nursing care plan often emphasizes interventions and outcomes in efforts to reduce the inherent risks in this clinical environment. Meanwhile, patients expect and deserve care that addresses their unique needs. Furthermore, a number of regulatory and accrediting bodies, including the Joint Commission on Accreditation of Healthcare Organizations, require evidence of care planning that is individualized to the patient and the clinical situation.

One approach to address the patient's unique cultural, ethnic, and individual needs is through the identification of nursing diagnoses specific for each patient. For example, a patient may be unable to communicate with the nurse and other members of the health care team. Based on assessment data, the nurse may identify a nursing diagnosis of impaired verbal communication. To meet the patient's needs, the nurse would select nursing interventions such as identifying the barriers to communication and assessing coping mechanisms. The nurse might determine a need for, and subsequently obtain, an interpreter to assist. The nursing diagnosis of impaired communication is not a common patient problem. When patients do experience the problem and when the nursing diagnosis is made, however, interventions can be selected to ensure achieving goals related to patient communication.

This edition of PNDS includes a list of nursing diagnoses that are potentially related to each outcome statement. Experts in perioperative nursing, as well as others,[9,10] have struggled in their efforts to link nursing diagnoses to outcomes and interventions. Outcomes can be linked to diagnoses, and interventions can be linked to outcomes. Establishing distinct relationships between all three nursing data elements, however, has presented clinicians and researchers with a number of issues. Each outcome statement in the PNDS is specifically linked to one or more nursing interventions. The listing of nursing diagnoses, however, simply provides examples of specific nursing diagnoses that might be associated with an outcome.

Nursing Interventions

Nursing interventions decribe actions performed to benefit patients.[11] Nursing interventions help the patient achieve a desired outcome. The PNDS interventions related to assessment use action verbs including *assesses, determines, identifies, monitors, notes, observes*, *recognizes*, *screens*, and *verifies*. Direct care interventions are indicated by terms such as *administers, applies, collaborates, implements, manages, performs,* and *provides*. Evaluation interventions that assess the effectiveness of care are indicated by the verb *evaluates*. Each of the action verbs, carefully chosen during the development of the PNDS, indicates the scope of perioperative professional nursing practice.

Each PNDS intervention has a specific definition and a list of activities. For example, one of the nursing interventions related to the prevention of chemical injury outcome relates to latex allergies. The intervention statement is **"Implements latex allergy precautions as needed (I139)."**[12-15] The definition is "Protects latex-sensitive patients from exposure to natural rubber." The activities statements include
- stores essential non-natural-rubber supplies in a quick access location,
- assesses/monitors for latex allergy response,
- initiates approved latex precautions protocol as needed, and
- evaluates effectiveness of precautions taken.

The intervention and its unique identifier are printed in bold. The definition clarifies the scope of the intervention. The activity statements describe nursing actions related to a specific nursing intervention.

Most interventions appear to contribute to only one PNDS outcome; however, occasionally there are exceptions. For example, the intervention "verifies allergies" relates to the outcome for prevention of medication injuries as well as the outcome that addresses knowledge of medication administration. Any intervention that is related to more than one outcome will have the same unique identifier.

THE VALUE OF THE PNDS

The PNDS is a data set of terms and phrases that represents perioperative nursing diagnoses, nursing interventions, and patient outcomes. It is an inductively derived, empirically validated, and standardized method of describing professional nursing care. Aggregated data derived from naming, defining, and coding nursing care provides a foundation for examining and evaluating the quality and effectiveness of that care. Administrators, clinicians, educators, researchers, and informaticists can use this structured vocabulary for communication, documentation, reporting, care planning, or teaching other clinicians and students.

Many policy makers, health care consumers, hospital administrators, and other nurses have voiced a limited understanding about the contributions of perioperative nurses. Some have even questioned whether perioperative nurses provide professional or technical care and expertise. Eliminating perioperative content from the curricula of basic nursing programs supports the premise that perioperative nurses have difficulty articulating how they implement the nursing process.[16]

CRITERIA FOR ADDING NEW NURSING DIAGNOSES, INTERVENTIONS, AND OUTCOMES

As new perioperative nursing diagnoses, interventions, and outcomes are identified, they will be assigned to one of the four domains using the "goodness-of-fit" test. This goodness-of-fit will be determined through a careful analysis and by comparing the diagnosis to the definitions of the domains. The defined interventions required to address the diagnosis or achieve the outcome will be linked appropriately and included in the domain.

Domain Definitions

Domain	Definition
Safety	The absence of signs and symptoms of physical injury unrelated to the intended therapeutic effects of an operative or other invasive procedure.
Physiologic responses	The physical, biochemical, and functional responses to the intended therapeutic effects of an operative or other invasive procedure.
Behavioral responses— Individual and family	The psychological, sociological, and spiritual responses of patients and their families to the operative or other invasive procedure. Also includes the standards of professional nursing practice and the related expected outcomes of the operative or other invasive procedure.
Health system	Structural data elements that exist in the perioperative environment or health system.

Data suggest that perioperative nurses, themselves, believe they work in a different world from other nurses.[17] Nurses frequently report that they feel the need to defend their practice as "real nursing" and have difficulty describing their role in nursing terminology. Indeed, perioperative nurses seem to struggle with the issue of whether perioperative nursing fits into the traditional definition of nursing. The PNDS addresses these issues and answers the questions about whether a professional RN is required in perioperative settings.

The PNDS describes and defines the professional skills and knowledge required to care for patients before, during, and after surgery. Using the PNDS and the Perioperative Patient Focused Model (see **Exhibit 2-A**) perioperative nurses can now describe four areas of concern for a patient undergoing surgery—safety, physiologic responses, behavioral responses, and the health system factors. Nurses can identify expected outcomes for each patient and the nursing interventions that contribute to achievement of those outcomes. The PNDS provides the communication tool needed to describe how professional nursing is practiced with the four walls of the OR and across the surgical continuum.

FUTURE CONSIDERATIONS

The PNDS must remain inherently flexible and undergo a process of continuous refinement. Changes in clinical practice and new knowledge will necessitate continuous review, revision, deletions, and additions to reflect newly identified phenomena, interventions, and outcomes. Clinical validation projects also will contribute to future developments and further refinements of the language.

Even at the time of the publication of this revised second editon, certain issues remain apparent and will influence ongoing review and subsequent revisions.
- Changes in technology, such as robotics and genetic engineering, will result in the identification and explication of new concepts that will need to be addressed within the PNDS of the future.
- To be useful, outcomes should be observable, measurable, and attainable and focus on patients' responses rather than the nurses' actions. Although written in a patient outcome format, many of the PNDS outcomes that relate to patient rights and ethics reflect nursing actions rather than patients' responses. For example, "The patient is the recipient of competent and ethical care within legal standards of

practice" actually describes core components of professional nursing practice such as competence and ethical practice. This outcome statement obviously does not relate to patient outcomes, but rather to standards of clinical practice. So the question remains, if this and related outcome statements are eventually moved to the health systems domain, where do the nursing interventions that currently relate to those outcomes fit?
- A recognized limitation of the Perioperative Patient Focused Model is the absence of fully developed concepts and definitions within the health systems domain. The Association of Anesthesia Clinical Directors glossary of times[18] provides some helpful terms. Ongoing theoretical explorations and collaborative efforts are required to more fully develop this health system component of the model. Questions that must be addressed include the following.
- Should structural elements documented on the clinical record (eg, time and the risk of infection) be addressed in a patient-centered domain or in the health systems domain?
- If structural elements can be located in both patient-centered and health system domains, does the Perioperative Patient Focused Model need to be adapted?

Fortunately, each revision is considered a scheduled step in the development of the PNDS vocabulary. Suggestions, recommendations, and proposals for change are encouraged. Major efforts continue from the organizational perspective to refine this perioperative nursing data set, disseminate information to AORN members, and create a national perioperative database.

In our current health care environment, perioperative nurses must have an organized approach to collect, organize, classify, and capture clinical nursing data to communicate nursing practice. The PNDS is a specialty nursing language that provides a systematic method of collecting the basic elements of perioperative nursing care. These data will allow nurses to predict costs, determine necessary resources, and validate nursing practice in perioperative settings.

The Perioperative Nursing Data Set reflects the expertise of many AORN members. As a clinically relevant and empirically validated standardized language, it is a beginning point to help perioperative

RNs document the care they provide and evaluate their contributions. The data set relates to the delivery of care in the perioperative setting during any time frame of the surgical experience and is appropriate for use in any perioperative setting. Clinical validation and further empirical testing of this standardized data set are essential for its further development and refinement.

References

1. AORN, Inc, *Perioperative Nursing Data Set,* first edition (Denver: AORN, Inc, 2000).

2. S V M Kleinbeck, "Revising the Perioperative Nursing Data Set," *AORN Journal* 75 (March 2002) 602.

3. A Donabedian, *The Methods and Findings of Quality Assessment and Monitoring* Vol 3 (Ann Arbor, Mich: Health Administration Press, 1985).

4. S V M Kleinbeck, M McKennett, "Challenges of measuring intraoperative patient outcomes," *AORN Journal* 72 (November 2000) 845-853.

5. O L Strickland, "Challenges in measuring patient outcomes," *Nursing Clinics of North America* 32 (September 1997) 495-512.

6. L I Iezzoni, *Risk Adjustment for Measuring Healthcare Outcomes,* second ed (Chicago: Health Administration Press, 1997.

7. B M Jennings, N Staggers, "The language of outcomes," *Advances in Nursing Science* 20 (June 1998) 72-80.

8. P W Shaughnessy et al, "Outcomes across the care continuum: Home health care," *Medical Care* 35 (November 1997) Suppl NS 115-123; "Comment," *Medical Care* 35 (December 1997) 1225-1226.

9. M L Maas, M Johnson, S Moorhead, "Classifying nursing-sensitive patient outcomes," *Journal of Nursing Scholarship* 28 (Winter 1996) 295-301.

10. M Johnson et al, *Nursing Diagnoses, Outcomes, & Interventions* (St Louis: Mosby, 2001).

11. G Bulecheck, J C McCloskey, *Nursing Interventions: Essential Nursing Treatments,* second ed (Philadelphia: W B Saunders, 1992).

12. American Society of Anesthesiologists, *Natural Rubber Latex Allergy: Considerations for anesthesiologists* (Park Ridge, Ill: American Society of Anesthesiologists, 1999) 1-33.

13. G L Sussman, "Latex allergy: An overview," *Canadian Journal of Allergy and Clinical Immunology* 5 no 8 (2000) 317-321.

14. M C Swanson, D W Olson, Latex allergen affinity for starch powders applied to natural rubber gloves and released as an aerosol," *Canadian Journal of Allergy and Clinical Immunology* 5 no 8 (2000) 328-336.

15. K J Kelly, "Latex allergy: Where do we go from here?" *Canadian Journal of Allergy and Clinical Immunology* 5 no 8 (2000) 337-340.

16. V D Wagner, C C Kee, D P Gray, "A historical decline of educational perioperative clincial experiences," *AORN Journal* 62 (November 1995) 771-782.

17. H O Sigurdsson, "The meaning of being a perioperative nurse," *AORN Journal* 74 (August 2001) 202-217.

18. Association of Anesthesia Clinical Directors, "Procedural times glossary—glossary of times used for scheduling and monitoring of diagnostic and therapeutic procedures," *Surgical Services Management* 3 (September 1997) 11-15.

EXHIBIT 2-A
The Perioperative Patient Focused Model

The Perioperative Patient Focused Model (**Figure 2-A** and inside front cover) is the conceptual framework for the PNDS and the model for perioperative nursing practice. The patient and his or her family, at the core of the model, provide the focus of perioperative nursing care. Within the model, concentric circles expand beyond the patient and family representing the perioperative nursing domains and elements. The model illustrates the relationship between the patient, family, and care provided by the perioperative professional nurse.

The model is divided into four quadrants, three representing patient-centered domains:
- safety of the patient,
- patient physiologic responses to surgery, and
- patient and family behavioral responses to surgery.

The fourth quadrant represents the health system in which the perioperative care is delivered. The health system domain designates administrative concerns and structure elements (ie, staff, equipment, environmental factors, supplies) essential to successful surgical intervention.

The model is patient focused. The patient is at the center of the model, which clearly represents the true focus of perioperative patient care. Regardless of practice setting, geographic location, or nature of the patient population, there is nothing more important to the practicing perioperative nurse than his or her patient. This model makes this concept of patient care "visible" in and between all other variables in the surgical setting.

The model focuses on outcomes. This is important, as nursing theories and models should embrace and represent all elements of the nursing process, including outcomes. AORN's model represents the outcomes focus of perioperative nurses by placing outcomes immediately adjacent to the patient care domains. An individualized patient assessment guides the identification of nursing diagnoses and selection of nursing interventions for each patient.

The model represents the "real world" for practicing perioperative nurses and has utility for practicing nurses, educators, and researchers. A simultaneous simplicity and elegance is reflected in this model. The interrelationships of the domains and concepts provide a picture of the building blocks of perioperative nursing practice in a way that instructs and educates the student, guides nursing practice, and offers infinite opportunities for testing and further validation through research.

The model as a whole illustrates the dynamic nature of the perioperative patient experience and the nursing presence throughout that process. Working in a collaborative manner with other members of the health care team and the patient, the nurse establishes outcomes, identifies nursing diagnoses, and provides nursing care. The nurse intervenes within the context of the health care system to assist the patient to achieve the highest attainable health outcomes (ie, physiological, behavioral, and safety) throughout the perioperative experience.

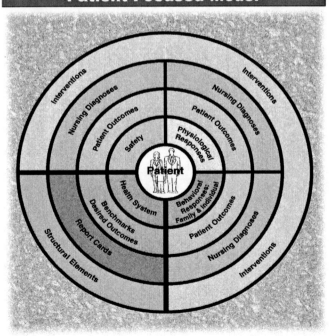

FIGURE 2-A: The Perioperative Patient Focused Model

## Chapter Three

The Conceptual Framework of the PNDS

The PNDS contains definitions of nursing domains, outcomes, interventions, and activities performed by the perioperative registered nurse when caring for a patient before, during, or after an invasive or operative procedure. The terms and statements in this dictionary are divided into domains with explanatory domain extensions:

- Safety: Freedom from acquired physical injury;
- Physiologic responses: Physiologic responses to surgery are as expected;
- Behavioral responses A: Knowledge about the perioperative process; and
- Behavioral responses B: Patient rights and ethics are supported.

Each domain has desired perioperative outcomes with detailed definitions, interpretive statements, outcome indictors, examples of interim outcome statements, potentially applicable nursing diagnoses, and nursing interventions with activities to accomplish each intervention. All of the PNDS elements are assigned a unique identifier which consists of a letter plus a number. For example, the outcome "Freedom from signs and symptoms of position injury" is coded O5, and the intervention "Performs required counts" is coded I94. Coded elements may not be edited or changed for clinical use. Other components of the PNDS, such as nursing activities and interim outcomes, are not coded and may be adapted for use in an individual facility.

The PNDS dictionary is not organized alphabetically or by nursing diagnoses. Instead, data elements and statements are linked under the appropriate expected outcome of delivered nursing care. For example, interventions that address positioning are found under the outcome "Freedom from signs and symptoms of positioning injury." Searches for data elements may be accomplished by

- locating the outcome being addressed and reading the content to identify the topic of interest,
- using the "Table of Contents," or
- using the index.

PNDS Domains		
Domain	*Domain Extension*	*Domain Definition*
1. Safety	Freedom from acquired physical injury.	The absence of signs and symptoms of physical injury unrelated to the intended therapeutic effects of an operative or other invasive procedure.
2. Physiologic Responses	Physiologic responses to surgery are as expected.	The physical, biochemical, and functional responses to the intended therapeutic effects of an operative or other invasive procedure.
3-A. Behavioral Responses: Patient and Family	Knowledge about the perioperative process.	The psychologic, sociologic, and spiritual responses of patients and their families to the operative or other invasive procedure.
3-B. Behavioral Responses: Patient and Family	Patient rights and ethics are supported.	The standards of professional nursing practice and the related expected outcomes of the operative or other invasive procedure.
4. Health system	The environment of perioperative settings.	Structural data elements that exist in the perioperative environment or health system.

Domains and Nursing Diagnoses

Domain Related nursing diagnoses	Domain Related nursing diagnoses
Safety	**Behavioral responses**

Safety
  Aspiration, risk for
  Bed mobility, impaired
  Body temperature, risk for imbalance
  Falls, risk for
  Infection, risk for
  Injury, risk for
  Mobility, impaired physical
  Perioperative positioning injury, risk for
  Peripheral neurovascular dysfunction, risk for
  Protection, ineffective
  Sensory perception, disturbed
  Skin integrity, impaired
  Skin integrity, risk for impaired
  Tissue integrity, impaired
  Transfer ability, impaired

Physiologic responses
  Activity intolerance
  Airway clearance, ineffective
  Aspiration, risk for
  Breathing pattern, ineffective
  Cardiac output, decreased
  Fatigue
  Fluid volume, deficient
  Fluid volume, excess
  Fluid volume, risk for deficiency
  Fluid volume, risk for imbalance
  Gas exchange, impaired
  Hyperthermia
  Hypothermia
  Intracranial adaptive capacity, decreased
  Latex allergy response
  Latex allergy response, risk for
  Nausea
  Nutrition; less than body requirements, imbalanced
  Nutrition; more than body requirements, imbalanced
  Pain, chronic
  Thermoregulation, ineffective
  Tissue perfusion, ineffective
  Urinary elimination, impaired
  Urinary retention
  Ventilation, impaired spontaneous

Behavioral responses
  Anticipatory grieving
  Anxiety
  Body image disturbance
  Caregiver role strain
  Caregiver role strain, risk for
  Confusion, acute
  Coping, defensive
  Coping, ineffective
  Decisional conflict
  Delayed surgical recovery
  Denial, ineffective
  Family coping, compromised
  Family processes, interrupted
  Fear
  Growth and development, delayed
  Health maintenance, ineffective
  Home maintenance, impaired
  Hopelessness
  Knowledge, deficient
  Noncompliance
  Pain
  Parental role conflict
  Patient/infant/child attachment, risk for impaired
  Post-trauma response
  Powerlessness
  Rights
  Role performance, ineffective
  Self-esteem, low
  Sexual dysfunction
  Sexuality patterns, ineffective
  Sleep pattern, disturbed
  Social isolation
  Spiritual distress
  Therapeutic regimen, management ineffective
  Thought process, disturbed
  Verbal communication, impaired

PNDS Unique Coding Document	
DOMAINS:	
D1	Safety
D2	Physiologic Responses
D3-A	Behavioral Responses—Patient and Family: Knowledge
D3-B	Behavioral Responses—Patient and Family: Rights/Ethics
D4	Health System
OUTCOMES:	**D1: SAFETY**
	Freedom from acquired physical injury.
O2	The patient is free from signs and symptoms of injury caused by extraneous objects.
O3	The patient is free from signs and symptoms of chemical injury.
O4	The patient is free from signs and symptoms of electrical injury.
O5	The patient is free from signs and symptoms of injury related to positioning.
O6	The patient is free from signs and symptoms of laser injury.
O7	The patient is free from signs and symptoms of radiation injury.
O8	The patient is free from signs and symptoms of injury related to transfer/transport.
O9	The patient receives appropriate medication(s), safely administered during the perioperative period.
	D2: PHYSIOLOGIC RESPONSES
	Physiologic responses to surgery are as expected.
O10	The patient is free from signs and symptoms of infection.
O11	The patient has wound/tissue perfusion consistent with or improved from baseline levels established preoperatively.
O12	The patient is at or returning to normothermia at the conclusion of the immediate postoperative period.
O13	The patient's fluid, electrolyte, and acid-base balances are consistent with or improved from baseline levels established preoperatively.
O14	The patient's respiratory status is consistent with or improved from baseline levels established preoperatively.
O15	The patient's cardiac status is consistent with or improved from baseline levels established preoperatively.
O30	The patient's neurological status is consistent with or improved from baseline levels established preoperatively.
O29	The patient demonstrates and/or reports adequate pain control throughout the perioperative period.
	D3-A: BEHAVIORAL RESPONSES—PATIENT AND FAMILY: KNOWLEDGE
	Knowledge about the perioperative process.
O31	The patient demonstrates knowledge of the expected responses to the operative or other invasive procedure.
O18	The patient demonstrates knowledge of nutritional requirements related to the operative or other invasive procedure.
O19	The patient demonstrates knowledge of medication management.
O20	The patient demonstrates knowledge of pain management.
O21	The patient participates in the rehabilitation process.
O22	The patient demonstrates knowledge of wound healing.
	D3-B: BEHAVIORAL RESPONSES—PATIENT AND FAMILY: RIGHTS/ETHICS
	Patient rights and ethics are supported.
O23	The patient participates in decision making affecting the perioperative plan of care.
O24	The patient's care is consistent with the perioperative plan of care.
O25	The patient's right to privacy is maintained.
O26	The patient is the recipient of competent and ethical care within legal standards of practice.

PNDS Unique Coding Document	
O27	The patient receives consistent and comparable levels of care from all caregivers regardless of the situation or setting.
O28	The patient's value system, lifestyle, ethnicity, and culture are considered, respected, and incorporated in the perioperative plan of care as appropriate.

NURSING DIAGNOSES:

X1	Activity intolerance
X2	Airway clearance, Ineffective
X3	Anticipatory grieving
X4	Anxiety
X5	Aspiration, Risk for
X6	Body image, Disturbed
X7	Breathing pattern, Ineffective
X8	Cardiac output, Decreased
X9	Caregiver role strain
X10	Caregiver role strain, Risk for
X11	Confusion, Acute
X12	Decisional conflict
X13	Denial, Ineffective
X14	Family coping, Compromised
X15	Family processes, Interrupted
X16	Fear
X17	Fluid volume, Deficient
X18	Fluid volume, Risk for deficient
X19	Fluid volume, Excess
X20	Fluid volume, Risk for imbalance
X21	Gas exchange, Impaired
X22	Growth and development, Delayed
X23	Home maintenance, Impaired
X24	Hopelessness
X25	Hyperthermia
X26	Hypothermia
X28	Infection, Risk for
X29	Injury, Risk for
X30	Knowledge, Deficient
X31	Latex allergy response
X32	Latex allergy response, Risk for
X33	Therapeutic regimen management, Ineffective
X34	Physical mobility, Impaired
X35	Noncompliance
X36	Nutrition, Imbalanced: Less than body requirements
X37	Nutrition, Imbalanced: More than body requirements
X38	Pain, Acute
X39	Parent/infant/child attachment, Risk for Impaired
X40	Perioperative positioning injury, Risk for
X41	Peripheral neurovascular dysfunction, Risk for
X42	Post-trauma syndrome
X43	Powerlessness
X44	Protection, Ineffective
X45	Role performance, Ineffective
X46	Self-esteem, Low
X47	Sensory perception, Disturbed
X48	Sexual dysfunction
X49	Sexuality patterns, Ineffective

	PNDS Unique Coding Document
X50	Skin integrity, Impaired
X51	Skin integrity, Risk for impaired
X52	Sleep pattern, Disturbed
X53	Social isolation
X54	Spiritual distress
X55	Ventilation, Impaired spontaneous
X56	Surgical recovery, Delayed
X57	Body temperature, Risk for imbalanced
X58	Thermoregulation, Ineffective
X59	Thought process, Disturbed
X60	Tissue integrity, Impaired
X61	Tissue perfusion, Ineffective
X62	Urinary elimination, Impaired
X63	Urinary retention
X64	Verbal communication, Impaired
X65	Bed mobility, Impaired
X66	Parental role conflict
X67	Coping, Defensive
X68	Coping, Ineffective
X69	Falls, Risk for
X70	Fatigue
X71	Health maintenance, Ineffective
X72	Intracranial adaptive capacity, Decreased
X73	Nausea
X74	Pain, Chronic
X75	Transfer ability, Impaired

INTERVENTIONS

I1	**Acts as a patient advocate by protecting the patient from incompetent, unethical, or illegal practices.** Respects the Patient's Bill of Rights, complies with facility policies of competent performance, complies with federal regulations (eg, OSHA), state nurse practice acts, accrediting agencies (eg, JCAHO), and adheres to professional standards of practice (eg, AORN), and confirms clinician's privileges and credentials. Intervenes to protect the patient's safety.
I2	**Administers blood product therapy as prescribed.** Arranges for availability and the administration of blood products or blood recovery per physician order.
I3	**Administers care to invasive device sites.** Examines and compares the characteristics of site, drainage, and patency of invasive devices (eg, urinary drainage systems, endotracheal tube, tracheostomy tube, drainage tube, percutaneous catheter, vascular access devices) and provides appropriate wound care.
I4	**Administers care to wound sites.** Examines characteristics of wound sites and provides appropriate wound care.
I5	**Administers electrolyte therapy as prescribed.** Administers medications related to electrolyte balance and monitors for complications resulting from abnormal serum electrolyte levels.
I7	**Administers prescribed antibiotic therapy and immunizing agents as ordered.** Verifies physician orders for antibiotic therapies and immunizing agents and safely administers.
I8	**Administers prescribed medications and solutions.** The correct prescribed medication or solution is administered to the right patient, at the right time, in the right dose, via the right route.

PNDS Unique Coding Document

I9	**Administers prescribed medications based on arterial blood gas results.** Safely administers prescribed medications related to acid-base balance and monitors for complications resulting from acid-base imbalance.
I10	**Administers prescribed prophylactic treatments.** Confirms and safely administers ordered treatments including dietary regimens, douche, enema, and bowel preparation as ordered.
I11	**Applies safety devices.** Prepares, applies, attaches, uses, and removes devices (eg, restraints, padding, support devices) and takes action to minimize risks.
I15	**Assesses factors related to risks for ineffective tissue perfusion.** Collects data to evaluate the patient's risk for ineffective tissue perfusion (eg, presence of diabetes, immunosuppression).
I16	**Assesses pain control.** Uses validated pain scale to assess pain control.
I17	**Assesses psychosocial issues specific to the patient's medication management.** Identifies any variances in medication plan related to psychosocial status.
I18	**Assesses psychosocial issues specific to the patient's nutritional status.** Identifies any variances in nutritional plan related to psychosocial status.
I21	**Assesses susceptibility for infection.** Evaluates the patient's risks for infection related to microbial contamination.
I22	**Classifies surgical wound.** Designates the appropriate wound classification category for each surgical wound site according to the Centers for Disease Control and Prevention.
I23	**Collaborates in fluid and electrolyte management.** Collaborates with other members of health care team to monitor and implement prescribed treatments (eg, autotransfusion, IV fluids, blood products, medications).
I24	**Collaborates in initiating patient-controlled analgesia.** Identifies and collaborates in identifying patients who will benefit from patient-controlled analgesia.
I26	**Confirms identity before the operative or invasive procedure.** Verifies verbally and visually the identity of the individual undergoing the operative or invasive procedure.
I27	**Ensures continuity of care.** Provides for a continuum of care throughout the perioperative phases of care.
I30	**Develops individualized plan of care.** Considers all assessment information including patient's preferences and unique needs when developing an individualized nursing care plan.
I32	**Elicits perceptions of surgery.** Assesses responses to the procedure and ensures access to correct information.
I33	**Encourages deep breathing and coughing exercises.** Encourages use of incentive spirometry (per physician order), diaphragmatic breathing, and coughing.
I34	**Establishes IV access.** Establishes and maintains peripheral IV access to administer IV fluids, medications, and blood products per physician order.
I35	**Evaluates environment for home care.** Identifies needs after discharge by identifying those at risk and the presence of any physical barriers and potential hazards in the home and by collaborating with the patient, family members, and discharge coordinators about home care needs.
I36	**Evaluates for signs and symptoms of chemical injury.** Observes for allergic reactions, burns, rashes, blistering, respiratory distress, or other signs and symptoms of a chemical injury.

	PNDS Unique Coding Document
I37	**Evaluates for signs and symptoms of electrical injury.**
	Observes for redness, blistering, or burn to the skin.
I38	**Evaluates for signs and symptoms of injury as a result of positioning.**
	Observes for signs and symptoms of injury to integumentary, neuromuscular, and cardiopulmonary systems as a result of the patient's position during the procedure.
I40	**Evaluates for signs and symptoms of laser injury.**
	Observes for injury unrelated to the intended therapeutic effects of laser therapy.
I42	**Evaluates for signs and symptoms of skin and tissue injury as a result of transfer or transport.**
	Observes for signs and symptoms of injury to skin and tissue related to transfer or transport.
I43	**Evaluates for signs of radiation injury to skin and tissue.**
	Observes for signs and symptoms of injury to skin and tissue unrelated to the intended diagnostic or therapeutic effects of radiation.
I44	**Evaluates postoperative cardiac status.**
	Observes and monitors cardiac status throughout postoperative phase of care.
I45	**Evaluates postoperative respiratory status.**
	Observes and monitors respiratory status throughout postoperative phase of care.
I46	**Evaluates postoperative tissue perfusion.**
	Assesses tissue perfusion throughout postoperative phase of care.
I47	**Evaluates psychosocial response to plan of care.**
	Determines effectiveness of plan and psychosocial responses of patient/family members and modifies plan as indicated.
I48	**Evaluates response to instruction about prescribed medications.**
	Evaluates understanding of medication instruction by listening to explanations and observing return demonstrations of activities related to the administration and management of medications.
I49	**Evaluates response to instruction about wound care and phases of wound healing.**
	Evaluates understanding of instruction about wound healing and wound care by listening to explanations and observing return demonstrations.
I50	**Evaluates response to instructions.**
	Evaluates patient's/family member's understanding of instructions regarding perioperative experience and ongoing care.
I51	**Evaluates response to medications.**
	Observes for response and adverse reactions to medications administered.
I52	**Evaluates response to nutritional instruction.**
	Evaluates understanding of nutritional instruction by listening to explanations and observing return demonstrations.
I53	**Evaluates response to pain management instruction.**
	Evaluates understanding of pain management instruction by listening to explanations and observing return demonstrations.
I54	**Evaluates response to pain management interventions.**
	Assesses patient's responses to pain management interventions including physiological parameters and subjective and objective findings.
I55	**Evaluates response to thermoregulation measures.**
	Observes and verifies body temperature and responses to thermoregulation measures, and monitors for adverse effects.
I56	**Explains expected sequence of events.**
	Describes routines and protocols related to perioperative care.
I57	**Identifies and reports philosophical, cultural, and spiritual beliefs and values.**
	Assesses philosophical, cultural, and spiritual factors valued by the patient. Incorporates pertinent information in the plan of care and reports to other members of the health care team as appropriate.

PNDS Unique Coding Document

I58	**Identifies and reports the presence of implantable cardiac devices.** Verifies presence of pacemaker and/or automatic implantable cardioverter-defibrillator and notifies appropriate members of health care team.
I59	**Identifies baseline cardiac status.** Assesses blood pressure, heart rate and rhythm, SaO_2, and other parameters as appropriate.
I60	**Identifies baseline tissue perfusion.** Assesses tissue perfusion and identifies any impairments or risk factors prior to an operative or invasive procedure.
I61	**Identifies cultural and value components related to pain.** Provides pain control considering cultural factors and manifestations of values (eg, stoicism, alternative therapy, verbalization, meditation).
I62	**Identifies expectations of home care.** Identifies home care needs relative to performing the activities of daily living, managing self-care, and returning to usual activities.
I63	**Identifies individual values and wishes concerning care.** Assesses values, beliefs, and preferences and includes in plan of care.
I64	**Identifies physical alterations that require additional precautions for procedure-specific positioning.** Determines those at risk for positioning injury and implements appropriate precautions.
I66	**Identifies physiological status.** Assesses current physiological status and reports variances to appropriate members of health care team.
I68	**Identifies psychosocial status.** Assesses the psychosocial factors that influence that patient's care and develops and implements plan of care to address those needs.
I69	**Implements alternative methods of pain control.** Uses diversified activities, therapeutic touch, meditation, breathing, and positioning to augment pain control methods.
I70	**Implements aseptic technique.** Initiates the actions necessary related to risks associated with disease-causing microorganisms by creating and maintaining a sterile field, preventing contamination of open wounds, and isolating the operative site from the surrounding nonsterile physical environment.
I71	**Implements pain guidelines.** Provides care consistent with clinical practice guidelines related to pain assessment and management
I72	**Implements protective measures to prevent injury due to electrical sources.** Prevents injury secondary to dispersive electrode placement, active electrode handling, electrosurgical unit use, or stray radiofrequency current.
I73	**Implements protective measures to prevent injury due to laser sources.** Provides safety equipment and protective measures during a procedure using laser sources.
I74	**Implements protective measures to prevent injury due to radiation sources.** Provides safety equipment and protective measures such as gonadal protection for diagnostic and therapeutic uses of radiation.
I75	**Implements protective measures to prevent skin and tissue injury due to chemical sources.** Prevents skin and tissue trauma secondary to chemical agents including antimicrobial agents, chemical disinfectants, liquid sterilants, irrigation solutions, ethylene oxide, methylmethacrylate, and tissue preservatives.
I76	**Implements protective measures to prevent skin or tissue injury due to thermal sources.**

PNDS Unique Coding Document

I77	Prevents skin and tissue trauma secondary to thermal sources including hot instruments, solutions, casting materials, thermal regulation devices, and light sources. **Implements protective measures to prevent skin/tissue injury due to mechanical sources.** Prevents skin and tissue trauma secondary to mechanical sources including the use of devices such as positioning equipment, tourniquets, sequential compression devices, razors, clippers. tape, and the OR bed.
I78	**Implements thermoregulation measures.** Initiates thermoregulation measures and applies devices to cool or warm the patient as indicated.
I79	**Includes family members in preoperative teaching.** Identifies family members' knowledge and provides education and support.
I80	**Includes patient and family members in discharge planning.** Reviews with patient/family members the patient's capabilities, anticipated plan for care, and resources available to facilitate the rehabilitation process.
I81	**Initiates traffic control.** Restricts access to patient care area to authorized individuals only.
I83	**Manages culture specimen collection.** Collects, identifies, labels, stores, preserves, and transports specimens for microbiological testing.
I84	**Manages specimen handling and disposition.** Collects, identifies, labels, processes, stores, preserves, and transports specimens.
I85	**Minimizes the length of invasive procedure by planning care.** Contributes to minimizing operative time by anticipation and advanced preparation, coordinates team members' efforts to set priorities, and efficiently accomplishes the tasks necessary to achieve a common goal.
I86	**Monitors body temperature.** Inserts, attaches, or applies temperature-monitoring devices.
I87	**Monitors changes in respiratory status.** Assesses respiratory status and monitors for changes in respiratory status.
I88	**Monitors for signs and symptoms of infection.** Observes for manifestations of tissue reaction due to pathogenic microorganism invasion of the body.
I89	**Monitors physiological parameters.** Monitors physiological parameters including intake and output, arterial blood gases, electrolyte levels, hemodynamic status, and SaO_2.
I90	**Notes sensory impairments.** Determines the patient's ability to see and hear without corrective devices.
I92	**Obtains consultation from the appropriate health care providers to initiate new treatments or change existing treatments.** Involves and/or consults other members of health care team if the patient's condition or planned procedure changes.
I93	**Performs required counts.** Ensures that the patient is free from injury related to retained sponges, instruments, and sharps.
I94	**Performs skin preparations.** Carries out necessary actions to prepare the epidermis for an operative or invasive procedure.
I95	**Performs venipuncture.** Obtains diagnostic blood samples.
I96	**Positions the patient.** Determines the need for, prepares, applies, and removes devices designed to enhance operative exposure, prevent neuromuscular injury, maintain skin and tissue integrity, and maintain body alignment and optimal physiological functioning.

	PNDS Unique Coding Document
I97	**Preserves and protects the patient's autonomy, dignity, and human rights.** Confirms consent, implements facility advance directive policy, and supports patient's participation in decision making.
I98	**Protects from cross-contamination.** Applies methodologies that prevent patient exposure to infective agents from endogenous sources (as from one tissue to another within the patient) and from exogenous sources (as acquired from objects, personnel, or other patients).
I99	**Provides care in a nondiscriminatory, nonprejudicial manner regardless of the setting in which care is given.** Adheres to AORN, Joint Commission, and other standards of care. Provides comparable levels of care regardless of the setting in which care is given (eg, inpatient, outpatient, public, private, home, emergency department).
I100	**Provides care respecting the worth and dignity regardless of diagnosis, disease process, procedure, or projected outcome.** Provides for spiritual comfort, arranges for substitute nursing care when personal values conflict with required care, and respects patient's decision for surgery.
I102	**Provides care without prejudicial behavior.** Applies standards of nursing practice consistently and without bias (eg, disability, economic background, education, culture, religion, race, age, and gender).
I103	**Provides information and explains Patient Self-Determination Act.** Assesses current knowledge of the Patient Self-Determination Act (eg, the living will, power of attorney for health care, do not resuscitate, informed consent, organ procurement) and provides a copy of resources/referral related to the Patient Self-Determination Act.
I104	**Provides instruction about prescribed medications.** Provides information about prescribed medications, such as purpose; administration; and desired, side, and adverse effects.
I105	**Provides instruction about wound care and phases of wound healing.** Provides necessary information about the phases of wound healing, techniques of wound care, and signs and symptoms to report.
I106	**Provides instruction based on age and identified needs.** Provides perioperative instructional activities that promote rehabilitation based on age and developmental and situation-specific needs.
I107	**Provides instruction regarding dietary needs.** Explains dietary needs or restrictions.
I108	**Provides pain management instruction.** Provides information about the purpose; administration; and desired, side, and adverse effects of prescribed medications and non-pharmacological techniques for managing pain.
I109	**Provides status reports to family members.** Reports progress to family members by telephone or in person.
I110	**Recognizes and reports deviation in arterial blood gas studies.** Identifies critical variances in acid-base balance and notifies appropriate members of health care team.
I111	**Recognizes and reports deviation in diagnostic study results.** Identifies critical variances in fluid, electrolyte, and acid-base balances and notifies appropriate members of health care team.
I112	**Records devices implanted during the operative or invasive procedure.** Verifies and records the placement of implants, manufacturer, lot number, type, size, and other identifying information in compliance with federal regulations for tracking implantable devices.
I113	**Screens for physical abuse.** Identifies defining characteristics for actual or risks for physical abuse and offers appropriate referrals.

PNDS Unique Coding Document

I114	**Screens for substance abuse.** Assesses for past or present substance abuse, monitors for and reports defining characteristics of substance abuse or withdrawal, and makes appropriate referrals.
I115	**Secures patient's records, belongings, and valuables.** Protects patient's clinical records and personal property. Releases belongings and valuables to patient or designated individual.
I116	**Shares patient information only with those directly involved in care.** Protects patient information by completing operative record accurately and shares information in a manner that ensures patient confidentiality.
I118	**Transports according to individual needs.** Ensures transfer without tissue injury; altered body temperature; ineffective breathing patterns; altered tissue perfusion; and undue discomfort, pain, or fear.
I119	**Uses a clinical pathway.** Actions performed are consistent with predetermined clinical pathway.
I120	**Uses monitoring equipment to assess cardiac status.** Assesses blood pressure, heart rate and rhythm, SaO_2, and other parameters as appropriate.
I121	**Uses monitoring equipment to assess respiratory status.** Assesses respiratory status and SaO_2.
I122	**Uses supplies and equipment within safe parameters.** Ensures that use of supplies, equipment, and instruments does not compromise patient safety.
I123	**Verifies allergies.** Identifies allergies, idiosyncrasies, and sensitivities to medications, latex, chemical agents, foods, and/or adhesives.
I124	**Verifies consent for planned procedure.** Determines that informed consent has been granted for planned operative or invasive procedure and any related activities (eg, photographs, investigational studies).
I127	**Verifies presence of prosthetics or corrective devices.** Identifies presence of or use of prosthetics or corrective devices and modifies nursing care as indicated for planned procedure.
I128	**Maintains continuous surveillance.** Acquires, interprets, and synthesizes patient data so as to detect and prevent potential adverse clinical events.
I129	**Functions as first assistant during surgical incision, excision, and repair of pathology (RNFA).** Functions as first assistant during an operative or other invasive procedure.
I130	**Evaluates progress of wound healing.** Assesses skin condition, tissue perfusion, and healing progress of surgical wound.
I131	**Assesses risk for inadvertent hypothermia.** Determines patients at risk for loss of body heat and plans appropriate interventions.
I132	**Identifies factors associated with an increased risk for hemorrhage or fluid and electrolyte loss.** Identifies individuals at risk for hemorrhage or hypovolemia including those with recent traumatic injury, abnormal bleeding or clotting time, extensive surgical procedure, complicated renal/liver disease, and major organ transplant.
I133	**Implements hemostasis techniques.** Provides supplies, instrumentation, and appropriate surgical techniques as needed to control hemorrhage.
I134	**Identifies barriers to communication.** Assesses factors that could affect ability to communicate, comprehend, and demonstrate understanding of new information.

PNDS Unique Coding Document	
I135	**Determines knowledge level.** Assesses knowledge and comprehension of new information and ability to apply in self-care activities.
I136	**Assesses readiness to learn.** Evaluates factors that may affect abilities to learn or demonstrate knowledge.
I137	**Assesses coping mechanisms.** Assesses the influence of coping practices and availability of support from family members.
I138	**Implements protective measures prior to operative or invasive procedure.** The patient, equipment, and environment are prepared to ensure safety during operative or other invasive procedure.
I139	**Implements latex allergy precautions as needed.** Protects patients with risks for or latex-sensitivity from exposure to natural rubber.
I140	**Applies chemical hemostatic agents (RNFA).** Uses chemical hemostatic agents to control bleeding within the surgical wound.
I141	**Prescribes medications within scope of practice (RNFA).** Prescribes medications in accordance with state and federal rules and regulations and facility policies.
I142	**Assesses history of previous radiation exposure.** Assesses patient's history of radiation exposure for therapeutic and diagnostic purposes.
I143	**Verifies operative procedure, surgical site, and laterality.** Verifies patient's/family member's understanding by listening to their explanations of procedure to be performed, site, and laterality.
I144	**Assess baseline neurological status.** Collects data to evaluate patient's current neurological status.
I145	**Implements protective measures during neurosurgical procedures.** Protects patient form harm caused by equipment, supplies, or positioning specific to neurosurgical procedures.
I146	**Evaluates postoperative neurological status.** Assesses and monitors neurological status throughout postoperative phase of care.
I147	**Implements measures to provide psychological support.** Offers assistance, advocates for patient, and provides psychological support during perioperative phases of care.
I148	**Assesses nutritional habits and patterns.** Identifies usual dietary intake, habits, and patterns.
I149	**Assesses knowledge regarding wound care and phases of wound healing.** Determines knowledge level about wound care and wound healing process.
I150	**Maintains patient's dignity and privacy.** Protects the patient's privacy (eg, keeps OR doors closed, only exposes body as needed for care). Treats the deceased patient with respect and provides privacy area for family viewing of the deceased.
I151	**Maintains patient confidentiality.** Limits access of patient information to appropriate members of health care team.
I152	**Evaluates for signs and symptoms of physical injury to skin and tissue.** Observes for signs and symptoms of physical injury to skin and tissue acquired from extraneous objects.
I153	**Evaluates response to administration of fluids and electrolytes.** Observes for signs and symptoms of fluid and electrolyte imbalances.

The Perioperative Nursing Data Set

Explanation of PNDS Layout		
Patient outcome.	→	**OUTCOME O7:** The patient is free from signs and symptoms of radiation injury.
Definition provides further explanation of the outcome.	→	**OUTCOME DEFINITION:** The patient is free from signs or symptoms of injury related to use of radiation. Radiation exposure is limited to the target site.
Interpretive statement describes the scope of the current problem or need.	→	**INTERPRETIVE STATEMENT:** Prevention of radiation injury requires the application of principles of physics and radiologic safety standards. Policies addressing education, credentialing, and radiologic safety and maintenance must be in accordance with national regulatory standards and manufacturers' documented instructions. Preexisting patient conditions (eg, length of and/or previous exposure) can influence the patient's susceptibility to radiologic injury.
Outcome indicators are derived from assessment data and provide a framework for evaluating the patient's progress or a clinical standard. *(This is not intended to be an all-inclusive list.)*	→	**OUTCOME INDICATORS:** • Skin condition (general): smooth, intact, and free from unexplained edema, redness, blistering, or tenderness in nontargeted areas. • Cognition: responds appropriately to questioning; memory intact.
Examples of interim outcome statements provide outcomes that reflect a patient's family member's* status at a specific point and time across the surgical continuum. *(This is not intended to be an all-inclusive list.)*	→	**EXAMPLES OF INTERIM OUTCOME STATEMENTS:** The patient's skin remains smooth, intact, and free from unexplained redness, blistering, or tenderness in targeted areas between admission and discharge from the OR.
Nursing diagnoses are linked to each outcome and provide possible human responses linked with surgical experiences. *(This is not intended to be an all-inclusive list.)*	→	**POTENTIALLY APPLICABLE NURSING DIAGNOSES:** • Risk of impaired skin integrity (X51) • Impaired skin integrity (X50) • Acute confusion (X11)
Nursing intervention statements are in bold print; each has a definition and is generally the data element that is documented. Activity statements are the bulleted points under interventions. Activities support interventions, but do not necessarily need to be documented. *(This is not intended to be an all-inclusive list.)*	→ →	**NURSING INTERVENTIONS AND ACTIVITIES:** **Implements protective measures to prevent injury due to radiation sources.** Provides safety equipment such as gonadal protection for diagnostic and therapeutic uses of radiation. • Assembles proper protective equipment. • Limits exposure to radiation to therapeutic levels (eg, fluoroscope is off when not in use, radioactive elements remain in lead-lined containers until ready for implantation). • Provides shields to protect body areas from scatter radiation or focused beam whenever possible (fetus/gonadal shields, thyroid/sternal shields, lead aprons, lead gloves). • Implements appropriate procedures for handling of radiated tissue specimens. • Implements measures to protect the patient from direct and scatter radiation. • Manages body fluids and tissue removed from patients who have undergone recent diagnostic studies using radioactive materials according to recommendations of the radiation safety department. • Documents protective measures on clinical record.

*Family member—AORN defines *family* as the person or people that the patient identifies as his or her family. *Family member* replaces the terms *support person* and *significant other* but indicates the same meaning.

ALPHABETICAL INDEX TO PNDS OUTCOMES

NOTE: For a list of interventions associated with each outcome, see pages 235–239 in the Index.
For the complete coding document containing the PNDS Domains, Outcomes, Nursing Diagnoses,
and Interventions in numerical order, see Chapter 3, "The Conceptual Framework of the PNDS."

EXTRANEOUS OBJECTS

OUTCOME O2   **The patient is free from signs and symptoms of injury caused by extraneous objects.**

OUTCOME DEFINITION: The patient is free from signs or symptoms of injury due to equipment, instrumentation, sponges, or sharps.

INTERPRETIVE STATEMENT: Performance of an operative or other invasive procedure requires the use of a variety of equipment (eg, IVs, tracheostomy tubes, pneumatic tourniquet, thermal blanket, and sequential compression devices). Prevention of injury requires application of knowledge regarding each item used during the operative or invasive procedure. Care must be taken to ensure the proper use, function, and coordination of these items so they serve their intended therapeutic purposes.

OUTCOME INDICATORS:

- **Skin condition (general):** smooth, intact, and free from ecchymosis, cuts, abrasions, shear injury, rash, or blistering.
- **Skin condition (IV site):** free from discoloration, swelling, or induration.
- **Neuromuscular status:** flexes and extends extremities without assistance; denies numbness or tingling of extremities.
- **Cardiovascular status:** heart rate and blood pressure within expected ranges; peripheral pulses present and equal bilaterally; skin warm to touch.

EXAMPLES OF INTERIM OUTCOME STATEMENTS:

- Patient's skin condition other than incision is unchanged between admission and discharge from the operating room (OR).
- The patient is free from unplanned retained objects following surgery.
- The patient's peripheral pulses distal to the operative tourniquet are equal to or improved from baseline.
- Skin distal to skeletal immobilizing device (cast, brace) is warm to touch and capillary refill less than 3 seconds at time of discharge from OR.

POTENTIALLY APPLICABLE NURSING DIAGNOSES:

- Risk for injury (X29)
- Risk for impaired skin integrity (X51)
- Impaired skin integrity (X50)
- Disturbed sensory perception (X47)
- Risk for peripheral neurovascular dysfunction (X41)
- Ineffective protection (X44)
- Impaired physical mobility (X34)

NURSING INTERVENTIONS AND ACTIVITIES:

Implements protective measures prior to operative or invasive procedure (I138).
The patient, equipment, and environment are prepared to ensure safety during operative or other invasive procedure.
- Reviews preoperative checklist for evidence of preparedness for procedure (eg, lab testing, history and physical on record). For pediatric patient includes birth history, developmental stages, and parent/child interactions.
- Confirms/establishes preoperative assessment of physical status.
- Collaborates with health care provider to obtain required/indicated diagnostic testing prior to surgical procedure.
- Refers variances from preoperative testing norms to appropriate health care provider.

- Introduces self to patient and explains perioperative role.
  - Identifies purpose of assessment to patient.
  - Identifies barriers to communication.
  - Determines knowledge level.
  - Verifies patient's ability or inability to understand information.
  - Obtains interpreter if needed.
- Verifies NPO status.
  - Asks when patient last ate food or drank liquids.
  - Asks what medications were taken day of procedure and dose and time.
  - Asks same questions of family member if patient is unable to respond.
  - Requests detailed list of food or fluid if patient has the ingested day of procedure, including time and amount.
  - Shares information with members of health care team for patient reevaluation as indicated.
- Reviews surgical consent form for completeness and accuracy (procedure, laterality, date).
  - Determines that physician's notations on health record are consistent with surgical consent.
  - Encourages patient, family member to describe understanding of intended procedure.
- Informs surgeon and/or administrative authority of any discrepancy.
- Assures that vacuum system is operative prior to induction.
- Checks OR light for function.
- Removes environmental hazards (eg, remove unnecessary equipment, provide appropriate waste receptacles).

Confirms identity before the operative or invasive procedure (I26).
Verifies verbally and visually the identity of the individual undergoing the operative or invasive procedure.

<u>Alert and oriented patient</u>
- Greets patient using his/her full name, introduces self, and asks patient to state name and the operative procedure to be performed.
- Verifies name and hospital number on the transfer slip with the patient's identification bracelet.
- Verifies and patient identification bracelet with patient's chart.
- Verifies that consent form coincides with procedure identified by patient.

<u>Child</u>
- Follows steps delineated above.
- Establishes contact with child and parent or legal guardian.
- Asks parent/legal guardian child's name and procedure being performed.
- Asks the same of child, if appropriate.
- Relies on unit nursing staff to identify patient in absence of parent/legal guardian.

<u>Comatose and disoriented patient</u>
- Verifies patient's identification bracelet and patient's chart.
- Asks family member, if present, to identify patient.
- Relies on unit nursing staff to identify patient in absence of any family member.

Verifies operative procedure, surgical site, and laterality (I143).
Verifies patient's/family member's understanding by listening to their explanations of procedure to be performed, site, and laterality.
- Reviews surgery schedule.
- Reviews surgical consent form for completeness, accuracy, and congruency with patient's statements.
- Determines that physician's notations on health record are consistent with surgical consent.
- Visually inspects patient identification band to verify correct name and number.
- Encourages patient/family member to verbalize identity.
- Encourages patient/family member to describe understanding of intended procedure, site, and laterality.
- Encourages patient/family member to indicate site and laterality.

- Informs surgeon and/or administrative authority of any discrepancy.
- Follows facility policies regarding verification of site and laterality.
- Evaluates patient's responses.

Applies safety devices (I11).
Prepares, applies, attaches, uses, and removes devices (eg, restraints, padding, support devices) and takes action to minimize risks.
- Examines the surgical environment for equipment or conditions that pose a safety risk and takes corrective action.
- Selects safety devices based on patient's needs and the planned operative or invasive procedure.
- Applies safety devices to patient according to the plan of care, applicable practice guidelines, facility policies, and manufacturers' documented instructions.
- Ensures that safety devices are readily available, clean, free of sharp edges, padded as appropriate, and in working order prior use.

Implements protective measures to prevent skin or tissue injury due to thermal sources (I76).
Prevents skin and tissue trauma secondary to thermal sources including hot instruments, solutions, casting materials, thermal regulation devices, and light sources.
- Assesses patient's risk for skin injury related to thermal hazards.
- Identifies nursing diagnoses that describe the patient's degree of risk for skin injury related to thermal hazards.
- Inspects skin periodically during and after using thermoregulation devices.
- Plans interventions to protect and maintain skin integrity.
- Monitors temperature when using thermoregulation devices.
- Protects patient from injury related to application of plaster.
  - Provides adequate padding, stockinette, roll padding, or felt to protect skin.
  - Dips casting materials in lukewarm, not hot, water (70° to 80° F).
  - Allows cast to remain uncovered to cool and dry.
- Monitors active electrode of electrosurgical unit during procedure.
  - Places active electrode in clean, dry, nonconductive, highly visible area during procedure.
  - Prevents active electrode from contacting metal clamps.
  - Prevents active electrode from lying on patient during procedure.
  - Insures alarms are active and functioning.
- Monitors function of dispersive electrode of electrosurgical unit during procedure.
  - Places dispersive electrode close as possible to surgical site.
  - Sets dysfunction alarm to audible status.
- Evaluates temperature safety of irrigating/infusion solutions immediately prior to administration.
- Protects skin and internal organs from heat transfer by endoscopes or other hot instruments.

Implements protective measures to prevent skin/tissue injury due to mechanical sources (I77).
Prevents skin and tissue trauma secondary to mechanical sources including the use of devices such as positioning equipment, tourniquets, sequential compression devices, razors, clippers, tape, and the OR bed.
- Assesses patient's risk for skin injury related to mechanical hazards.
- Assesses skin for injury from invasive devices (tubes, drains, indwelling catheters, cables).
- Identifies the nursing diagnoses that describe patient's degree of risk for skin injury related to mechanical hazards.
- Plans interventions to protect and maintain skin integrity.
- Selects safest method of hair removal (if indicated) that preserves skin integrity.
  - Provides adequate lighting.
  - Inquires about allergies.
  - Observes for scars, moles, skin lesions, or raised areas.
  - Avoids traumatizing skin lesions or raised areas on the skin surface (melanomas, basal cell carcinomas, moles) or other lesions erupting through the skin.
  - Removes hair, if necessary, as close to time of surgery as possible.
  - Uses electric or battery powered clippers, with disposable clipper head, or, if reusable, disinfected clipper head as first choice for hair removal.

- Uses disposable razor or razor that has been terminally sterilized and wet shave method for hair removal if clippers or depilatories cannot be used.
- Reassess skin immediately after hair removal observing for redness, razor or clipper nicks, or skin abrasions.
- Evaluates skin postoperatively for redness, razor or clipper nicks, or skin abrasions.
- Applies casting materials and immobilizing devices. *(RNFA)*
- Provides cast care to patients with fresh plaster cast to prevent injury to skin.
  - Pads and/or covers rough edges of plaster cast.
  - Holds cast with outstretched palm to prevent undue pressure on skin.
  - Places fresh casted extremity on pillow to protect cast from rough surfaces or excessive pressure that may cause denting.
  - Monitors circulation and color of exposed digits on casted extremity (includes capillary refill).
  - Monitors patient for increased pain and/or change in sensation after cast application.
- Cleans and dries skin around incision site before applying dressing.
- Secures dressing with tape without stretching the skin.
- Inspects, tests, and uses powered surgical instruments according to manufacturers' documented instructions.
  - Tests device before use.
  - Places triggers/handles in safety position when changing attachments.
  - Sets and runs pneumatically powered instruments at manufacturer-recommended pounds per square inch (psi).
- Uses tourniquet according to procedural need.
  - Selects cuff according to dimensions of patient's extremity and manufacturers' documented instructions.
  - Checks cuff for function and integrity.
  - Applies wrinkle-free padding to extremity at cuff site unless contraindicated by manufacturer.
  - Positions the cuff according to procedure to be performed.
  - Secures cuff.
  - Avoids rotating cuff after application.
  - Applies impervious barrier around cuff during skin preparation for procedure.
  - Avoids allowing prep solution to seep under cuff. Removes cuff, dries extremity, and replaces cuff with dry cuff if solution has wet cuff.
  - Avoids damaging cuff with perforating towel clip or other sharp object.
  - Inflates and deflates cuff as instructed by the surgeon.
  - Confirms requested change in tourniquet pressure.
  - Keeps tourniquet pressure gauge clearly visible during use.
  - Maintains record of tourniquet use duration and informs surgeon of tourniquet time at established intervals.
  - Inspects skin after cuff removal for signs of bruising, blistering, pinching, and/or necrosis.

Performs required counts (I93).
Ensures that the patient is free from injury related to retained sponges, instruments, and sharps.

Sponges
- Counts sponges before the procedure to establish a baseline, at the time of permanent relief of either the scrub person or the circulating nurse, before closure of a cavity within a cavity, before wound closure begins, and at skin closure or end of procedure.
  - Counts audibly and concurrently with team counterpart (scrub person or circulating nurse).
  - Separates sponges when counting.
  - Uses only x-ray-detectable sponges during the procedure.
  - Examines wound for sponges prior to required counts. *(RNFA)*
  - Counts sponges in units of five or 10, according to packaging.
  - Removes packages of sponges that contain more or less than expected packaged number from the operative field.
  - Keeps sponges, linen, and trash in the OR during entire procedure.
  - Maintains knowledge of sponge locations on sterile field.

- Discards used sponges in a fluid-impervious lined container.
- Places counted sponges in clear plastic bags in groups of five or 10 as they are accumulated.
- Labels bag with number of sponges and initials bag according to facility policy.
- Reports count results to surgeon.
- Documents count on patient record according to policy.

Sharps
- Counts sharps before the procedure to establish a baseline, at the time of permanent relief of either the scrub person or the circulating nurse, before closure of a cavity within a cavity, before wound closure begins, and at skin closure or end of procedure.
  - Counts audibly and concurrently with team counterpart (ie, scrub person or circulating nurse).
  - Counts needles according to number indicated on package.
  - Verifies number of needles with circulating nurse when package is opened.
  - Retains sharps in OR during procedure.
  - Maintains knowledge of location of sharps on sterile field.
  - Exercises caution to prevent injury when handling used sharps.
  - Implements "hands-free" techniques for exchange of all sharps.
  - Accounts for all pieces of broken sharps.
  - Examines wound for needles/sharps prior to required counts. *(RNFA)*
  - Reports count results to surgeon.
  - Documents count on patient record according to policy.

Instruments
- Counts instruments before the procedure to establish a baseline, at the time of permanent relief of either the scrub person or the circulating nurse, and before wound closure begins.
  - Counts audibly and concurrently with team counterpart (ie, scrub person or circulating nurse).
  - Maintains knowledge of location of instruments on and off the sterile field.
  - Isolates and accounts for all removable instrument parts and all pieces of broken instruments.
  - Exercises caution to prevent injury when handling used instruments
  - Examines wound for instruments prior to required counts. *(RNFA)*
  - Reports count results to surgeon.
  - Documents count on patient record according to policy.

Unresolved counts
- Notify surgeon of unresolved counts.
- Resolves count according to facility policy.
- Implements documentation procedures according to facility policy.

Manages specimen handling and disposition (I84).
Collects, identifies, labels, processes, stores, preserves, and transports specimens.
- Establishes chain of custody for cultures and tissue specimens.
- Provides supplies and equipment needed for collection of cultures and specimens.
- Labels culture and tissue specimen containers.
- Completes laboratory slips.
- Documents collection of cultures and specimens on the patient's operative record.
- Obtains and processes frozen sections for pathology examination as quickly as possible.
- Prepares surgical specimens for disposition according to hospital policy.
- Directs transfer of cultures and specimens to laboratory.
- Communicates intraoperative pathology reports to physician.

Uses supplies and equipment within safe parameters (I122).
Ensures that use of supplies, equipment, and instruments does not compromise patient safety.
- Obtains necessary supplies and equipment for procedure.
- Consults manufacturers' documented instructions for use of supplies, equipment, and instruments.
- Operates equipment according to manufacturers' documented instructions.

- Verifies safety/biotechnology inspections are current on all equipment.
- Isolates malfunctioning equipment and defective supplies.
- Checks for manufacturer outdates before using packaged items.
- Provides care using the principles of aseptic technique and transmission-based precautions.
- Opens supply packages according to manufacturers' documented instructions, principles of aseptic technique, and facility policy and procedure.
- Discards contaminated packages.

Records devices implanted during the operative or invasive procedure (I112).
Verifies and records the placement of implants, manufacturer, lot number, type, size, and other identifying information in compliance with federal regulations for tracking implantable devices.
- Complies with federal regulations for tracking implantable devices.
- Completes required internal and external paperwork.
- Notifies appropriate personnel, facility, or manufacturer of implant defects or failure.
- Provides patient with implant identification documentation/card.

Performs venipuncture (I95).
Obtains diagnostic blood samples.
- Collects appropriate supplies for procedure.
- Verifies order for venipuncture.
- Reviews chart for allergies, laboratory results, and patient history.
- Assesses barriers to communication.
- Assesses patient's ability to understand information.
- Provides information about procedure to be completed and offers emotional support.
- Reviews with patient presence of allergies, clotting problems, or medications that may affect clotting.
- Maintains aseptic technique throughout procedure.
- Applies warm compresses to dilate venous system as appropriate.
- Applies tourniquet above insertion site.
- Cleanses area with appropriate solution per facility policy or protocol.
- Inserts needle per appropriate policy or protocol.
- Observes for blood in flash chamber/blood collection tube.
- Evaluates patient's response to procedure.

Maintains continuous surveillance (I128).
Acquires, interprets, and synthesizes patient data so as to detect and prevent potential adverse clinical events.
- Continually monitors physiological and psychological indicators to detect discrete changes in overall condition.
- Utilizes critical thinking.
- Recognizes patients at high risk for complications.
- Communicates information about patient's risk status to appropriate member(s) of health care team.
- Monitors and controls clinical environment for safety or infection risks and other potential hazards.
- Prioritizes nursing actions based on clinical situation and patient's condition.
- Monitors patient for changes in status that requires immediate nurse attention.
- Institutes appropriate care utilizing clinical practice guidelines.
- Notes type and amounts of effluent from drainage tube and notifies appropriate member of health care team regarding significant changes.
- Troubleshoots surgical equipment and clinical systems.

Evaluates for signs and symptoms of physical injury to skin and tissue (I152).
Observes for signs and symptoms of physical injury to skin and tissue acquired from extraneous objects.
- Verifies preoperative nursing assessment.
- Assesses skin postoperatively for razor or clipper nicks, or skin abrasions.
- Inspects entire area prepped with antimicrobial solution for signs of redness, rash, abrasion, or blisters.
- Inspects skin for signs of bruising, blistering, pinching, and necrosis after removal of tourniquet cuff.
- Observes extremities for ability to move fingers/toes after removal of tourniquet.
- Assesses peripheral sensation after removal of tourniquet.

- Evaluates skin integrity after electrocautery use, paying close attention to any imprint on the dispersive pad itself, areas under dispersive electrode, skin under the electrocardiogram (ECG) leads, and at temperature probe entry sites.
- Assesses circulation, sensation, and motion of extremities:
  - Inspects color, size, and shape;
  - Palpates for warmth, dryness, and capillary refill;
  - Palpates for quality and volume of pulses;
  - Assesses for complaints of pain or discomfort in areas other than surgical incision; and
  - Reports variances from expected findings to appropriate health care providers.

CHEMICAL INJURY

OUTCOME O3   **The patient is free from signs and symptoms of chemical injury.**

OUTCOME DEFINITION: The patient remains free from signs or symptoms of injury related to chemical hazards.

INTERPRETIVE STATEMENT: Hazards arise from the use of a variety of chemicals in the perioperative environment. Prevention of chemical injury requires application of knowledge of the proper use of each chemical compound. Preexisting patient conditions (eg, open wounds, skin condition, immune status, previous chemical exposure) can influence patient susceptibility to chemical injury. Length of exposure to a chemical may increase the likelihood of injury. These chemicals include, but are not limited to:
- cleaning solutions,
- skin prep solutions,
- pharmaceuticals (eg, irrigation solutions),
- methylmethacrylate, and
- tissue preservatives (eg, formalin).

OUTCOME INDICATORS:

- **Skin condition (wound):** skin prepared for surgical incision is free from redness, rash, abrasion, or blistering.
- **Skin condition (general):** smooth, intact, and free from ecchymosis, redness, cuts, abrasions, shear injury, hives, rash, or blistering.
- **Respiratory status:** respirations free from dyspnea, wheezing, or stridor; SaO_2 within expected range.
- **Cardiovascular status:** heart rate and blood pressure within expected ranges; peripheral pulses present and equal bilaterally; skin warm to touch.
- **Gastrointestinal status:** free from nausea, vomiting, or diarrhea following exposure to chemical agents.

EXAMPLES OF INTERIM OUTCOME STATEMENTS:

- The patient's skin condition, other than incision, is unchanged between admission and discharge from the OR.
- The patient is breathing spontaneously on room air without assistance at discharge from the OR.
- The patient's vital signs are stable at discharge from the OR.

POTENTIALLY APPLICABLE NURSING DIAGNOSES:

- Risk for impaired skin integrity (X51)
- Impaired skin integrity (X50)
- Ineffective breathing pattern (X7)
- Risk for allergic response to latex (X32)
- Allergic response to latex (X31)
- Nausea (X73)
- Decreased cardiac output (X8)

NURSING INTERVENTIONS AND ACTIVITIES:

Implements protective measures to prevent skin and tissue injury due to chemical sources (I75).
Prevents skin and tissue trauma secondary to chemical agents including antimicrobial agents, chemical disinfectants, liquid sterilants, irrigation solutions, ethylene oxide, methylmethacrylate, and tissue preservatives.
- Assesses the patient's risk for skin injury related to chemical hazards during the perioperative period.
- Identifies nursing diagnoses that describe the patient's degree of risk for skin injury related to chemical hazards.
- Plans interventions to protect and maintain skin integrity.

- Follows manufacturers' documented instructions regarding skin testing and use of chemical depilatories when removing hair.
- Prepares skin with antimicrobial agents before surgical intervention in a manner that preserves skin integrity.
  - Selects antimicrobial agents based on patient's allergies and sensitivities, incision location, and skin condition.
  - Uses antimicrobial agent according to manufacturers' documented instructions.
  - Places sterile towels under the patient before skin preparation to prevent antimicrobial solutions from pooling beneath the patient.
  - Places impervious pads under extremities before skin preparation to prevent antimicrobial solutions from saturating bed linens.
  - Applies an impervious barrier around the tourniquet cuff before preparing skin to prevent antimicrobial solution from pooling beneath tourniquet cuff. If solutions seep under the cuff, removes the cuff, dries the limb and the cuff, and reapplies the cuff.
  - Allows antimicrobial solutions drying time.
  - Documents type of prep solution used and site prepped.
  - Observes skin for any allergic type responses to prep solutions.
  - Cleans remaining dried prep solution from around surgical site.
- Allows flammable solutions (eg, alcohol, acetone, fat solvents) to dry and fumes to evaporate before draping or activating electrosurgical or laser equipment.
- Observes patient's skin immediately postoperatively for redness, rash, abrasion, or blisters.
- Uses sterile water to thoroughly rinse items disinfected with chemical germicides prior to use in an invasive procedure.
- Prevents burns to patient's skin/tissue by completing full aeration cycle for gas-sterilized items/supplies before use.
- Protects patient from skin/tissue burn by completely rinsing high-level disinfectants solutions from the surface of equipment or devices.
- Prevents undiluted sterilant from touching patient by completing entire sterilization cycle when using low temperature liquid chemical sterilization methods.
- Cleans and dries skin around incision before applying dressing to prevent applying tape over dried preparation solutions.
- Evaluates skin/tissue for chemical injury.

Verifies allergies (I123).
Identifies allergies, idiosyncrasies, and sensitivities to medications, latex, chemical agents, foods, and/or adhesives.
- Queries patient about allergies or hypersensitivity reaction to adhesives, egg products, latex or iodine products.
- Queries patient about medications and foreign proteins that cause anaphylaxis (eg, antibiotics, opiates, insulin, vasopressin, protamine, allergen extracts, muscle relaxants, vaccines, local anesthetics, whole blood, cryoprecipitate, immune globulin, iodinated contrast media).
- Determines type of food, nutritional supplements or substance and type of reaction experienced, if any, as reported by the patient.
- Records and communicates to the anesthesia care provider a patient history of anaphylaxis, asthma, or other respiratory difficulties related to the presence of allergens, toxins, or antigens.

Implements latex allergy precautions as needed (I139).
Protects patients with risks for or latex-sensitivity from exposure to natural rubber.
- Stores essential non-natural-rubber supplies in a quick access location.
- Assesses/monitors for latex allergy response.
- Initiates approved latex precautions protocol as needed.
- Evaluates effectiveness of precautions taken.

Applies chemical hemostatic agents *(RNFA)* (I140).
Uses chemical hemostatic agents to control bleeding within the surgical wound.
- Assesses/monitors blood loss throughout procedure.
- Assesses blood flow to determine if chemical hemostatic agent is contraindicated. *(RNFA)*
- Assesses proximity of skin for appropriate use and placement of hemostatic agents. *(RNFA)*
- Evaluates response to chemical hemostatic agents.

Evaluates for signs and symptoms of chemical injury (I36).
Observes for allergic reactions, burns, rashes, blistering, respiratory distress, or other signs and symptoms of a chemical injury.
- Assesses skin for any allergic type responses to prep solutions.
- Inspects entire area prepped with solution(s) for signs of redness, rash, abrasion, or burns.
- Assesses dependent areas of skin for injury due to pooling of prep or irrigation solution.
- Assesses respiratory status for signs and symptoms such as dyspnea, shortness of breath, labored respirations, wheezing, or stridor.

ELECTRICAL INJURY

OUTCOME O4   **The patient is free from signs and symptoms of electrical injury.**

OUTCOME DEFINITION: The patient is free from any observable signs or reported symptoms of injury related to use of electrical devices.

INTERPRETIVE STATEMENT: Prevention of electrical injury requires application of principles of electrosurgical safety, routine maintenance, and knowledge of potential hazards. Performance of the operative or other invasive procedure relies on many electrical devices, notably the electrosurgical unit (ESU). Electrical equipment must be used according to manufacturers' documented instructions.

OUTCOME INDICATORS:

- **Skin condition (dispersive electrode sites and potential alternative ground injury):** smooth, intact, and free from ecchymosis, blisters, or redness.
- **Neuromuscular status:** flexes and extends extremities without assistance; denies numbness or tingling of extremities.
- **Cardiovascular status:** heart rate and blood pressure within expected ranges; peripheral pulses present and equal bilaterally; skin warm to touch.
- **Pain perception:** denies acute pain or discomfort at dispersive electrode ground site.

EXAMPLES OF INTERIM OUTCOME STATEMENTS:

- The patient's skin, other than incision, remains unchanged between admission and discharge from the OR.
- The patient's vital signs are stable at discharge from the OR.
- The patient reports comfort at the dispersive electrode site on admission to the postoperative unit.

POTENTIALLY APPLICABLE NURSING DIAGNOSES:

- Risk of impaired skin integrity (X51)
- Impaired skin integrity (X50)
- Acute pain (X38)

NURSING INTERVENTIONS AND ACTIVITIES:

Implements protective measures to prevent injury due to electrical sources (I72).
Prevents injury secondary to dispersive electrode placement, active electrode handling, electrosurgical unit use, or stray radiofrequency current.
- Implements general electrosurgery safety precautions.
  - Prevents electrosurgery use in the presence of flammable gases, flammable liquids, or flammable objects.
  - Limits electrosurgery use in oxygen enriched atmospheres, nitrous oxide (N_2O) atmospheres, or in the presence of other oxidizing agents.
  - Prevents accumulation of oxygen, other oxidizing gases (eg, N_2O), and flammable gases under surgical drapes or within areas where electrosurgery is performed.
  - Verifies that all oxygen circuit connections are leak-free before and during use of electrosurgery, especially in head and neck region of patient's body.
  - Prevents electrosurgery use in the presence of flammable (alcohol-based) skin prepping agents and tinctures.
  - Prevents pooling of prepping solutions and other fluids.
  - Recognizes that no dispersive electrode is needed for bipolar procedures.
- Implements dispersive patient electrode safety precautions.
  - Checks dispersive electrode package for outdate and package integrity.
  - Discards packages that have expired or have been compromised.

- Uses dispersive electrode according to the manufacturers' documented instructions.
- Inspects dispersive electrode before each use for wire breakage or fraying.
- Selects appropriate size dispersive electrode for patient (ie, neonate/infant, pediatric, adult).
- Does not cut dispersive electrode to accommodate patient size.
- Shaves, cleans, and dries application site as needed.
- Places dispersive electrode on positioned patient on a clean, dry skin surface over well-vascularized, convex area in close proximity to operative site.
- Avoids bony prominences, scar tissue, skin over an implanted metal prosthesis, hairy surfaces, pressure points, adipose tissue, and areas where fluid may pool.
- Applies finger pressure to adhesive border of the electrode and massages entire pad area to ensure adequate contact with the patient's skin.
- Follows manufacturers' guidelines for alarm system check prior to use.
- Uses only manufacturer-approved adapter to connect dispersive electrode to electrosurgical unit (ESU).
- Checks dispersive electrode connections to ascertain that they are clean, intact, and can make effective contact.
- Avoids skin to skin contact, such as fingers touching the patient's leg, when ESU is activated.
- Prevents dispersive electrode from tenting, gaping, and contacting liquids that interfere with adhesion.
- Removes dispersive electrode gently in manner to protect skin.
- Monitors status and function of dispersive electrode.

- Implements active electrode safety precautions.
  - Prevents electrosurgical active electrodes from being placed near or in contact with flammable materials such as gauze and surgical drapes.
  - Places active electrodes in a nonconductive holster designed to hold electrosurgical pencils and similar accessories when they are not in use.
  - Sets the generator activation tone at an audible level.
  - Checks both the active and the patient dispersive electrodes and their connections before increasing power settings.
  - Places both monopolar and bipolar accessories in the appropriate power output receptacles.
  - Activates electrode mode and function. *(RNFA)*
    - Assesses proximity of nerves and adjacent structures when activating electrode. *(RNFA)*
    - Determines appropriate mode (mono/bipolar) and function (cut or coagulation). *(RNFA)*
  - Keeps active electrode free from debris and eschar buildup.
  - Avoids using the suction coagulator as a tissue retractor during activation.

- Inspects insulation of active electrodes for cracks, breaks, and holes before use in minimally invasive surgery.
- Avoids using a hybrid cannula system (metal and plastic components) during minimally invasive surgery.
- Avoids coiling, bundling, or clamping active and patient dispersive electrodes.
- Avoids wrapping active electrode cords around a metal instrument.
- Removes all metal patient jewelry to prevent current diversion and to avoid contact with other metals.
- Reviews chart to determine special considerations (eg, pacemaker, AICD).
- Applies safety devices to patient according to manufacturers' documented instructions, plan of care, and applicable facility practice guidelines.
- Removes safety devices from patient when indicated.
- Inspects insulation on reusable and disposable electrodes.
- Encourages lowest possible power settings and verbally confirms settings with surgeon.
- Secures ESU cords to avoid displacement of pad.
- Records placement of dispersive electrode, identification number of unit, and settings used.

Evaluates for signs and symptoms of electrical injury (I37).
Observes for redness, blistering, or burn to the skin.
- Examines patient dispersive electrode site for any skin changes.
- Evaluates skin integrity, paying close attention to any imprint on the dispersive pad itself, areas under dispersive electrode, skin under the electrocardiogram (ECG) leads, and at temperature probe entry sites.
- Assesses skin at bony prominences or pressure sites for reddened or raised areas.

POSITIONING INJURY

OUTCOME O5

The patient is free from signs and symptoms of injury related to positioning.

OUTCOME DEFINITION: The patient remains free from signs and symptoms of injury related to positioning.

INTERPRETIVE STATEMENT: Prevention of positioning injury requires application of the principles of body mechanics, ongoing assessment throughout the perioperative period, and coordination with the entire health care team. Preexisting conditions (eg, poor nutritional status, extremes of age, vascular insufficiency, diabetes, impaired nerve function) may increase the patient's risk of injury. Other factors, independent of nursing care, (eg, type and length of procedure, type of anesthesia) can contribute to the risk of positioning injury.

OUTCOME INDICATORS:

- **Skin condition (general):** smooth, intact, and free from ecchymosis, cuts, abrasions, shear injury, or blistering.
- **Cardiovascular status:** heart rate and blood pressure within expected ranges; peripheral pulses present and equal bilaterally; skin warm to touch.
- **Neuromuscular status:** flexes and extends extremities without assistance; denies numbness or tingling of extremities.

EXAMPLES OF INTERIM OUTCOME STATEMENTS:

- The patient's pressure points demonstrate hyperemia for less than 30 minutes.
- The patient has full return of movement of extremities at time of discharge from the OR.
- The patient is unable to move lower extremities secondary to spinal anesthesia at time of transfer to PACU.
- The patient's peripheral tissue perfusion is consistent with preoperative status at discharge from the OR.
- The patient is free from pain or numbness associated with surgical positioning.

POTENTIALLY APPLICABLE NURSING DIAGNOSES:

- Risk for impaired skin integrity (X51)
- Impaired skin integrity (X50)
- Risk for perioperative positioning injury (X40)
- Impaired physical mobility (X34)
- Ineffective protection (X44)
- Ineffective tissue perfusion (X61)

NURSING INTERVENTIONS AND ACTIVITIES:

Identifies physical alterations that require additional precautions for procedure-specific positioning (I64).
Determines those at risk for positioning injury and implements appropriate precautions.
- Identifies individuals at risk for positioning injury (eg, those with implanted devices or amputations, the elderly, infants, the morbidly obese, and those who have limited mobility or incontinence).
- Reviews chart for information on patient's weight, preexisting medical conditions, and laboratory results.
- Interviews patient for history of implanted devices.
- Examines patient skin condition, LOC, perception of pain, presence of peripheral pulses, and mobility impairments.
- Assess external devices (eg, drains, catheters, orthopedic immobilizers).

- Applies antiembolism stockings in a manner to minimize friction injuries.
- Implements measures to prevent inadvertent hypothermia.
- Maintains safe transport environment through use of elevated bed rails, safety straps applied, additional devices secured (eg, oxygen tanks, IV poles, Foley catheter, chest tube).
- Supervises placement of equipment and/or surgical instruments on patient.
- Monitors patient for external pressures applied by members of health care team.

Verifies presence of prosthetics or corrective devices (I127).
Identifies presence of or use of prosthetics or corrective devices and modifies nursing care as indicated for planned procedure.
- Determines presence of metal and synthetic prostheses and implants, pacemakers, automated implanted cardioverter defibrillators (AICD), hearing augmentation devices, intraocular lenses, or plastic/fluid implants (eg, penile implants, testicular implants, breast implants) and notifies appropriate members of health care team.
- Individualizes plan of care to accommodate prosthetic or corrective devices.

Positions the patient (I96).
Determines the need for, prepares, applies, and removes devices designed to enhance operative exposure, prevent neuromuscular injury, maintain skin and tissue integrity, and maintain body alignment and optimal physiological functioning.
- Selects positioning devices based on patient's identified needs and the planned operative or invasive procedure.
- Positions patient on stretcher with side rails up and wheels locked when:
  - Awaiting admission to OR.
  - Procedure is completed on the stretcher.
- Determines that devices are readily available, clean, free of sharp edges, padded as appropriate, and in working order before placing patient on the OR bed.
- Modifies OR bed as necessary before attaching positioning devices.
- Reviews chart for information on patient's weight, preexisting medical conditions, previous surgeries, and laboratory results.
- Assesses functional limitations while patient is awake and responsive.
- Assesses patient for presence of skin conditions, LOC, perception of pain, presence of peripheral pulses, and mobility impairments while awake.
- Adapts positioning plan to accommodate limitations.
- Maintains body alignment.
- Maintains proper alignment of legs (uncrossed).
- Uses positioning devices to protect, support, and maintain patient position.
- Attaches padded arm boards to bed at less than 90° angle.
- Places patient's arms on boards with palms up and fingers extended or secures arms at patient's side in neutral position.
- Places fingers in position clear of table breaks or other hazards.
- Applies safety belt loosely so blood flow is not compromised.
- Protects body parts from contact with metal portions of OR bed.
- Protects patency of tubes, drains, and catheters.
- Prevents limbs from dropping below bed level to prevent compression of peripheral nerves.
- Rechecks body alignment, extremities, safety strap, and all padding if repositioning occurs.
- Removes positioning devices cautiously after surgery while maintaining body alignment and homeostatic status.

Evaluates for signs and symptoms of injury as a result of positioning (I38).
Observes for signs and symptoms of injury to integumentary, neuromuscular, and cardiopulmonary systems as a result of the patient's position during the procedure.
- Examines patient to assess peripheral pulses and/or neuromuscular impairments.
- Examines sites related to positional devices for signs and symptoms of skin/tissue injury.
- Examines pressure areas for signs of skin injury.
- Assesses and monitors vital signs.

LASER INJURY

OUTCOME O6   **The patient is free from signs and symptoms of laser injury.**

OUTCOME DEFINITION: The patient receives the minimal laser energy exposure needed to achieve the therapeutic purpose and has no contact with the laser beam other than for the intended purpose. The patient remains free from any observable signs or reported symptoms of laser injury.

INTERPRETIVE STATEMENT: Prevention of laser injury requires application of laser safety principles, coordination with the entire health care team, and knowledge of hazards. Policies that address credentialing of personnel, laser safety, and maintenance must be in accordance with national regulatory standards and manufacturers' documented instructions.

OUTCOME INDICATORS:

- **Skin condition (general):** smooth, intact, and free from unexplained edema, redness, or tenderness in nontargeted area.
- **Vision:** vision equal to preoperative status (nonopthalmologic patient); vision in nonoperative eye unaffected (ophthalmologic patient).
- **Pain perception:** denies corneal pain or discomfort in nontargeted areas.

EXAMPLES OF INTERIM OUTCOME STATEMENTS:

- The non-ophthalmologic patient reports vision unchanged from preoperative status at discharge from the OR.
- The patient reports comfort in all nontargeted areas at discharge from the OR.

POTENTIALLY APPLICABLE NURSING DIAGNOSES:

- Risk for impaired skin integrity (X51)
- Impaired skin integrity (X50)
- Acute pain (X38)
- Disturbed sensory perception (X47)

NURSING INTERVENTIONS AND ACTIVITIES:

Implements protective measures to prevent injury due to laser sources (I73).
Provides safety equipment and protective measures during a procedure using laser sources.
- Verifies that surgeon is credentialed to perform laser surgery.
- Assesses patient for mobility and comfort.
- Controls access to laser treatment area and laser equipment.
  - Identifies nominal hazard zone.
  - Secures laser operation key.
  - Places laser safety signs at all entrances to laser treatment areas.
  - Keeps doors closed.
  - Makes laser safety eyewear readily available when required.
  - Covers windows if indicated by type of laser device in use.
  - Limits access to health care personnel knowledgeable of laser safety precautions.
- Removes patient's makeup from surgical site.
- Coordinates distribution of appropriate laser safety eyewear that is labeled with appropriate optical density and wave length for the laser in use for staff (eg, glasses, goggles, and microscope or ophthalmoscope shutters) and the patient (eg, wet eyepads, laser protective eyewear, and laser specific eye shields).

- Protects skin and nontargeted tissues from unintended laser beam exposure.
    - Covers exposed area around surgical site with saline/water-saturated towels or sponges.
    - Uses anodized, dull, nonreflective, or matte-finished instruments.
    - Uses appropriate backstops or guards to prevent the laser beam from striking normal tissue.
    - Extends fiber 1 cm past the end of an endoscope when using a scope to deliver laser energy.
- Reduces exposure to smoke plume generated during laser surgery (eg, wall suction unit with in-line filter or appropriate smoke evacuator unit and high-filtration surgical masks).
- Implements fire protection measures.
    - Is prepared to operate the appropriate fire extinguisher which is immediately available.
    - Is prepared to turn off the free flow of oxygen.
    - Recognizes surgical materials that can serve as fuel for fire (eg, oxygen, skin prep solutions, oil-based lubricants, plastics such as plastic speculums or teeth protectors, paper or gauze materials, surgical drapes, adhesive or plastic tapes, and some endotracheal tubes).
    - Provides for ready availability of saline or water.
    - Removes pooled skin prep solutions that can retain laser heat and cause a tissue burn.
    - Moistens hair around surgical site and/or applies nonflammable water-based ointment to hair (oil-based petrolatum is flammable).
    - Drapes with fire-retardant materials or moist drapes surrounding the surgical incision.
    - Adapts surgical techniques to prevent fire in the presence of oxygen therapy especially in head and neck procedures. *(RNFA)*
    - Places laser in stand-by mode when not in use.
- Inspects equipment, including laser, for electrical hazards.

Evaluates for signs and symptoms of laser injury (I40).
Observes for injury unrelated to the intended therapeutic effects of the laser therapy.
- Inspects and assesses skin and adjacent tissue for discoloration, reddened raised or painful areas around surgical site.
- Instructs patient to report any complaints of visual problems postoperatively.
- Assesses for complaints of vision difficulty.

RADIATION INJURY

OUTCOME O7   **The patient is free from signs and symptoms of radiation injury.**

OUTCOME DEFINITION: The patient is free from signs or symptoms of injury related to use of radiation. Radiation exposure is limited to the target site.

INTERPRETIVE STATEMENT: Prevention of radiation injury requires the application of principles of physics and radiologic safety standards. Policies addressing education, credentialing, and radiologic safety and maintenance must be in accordance with national regulatory standards and manufacturers' documented instructions. Preexisting patient conditions (eg, length of and/or previous exposure) can influence the patient's susceptibility to radiologic injury.

OUTCOME INDICATORS:

- **Skin condition (general):** smooth, intact, and free from unexplained edema, redness, blistering, or tenderness in nontargeted areas.
- **Cognition:** responds appropriately to questioning; memory intact.

EXAMPLES OF INTERIM OUTCOME STATEMENTS:

- The patient's skin remains smooth, intact, free from unexplained redness, blistering, or tenderness in targeted areas between admission and discharge from the OR.

POTENTIALLY APPLICABLE NURSING DIAGNOSES:

- Risk of impaired skin integrity (X51)
- Impaired skin integrity (X50)
- Acute confusion (X11)

NURSING INTERVENTIONS AND ACTIVITIES:

Assesses history of previous radiation exposure (I142).
Assesses patient's history of radiation exposure for therapeutic and diagnostic purposes.
- Ensures that premenopausal women are aware of radiation risks associated with pregnancy.
- Delays, if possible, surgical procedure for 24 hours after radioactive diagnostic studies.
- Recognizes risk of compromised wound healing in patients who have received radiation in large doses preoperatively.

Implements protective measures to prevent injury due to radiation sources (I74).
Provides safety equipment and protective measures such as gonadal protection for diagnostic and therapeutic uses of radiation.
- Assembles proper protective equipment.
- Limits exposure to radiation to therapeutic levels (eg, fluoroscope is off when not in use, radioactive elements remain in lead-lined containers until ready for implantation).
- Provides shields to protect body areas from scatter radiation or focused beam whenever possible (fetus/gonadal shields, thyroid/sternal shields, lead aprons, lead gloves).
- Implements appropriate procedures for handling of radiated tissue specimens.
- Implements measures to protect the patient from direct and scatter radiation.
- Manages body fluids and tissue removed from patients who have undergone recent diagnostic studies using radioactive materials according to the recommendations of the radiation safety department.
- Documents protective measures.

Evaluates for signs of radiation injury to skin and tissue (I43).
Observes for signs and symptoms of injury to skin and tissue unrelated to the intended diagnostic or therapeutic effects of radiation.
- Follows facility policies, procedures, guidelines, or protocols for skin assessment.
- Monitors patient for skin changes (eg, redness, abrasions, bruising, blistering or edema).
- Reports variances from expected to appropriate members of health care team.

TRANSFER/TRANSPORT INJURY

OUTCOME O8   **The patient is free from signs and symptoms of injury related to transfer/transport.**

OUTCOME DEFINITION: The patient is free from signs or symptoms of injury associated with transfer/transport. Transfer/transport injuries may include skin damage from shearing, falls, fracture, or neuromuscular injury.

INTERPRETIVE STATEMENT: Prevention of patient injury during transfer/transport requires application of principles of body mechanics, knowledge of transfer/transport techniques and equipment, and coordination of the entire health care team. Appropriate restraints or safety devices are used in accordance with regulatory standards and manufacturers' documented instructions. The condition of the patient will determine the qualifications and number of health care providers necessary during transfer/transport to ensure safety.

OUTCOME INDICATORS:

- **Skin condition (general):** smooth, intact, and free from ecchymosis, cuts, abrasions, shear injury, or blistering.
- **Musculoskeletal status:** flexes and extends extremities with ease.
- **Pain perception:** reports comfort during and after transfer/transport.

EXAMPLES OF INTERIM OUTCOME STATEMENTS:

- The patient reports being comfortable when reclined on the transport stretcher.
- The patient is free from signs and symptoms of injury related to transfer/transport on discharge from the OR.

POTENTIALLY APPLICABLE NURSING DIAGNOSES:

- Risk for impaired skin integrity (X51)
- Impaired skin integrity (X50)
- Risk for falls (X69)
- Acute confusion (X11)
- Impaired bed mobility (X65)

NURSING INTERVENTIONS AND ACTIVITIES:

Transports according to individual needs (I118).
Ensures transfer without tissue injury; altered body temperature; ineffective breathing patterns; altered tissue perfusion; and undue discomfort, pain, or fear.
- Correctly identifies patient.
- Assesses mobility limitations.
- Explains what patient can expect prior to implementing transfer/transport.
- Adapts plan of care to address mobility impairments.
- Performs or directs patient transfer.
- Positions patient to maintain respiration and circulation.
- Maintains body alignment during transfer.
- Applies safety devices.
- Implements measures to prevent inadvertent hypothermia.
- Ensures adequate number and properly trained personnel for safe transfer.
- Plans for special needs during transport and transfer.

Evaluates for signs and symptoms of skin and tissue injury as a result of transfer or transport (I42).
Observes for signs and symptoms of injury to skin and tissue related to transfer or transport.
- Assesses patient for correct anatomical alignment by checking position of arms, legs, torso, and head and neck.
- Assesses pain/discomfort level using an approved pain scale.
- Visually inspects skin for areas of redness, bruising, abrasion, compression, and/or pressure related to transport.

MEDICATION ADMINISTRATION INJURY	
OUTCOME O9	**The patient receives appropriate medication(s), safely administered during the perioperative period.**

OUTCOME DEFINITION: The correct patient receives the correct medication(s) in accurate doses, at the correct time, and via the correct route throughout the surgical experience.

INTERPRETIVE STATEMENT: Medications administered must be within the defined scope of nursing practice. Safe administration of medications during the perioperative period requires knowledge of the intended purpose and side effects of each medication and the patient's condition and current medication usage. Documentation should reflect name, dose, route, time, and effects of all medications administered.

OUTCOME INDICATORS:

- **Clinical documentation:** Name, dose, route, time, and effects of medications are administered as ordered and recorded in a manner consistent with the facility's policy.
- **Cognition:** The patient states understanding of purpose, effects, and side effects of medications administered.

EXAMPLES OF INTERIM OUTCOME STATEMENTS:

- The patient receives correct medication(s) in accurate doses, at the correct time, and via the correct route throughout the surgical experience.

POTENTIALLY APPLICABLE NURSING DIAGNOSES:

- Risk for injury (X29)

NURSING INTERVENTIONS AND ACTIVITIES:

Verifies allergies (I123).
Identifies allergies, idiosyncrasies, and sensitivities to medications, latex, chemical agents, foods, and/or adhesives.
- Queries patient about allergies or hypersensitivity reaction to adhesives, egg products, latex or iodine products.
- Queries patient about medications and foreign proteins that cause anaphylaxis (eg, antibiotics, opiates, insulin, vasopressin, protamine, allergen extracts, muscle relaxants, vaccines, local anesthetics, whole blood, cryoprecipitate, immune globulin, iodinated contrast media).
- Determines type of food, nutritional supplements or substance and type of reaction experienced, if any, as reported by the patient.
- Records and communicates to the anesthesia care provider a patient history of anaphylaxis, asthma, or other respiratory difficulties related to the presence of allergens, toxins, or antigens.

Prescribes medications within scope of practice *(RNFA)* (I141).
Prescribes medications in accordance with state and federal rules and regulations and facility policies.
- Assesses current prescription, over the counter medication, and herbal supplement use.
- Collaborates with surgeon to establish medication protocols applicable to specific patient populations. *(RNFA)*
- Assesses allergies and/or any limitations to medications protocol. *(RNFA)*
- Prescribes medications when authorized by state rules and regulations and approved by facility policy. *(RNFA)*
- Instructs patients regarding side effects of self-administered medications, herbs, and food supplements.
- Evaluates response to prescribed medications.

Administers prescribed medications and solutions (I8).
The correct prescribed medication or solution is administered to the right patient, at the right time, in the right dose, via the right route.
- Reviews patient's history and assessment to identify potential allergies, medication interactions, and contraindications.
- Identifies patient's culturally based home health remedies and any influence on medication management.
- Identifies patient's over-the-counter self-medication use and herbal practices.

- Reviews medication orders and understands the medication actions, indications, contraindications, adverse reactions, and emergency management.
- Verifies patient identification, medication or solution, dose, route, and time for administration.
- Verifies the medication, the doses, and the route of administration with the physician and the scrub person before transferring medication to sterile field.
- Verifies patient's written consent before administration of experimental medications.
- Verifies verbal orders before administration.
- Questions orders that appear to be erroneous, illegible, or incomplete.
- Gathers prescribed medications/solutions and necessary supplies and equipment.
- Prepares and administers medications/solutions according to facility policy, manufacturers' documented instructions, and federal and state regulations.
- Ensures the five rights of medication administration are followed during medication administration:
  - Right patient,
  - Right medication,
  - Right dose,
  - Right route, and
  - Right time.
- Prepares a written label for all medications placed on the sterile field.
- Injects local anesthesia when within of scope of practice. *(RNFA)*
- Recognizes medication reactions, complications, and contraindications.
- Determines that specific antidotes and other emergency medication and equipment are available.
- Uses resources as needed (eg, product literature, medication bulletins, hospital formulary).
- Communicates with facility's pharmacist as needed.
- Offers instruction about medication actions to patient and family as appropriate.
- Maintains and follows policies, procedures, guidelines, and/or protocols for safe medication administration.

Administers prescribed antibiotic therapy and immunizing agents as ordered (I7).
Verifies physician orders for antibiotic therapies and immunizing agents and safely administers.
- Determines if physician orders for antibiotic therapy have been written.
  - Verifies physician orders and determines that orders are appropriate.
    - Consults with physician as needed.
    - Consults with pharmacist as needed.
  - Determines indications, doses, and intended effects of prescribed medications as well as interactions with other medications that the patient is receiving.
  - Confirms patient compliance with prescribed prophylactic therapies ordered to be self-administered.
  - Assesses patient before administering, delaying, or withholding medication if necessary.
  - Compares physician's order with label on medication container.
  - Confirms correct medication is administered to the right patient at the right dose via the right route at the right time.
  - Notes expiration date.
  - Safely administers antibiotic therapy as prescribed.
  - Recognizes and identifies adverse effects, toxic reactions, and medication allergies.
  - Evaluates the patient's response to medications administered.
- Assesses the patient's immunization history for recommended immunizations (eg, vaccines, antisera, immune globulins).
  - Obtains physician's order for any required immunizations as appropriate.
  - Follows above procedure for safely administering immunizing agents.
  - Safely administers immunization agent as prescribed.
  - Recognizes and identifies adverse effects, toxic reactions, and medication allergies.
  - Evaluates patient's response to medications administered.

Evaluates response to medications (I51).
Observes for response and adverse reactions to medications administered.
- Monitors patient for demonstrated signs of therapeutic effect.
- Monitors patient for signs of allergic effects.
- Monitors patient for signs and symptoms of medication toxicity, to include nausea or vomiting.
- Monitors patient who identifies significant home remedies/over-the-counter medications for potential complications and/or drug interactions.
- Reports signs or symptoms of adverse reaction to appropriate member of health care team.

INFECTION	
OUTCOME O10	**The patient is free from signs and symptoms of infection.**

OUTCOME DEFINITION: The patient is free from signs and symptoms of nosocomial surgical site infection such as pain, induration, foul odor, purulent drainage, and/or fever through 30 days following the perioperative procedure.

INTERPRETIVE STATEMENT: Prevention of infection requires the application of the principles of microbiology and aseptic practice. Measurement of this outcome is based on the stages of wound healing and the Centers for Disease Control and Prevention (CDC) guidelines defining surgical site infections as occurring 30 days postoperative and up to one year for transplant surgery. Preexisting patient conditions and other factors independent of nursing care can contribute to the development of infections. These factors include, but are not limited to:

- procedure type;
- organ systems involved;
- tissue trauma;
- wound class (ie, clean, clean contaminated, contaminated, dirty);
- presence of devices (eg, urinary catheters, IVs, invasive monitoring devices, endotracheal tubes);
- procedure length;
- implants;
- administration of prophylactic antibiotics;
- surgical technique; and
- practice setting.

OUTCOME INDICATORS:

- **Immune status:** afebrile; leukocyte count three to 30 days postoperative within expected range.
- **Skin condition (surgical wound):** incision well approximated and free from heat, redness, induration, swelling, or foul odor; drains covered with sterile dressing and/or connected to continuous drainage; wound class identified.
- **Medication regimen:** preoperative antibiotics given according to recommended guidelines; no antibiotic use three to 30 days postoperative.
- **Clinical documentation:** wound class and infection control interventions and measures documented according to facility policy.

EXAMPLES OF INTERIM OUTCOME STATEMENTS:

- The patient has a clean, primarily closed surgical wound covered with dry, sterile dressing at discharge from the OR.
- The patient's wound is intact and free from signs of infection 30 days following surgery.
- The patient's immune status remains within expected levels 5 days following surgery.
- The patient's white blood cell count remains within expected levels 5 days following surgery.
- The patient is afebrile and free from signs and symptoms of infection.
- The patient has a Class III wound covered with a dry, sterile dressing.
- The patient's wound is free from signs or symptoms of infection and pain, redness, swelling, drainage, or delayed healing at time of discharge.

POTENTIALLY APPLICABLE NURSING DIAGNOSES:

- Risk for infection (X28)
- Risk for impaired skin integrity (X51)
- Impaired skin integrity (X50)
- Delayed surgical recovery (X56)

NURSING INTERVENTIONS AND ACTIVITIES:

Implements aseptic technique (I70).

Initiates the actions necessary related to risks associated with disease-causing microorganisms by creating and maintaining a sterile field, preventing contamination of open wounds, and isolating the operative site from the surrounding nonsterile physical environment.

- Establishes and maintains sterile field.
- Applies principles of aseptic technique *(See Appendix V)*.
- Performs skin preparations.
- Ensures perioperative environmental sanitation.
- Adheres to standard and transmission-based precautions.
- Dresses wound at completion of procedure.
- Cares for incision sites, invasive-devices wound sites (ie, endotracheal tube, tracheostomy tube, drainage tube, percutaneous catheter, and vascular access device), urinary drainage systems, and other drainage systems.
- Monitors for wound contamination.
- Evaluates implementation of aseptic practices by health care team.

Assesses susceptibility for infection (I21).

Evaluates the patient's risks for infection related to microbial contamination.

- Identifies the patient's specific risk factors (ie, health problems and situations) for infection.
  - Identifies pathophysiological risk factors: chronic diseases (eg, cancer, renal failure, arthritis, HIV, hematological disorders, diabetes mellitus, hepatic disorders, respiratory disorders, collagen disorders, genetic conditions, renal disorders); alcoholism; immunosuppression; immunodeficiency; altered or insufficient leukocytes; blood dyscrasias; impaired circulation; altered integumentary system; periodontal disease; obesity; altered mental status; dysphasia; splenectomy; anatomic abnormality; and sleep deprivation.
  - Identifies treatment-related risk factors: medications (eg, antibiotics, steroids, antiviral agents, insulin, antifungal agents, tranquilizers, immunosuppressants, antacids); surgery; radiation therapy; dialysis; total parenteral nutrition; chemotherapy; presence of invasive lines (eg, circulatory, gastrointestinal, respiratory, urinary); intubation; enteral feedings; organ transplants; presence of implants and recent blood transfusions.
  - Identifies situational (personal, environmental) risk factors: history of infections; prolonged immobility; trauma (accidental, intentional); postpartum; exposure to contagious agents (nosocomial or community acquired); postoperative period; prolonged length of hospital stay; malnutrition; stress; bites (animal, insect, human); thermal injuries; moist skin areas; limited personal hygiene; lack of immunizations; smoking.
  - Identifies patients at high risk for transmitting nosocomial infections (individuals with antibiotic or medication resistant microorganisms, prion diseases, tuberculosis, and/or preoperative nasal colonization of *S. aureus*).
  - Identifies maturational risk factors: newborn—lack of maternal antibodies (dependent on maternal exposures), lack of normal flora, open wounds (umbilical, circumcision), and immature immune system; infant/child—lack of immunization; and elderly—debilitated, diminished immune response, and chronic diseases.
  - Identifies recent history of travel, within or outside the United States.
  - Notes ASA risk classification.
- Determines if the patient is at high risk for infection (ie, state in which an individual is at risk to be invaded by an opportunistic or pathogenic agent such as virus, fungus, bacteria, protozoa, or other parasite) from endogenous or exogenous sources.
- Identifies the individuals at high risk for nosocomial infections. Considers a person who has one or more contributing factors and one or more predictors to be at high risk.
  - Assesses for infection predictors (eg, procedure length, procedure type, presence of other devices or instruments).
  - Assesses for confounding factors (eg, age, nutritional status, health status).

Classifies surgical wound (I22).
Designates the appropriate wound classification category for each surgical wound site according to the Centers for Disease Control and Prevention.

- Class I/Clean wounds: Uninfected operative wounds in which no inflammation is encountered and the respiratory, alimentary, genital, or uninfected urinary tracts are not entered. Clean wounds are primarily closed, and if necessary, drained with closed drainage. Operative incisional wounds that follow nonpenetrating (blunt) trauma should be included in this category if they meet the criteria.
- Class II/Clean-contaminated wounds: Operative wounds in which the respiratory, alimentary, genital, or urinary tract is entered under controlled conditions and without unusual contamination. Specifically, surgical procedures involving the biliary tract, appendix, vagina, and oropharynx are included in this category, provided no evidence of infection or major break in technique is encountered.
- Class III/Contaminated wounds: Open, fresh, accidental wounds, surgical procedures with major breaks in sterile technique or gross spillage from the gastrointestinal tract, and incisions in which acute, nonpurulent inflammation is encountered.
- Class IV/Dirty-infected wounds: Old traumatic wounds with retained devitalized tissue and those that involve existing clinical infection or perforated viscera. This definition suggests that organisms causing postoperative infection were present in the operative field before the surgical procedure.

Performs skin preparations (I94).
Carries out necessary actions to prepare the epidermis for an operative or invasive procedure.

- Assesses patient's overall health status, including:
  - Age (eg, most pediatric patients are not shaved; skin of geriatric patient may be dry and lack resiliency).
  - Nutritional status (eg, malnourished, obese, hypovolemic or edematous patient may have altered skin texture and tone).
  - State of consciousness (eg, degree of alertness, which may make positioning difficult and require extra personnel for the semiconscious or unconscious patient).
  - Medical condition (eg, diabetes, which diminishes circulation to extremities; impaired healing ability, which requires extra caution exercised when shaving).
  - Previous surgery (eg, presence of scars, degrees of keloid formation; scars and keloids are fragile tissue and must be avoided when shaving).
  - Limitations of motion (eg, arthritis, amputation, contractures, attention given to comfortable positioning).
- Assesses patient's skin condition, including:
  - Color (eg, pallor, cyanosis, jaundice, pigmentation changes);
  - Vascularity (eg, evidence of bleeding or bruising; ulcers);
  - Obvious lesions (eg, allergy reaction, acne, pustule, psoriasis, traumatic injury);
  - Edema (eg, injury or underlying medical conditions);
  - Moisture (eg, dry or sweaty);
  - Temperature (eg, warm, hot, or cool);
  - Texture (eg, rough or smooth);
  - Thickness (eg, paper thin, fragile, or thick); and
  - Turgor (eg, decreased due to dehydration).
- Assesses patient for previous surgery sites (eg, presence of fragile tissue such as scars and/or keloid formation) and exercises caution when preparing the area.
- Assesses operative site before skin preparation.
  - Inspects for cleanliness, hair, and integrity.
  - Examines for presence of lesions such as moles or warts.
  - Examines for other skin conditions such as rash, skin eruption, or abrasion.
- Cleans operative site(s) and surrounding areas to remove soil, debris, and transient flora by any or all of the following methods:
  - Patient shower(s) and/or shampoo;
  - Washing operative site before arriving in practice setting; and
  - Washing operative site immediately before applying antimicrobial agent in the practice setting.
- Determines need for hair removal at the operative site based on:
  - Amount of hair present,
  - Location of the incision,

- Type of procedure to be performed,
- Physician orders, and
- Facility policy.
  - If hair is to be removed, hair is removed as close to the time of surgery as possible. Hair is removed outside of the room where the procedure will be performed.
- Provides for hair removal if indicated.
  - Provides adequate lighting (or positions patient to obtain adequate lighting).
  - Removes hair in a manner that preserves skin integrity, using one of the following methods:
    - Electric or battery powered clippers with disposable or reusable head that has been disinfected;
    - Chemical depilatory (if the patient is not allergic to such agents) applied before the patient's arrival in the practice setting, following the manufacturer's documented instructions regarding skin testing and use; or
    - Disposable razor or razor that has been terminally sterilized to shave (preferably the wet shave method) only when all other methods of hair removal are not available.
  - Removes hair in or around skin lesions or raised areas on skin surface (ie, melanomas, basal cell carcinomas, or lesions erupting through the skin) in a manner that does not inadvertently traumatize these areas. Trims hair on or close to lesions with scissors.
- Assembles all equipment and supplies on a sterile field. Equipment and supplies may include:
  - Containers for prep solutions.
  - Prep sponges of a size and shape differing from those to be used for the operative procedure. Prep sponges should be contained in a separated and isolated area until the end of the surgical procedure.
  - When surgical sponges are used for a portion of the surgical prep, those sponges are included in the facility count procedure.
- Prepares operative site and surrounding area with antimicrobial agent.
  - Selects broad spectrum antimicrobial agents that provide residual protection and are nontoxic (uses data provided by scientific literature, manufacturers' tests, and US Food and Drug Administration categories to select agent).
  - Selects antimicrobial agents based on patient sensitivity, incision location, and skin condition.
  - Uses antimicrobial agent in accordance with manufacturers' documented instructions.
  - Applies antimicrobial agents using sterile supplies and sterile gloves or using the no-touch technique (ie, the use of an extension such as a sponge forceps, rather than hands, to handle or touch contaminated items or to handle or touch sterile items).
- Implements skin preparation technique suitable for site and condition of skin.
  - Prepares skin by applying antimicrobial agents.
    - Uses friction.
    - Proceeds from incision site to the periphery.
    - Uses sponge or implement provided with preparation kit and discards same when the periphery has been reached.
    - Uses fresh sponge/implement to continue procedure.
    - Repeats process several times according to manufacturer's written instructions.

Monitors for signs and symptoms of infection (I88).
Observes for manifestations of tissue reaction due to pathogenic microorganism invasion of the body.
- Evaluates patient assessment data noting indications of infection including:
  - Fever: continuous or intermittent.
  - Previous infections: urinary tract, pneumonia, surgical wound, skin and soft tissues, reproductive tract, lower respiratory tract, blood, bone/joint, cardiovascular system, central nervous system, eye, ear, nose, throat, mouth, systemic, GI system.
  - Pain or swelling, generalized or local.
  - Presence of wounds including those that may be:
    - Surgical.
    - Trauma.
    - Burns.
    - Invasive devices (tracheotomy, IV, drains).
    - Self-induced.

- Reviews laboratory diagnostic tests for infection:
  - White blood cell count,
  - Urinalysis,
  - Cultures,
  - Serologies.
- Assesses for signs and symptoms of infection/inflammation.
  - Observes for local manifestations of inflammation:
    - Redness caused by hyperemia from vasodilation.
    - Heat caused by increased metabolism at inflammatory site.
    - Pain caused by change in pH; change in local ionic concentration; nerve stimulation by chemicals (eg, histamine, prostaglandins); pressure from fluid exudate.
    - Swelling caused by fluid shift to interstitial spaces; fluid exudate accumulation.
    - Loss of function caused by swelling and pain.
  - Observes for signs and symptoms of pulmonary infection:
    - Hypoxia.
    - Increasing temperature.
    - Increased production of secretions.
    - Change in color of secretions from clear or pale yellow to yellow or green.
- Contacts postoperative patients to determine signs and symptoms of postoperative infection.
- Reports occurrence of surgical wound infection according to approved policy.

Protects from cross-contamination (I98).

Applies methodologies that prevent patient exposure to infective agents from endogenous sources (as from one tissue to another within the patient) and from exogenous sources (as acquired from objects, personnel, or other patients).

- Establishes and/or participates in a formalized, multidisciplinary, infection control program.
  - Develops and/or contributes to specific written infection control policies and procedures for all services throughout the practice setting.
  - Develops and/or contributes to written policies defining indications for isolation precautions.
  - Establishes and/or participates in reporting, evaluating, and maintaining records of infections occurring in patients and personnel.
  - Defines nosocomial infections for surveillance purposes to provide early uniform identification and reporting of infections.
  - Conducts preventive surveillance and infection control procedures relating to the practice setting environment.
  - Determines practice setting infection rates.
  - Provides feedback about surgical wound infection rates to surgeons.
  - Collaborates with medical staff on action based on clinical use of antibiotics.
  - Reviews and evaluates all aseptic, standard transmission-based precautions, and environmental control techniques of the practice setting on an ongoing basis.
  - Reports breaks in infection control procedure(s) and initiates corrective action.
  - Orients new employees regarding personal hygiene and importance of infection control while caring for patients.
- Works with facility engineers and managers to provide for ventilation and air filtration systems that meet local, state, and federal regulations and recommendations.
  - Filters are designed to remove dust and aerosol particles from the air.
  - Air flow in ORs is unidirectional.
  - Air pressure gradient in each OR is positive in relation to surrounding areas.
  - Air filtration system is continuously monitored and maintenance performed on a regular basis.
  - Doors to the OR remain closed except for necessary patient/personnel traffic.
  - OR temperature and humidity are maintained according to local, state, and federal regulations and recommendations.
  - Use of additional protective measures (eg, laminar air flow systems, body exhaust suits) is weighed to determine benefit and achievable outcome.
- Promotes personnel health and hygiene.
  - Excludes personnel with acute infection or skin lesion from the practice setting. This includes individuals with:

- o   Upper respiratory infections,
- o   Fever,
- o   Skin lesions or draining wounds, and
- o   Any other type of infection.
  - ▪ Expects personnel to demonstrate good personal hygiene.
    - o   Encourages and demonstrates thorough and frequent handwashing. For most activities, a vigorous, rubbing together of all surfaces of lathered hands and wrists, followed by rinsing under a stream of water is recommended. If hands are visibly soiled more time may be required.
    - o   Limits use of waterless alcohol-based hand cleansers to facility-approved occasions.
    - o   Washes hands:
      - ◆ Before and after engaging in hand-to-nose, hand-to-mouth, or hand-to-eye activities (eg, eating, drinking, smoking, applying cosmetics or lip balm, handling contact lenses).
      - ◆ Before and after direct patient contact, even if gloves are worn.
      - ◆ Before and after contact with a source that is likely to be contaminated with virulent microorganisms or pathogens.
      - ◆ At first opportunity, if contaminated with blood or other body fluids containing blood or potentially infective material.
      - ◆ Before and after invasive procedures, even if gloves are worn.
      - ◆ Before and after touching wounds, whether surgical, traumatic, or associated with an invasive device, even if gloves are worn.
      - ◆ Immediately after glove removal.
- •   Helps contain contamination by developing and implementing appropriate traffic patterns based on design of surgical suite.

Equipment/Supplies
- ▪ Removes supplies and equipment from external shipping containers before transferring items into surgical suite.
- ▪ Separates movement of clean and sterile supplies from contaminated supplies and waste by space, time, and/or traffic patterns.
- ▪ Avoids entering elevator with contained or uncontained soiled items when patients, food, or clean/sterile items are present. Uses enclosed soiled linen and trash collection systems in areas separate from corridors, lounges, and other storage areas.
- ▪ Moves supplies from restricted area (if present) through ORs to semirestricted corridor. Prevents soiled materials from entering restricted area.
- ▪ Maintains unidirectional traffic pattern for items to be reprocessed within surgical suite. Moves items from decontamination area to processing area, and, after processing, to storage areas. Uses clearly identified work areas for each task to minimize cross-contamination.

Personnel
- ▪ Wears clean, dry, freshly laundered surgical attire intended for use in the surgical suite.
- ▪ Wears long-sleeved jacket that is snapped or buttoned closed when not scrubbed.
- ▪ Covers head and facial hair, including sideburns and neckline, when in semirestricted areas (which includes most of the peripheral support areas of the surgical suite that have storage areas for clean and sterile supplies) and restricted areas (where surgical procedures are performed and unwrapped supplies are sterilized) of surgical suite by wearing hat or hood that minimizes microbial dispersal.
- ▪ Wears single high-efficiency mask when there are open sterile supplies and equipment present or where scrubbed persons may be located.
  - o   Positions mask to cover nose and mouth and ties securely to minimize tenting.
  - o   Removes and discards masks after use handling only the ties.
- ▪ Confines or removes all jewelry and watches.
- ▪ Keeps fingernails short, clean, healthy, and free of artificial or acrylic nails.
- ▪ Wears shoe covers when gross contamination of the feet can be reasonably expected (eg, orthopedics, neurosurgery, obstetric surgery).
- ▪ Dons sterile gown and gloves after drying scrubbed hands and arms.

- Minimizes cross-contamination by understanding and implementing infection control practices when preparing instruments and supplies for use.
  - Uses Spaulding classification system to define necessary preparation.
    - Items that enter sterile tissue or the vascular system are categorized as critical and must be sterile (eg, surgical instruments, cardiac and urinary catheters, implants, needles).
    - Items that come in contact with nonintact skin or mucous membranes are considered semicritical and receive a minimum of high-level disinfection (eg, respiratory therapy equipment, anesthesia equipment, bronchoscopes, gastrointestinal endoscopes, thermometers).
    - Items that come in contact only with intact skin are considered noncritical items and receive intermediate-level or low-level disinfection or cleaning (eg, blood pressure cuffs, crutches, bedside tables, furniture).
  - Follows established protocols for high-level disinfection.
    - Cleans items thoroughly before disinfection.
    - Disassembles items with lumens, channels, crevices, and joints when design permits.
    - Uses enzymatic detergents as appropriate.
    - Rinses items to remove residual detergent.
    - Dries items before subjecting them to disinfection process.
    - Follows manufacturers' documented instructions when preparing disinfecting solutions and calculating expirations dates.
    - Uses chemical germicides according to manufacturers' documented instructions.
    - Completely immerses items in chemical germicide.
    - Rinses items thoroughly with sterile water after completing required exposure time.
    - Creates and maintains safe practice environment when using chemical germicides according to manufacturers' instructions.
  - Uses category-specific or disease-specific isolation precautions as necessary if infections other than bloodborne infections are diagnosed or suspected.
    - Recognizes hazards and consistently adheres to established control practices:
      - Implements aseptic technique.
      - Monitors sterile field.
      - Performs skin preparation.
      - Maintains perioperative environmental sanitation.
      - Adheres to universal, standard, and transmission-based precautions.
      - Dresses wound at completion of procedure.
      - Verifies prophylactic intervention.
    - Implements precautions specific to contagion present or suspected (eg, prion infections).

Minimizes the length of invasive procedure by planning care (I85).
Contributes to minimizing operative time by anticipation and advanced preparation, coordinates team members' efforts to set priorities, and efficiently accomplishes the tasks necessary to achieve a common goal.
- Collects and interprets patient data, identifying appropriate nursing diagnoses and desired outcomes.
- Plans individualized patient care (a dynamic process that is ongoing and continuous throughout the preoperative, intraoperative, and postoperative phases) based on patient assessment data and an understanding of OR systems, methodologies, and perioperative nursing interventions resulting in desired outcomes.
  - Applies perioperative nursing principles and knowledge when preparing the OR environment.
    - Uses preference lists, care guides, and knowledge of surgical procedures to ready room, supplies, and equipment.
    - Assembles proper instruments and suture for planned surgical procedure.
    - Checks equipment for proper functioning.
  - Plans and implements intraoperative nursing activities.
    - Organizes activities into logical sequence to minimize disruption of procedure flow.
    - Prioritizes nursing actions.
    - Communicates activities to health care team and patient's family as appropriate.
    - Makes supplies and equipment that may be needed readily available.

- Plans and implements postoperative activities.
  - o Reviews care plan in light of preoperative and intraoperative activities.
  - o Revises plan as indicated.
  - o Notes potential risk factors (eg, intraoperative tissue trauma, wound classification, length of surgical procedure, implants, the presence of indwelling catheters or drainage tubing).
- Maximizes surgeon's efficiency of movement within the surgical wound. *(RNFA)*
  - o Anticipates wound exposure needs by positioning retractors, controlling bleeding, suctioning, and counter traction techniques. *(RNFA)*
  - o Demonstrates manual dexterity when handling surgical instruments within the wound. *(RNFA)*
  - o Marks ostomy site in collaboration with surgeon, considering skin folds and body habitus. *(RNFA)*

Initiates traffic control (I81).
Restricts access to patient care area to authorized individuals only.
- Keeps doors to OR or procedure rooms closed except during movement of patients, personnel, supplies, and equipment.
- Restricts access to surgical suite to authorized personnel only.
- Records names of all individuals who participate in surgical procedure.

Administers prescribed prophylactic treatments (I10).
Confirms and safely administers orders including dietary regimens, douche, enema, bowel preparation, and/or antimicrobial prophylaxis as ordered.
- Determines if physician orders for prophylactic therapy have been written.
  - Confirms and implements physician orders.
  - Confirms patient compliance with prescribed prophylactic therapies to be patient-administered (eg, dietary restrictions, douche, enema, and/or bowel preparation).
- Seeks physician order for parenteral antimicrobial prophylactic therapy as indicated by CDC Guideline for Prevention of Surgical Site Infections (1999). Examples include:
  - Procedures with high risk of infection.
  - Procedures having severe or life-threatening consequences of infection even though infection risk may be low (eg, cardiovascular and/or orthopedic implant procedures).
- Ensures timing of antimicrobial administration achieves maximum effectiveness.
- Confirms physician order and discusses any questions with ordering physician.
  - Discourages use of prophylactic vancomycin to decrease risk factor for subsequent colonization and infection with antibiotic resistant organisms as recommended by the CDC.
  - Begins parenteral antimicrobial prophylaxis shortly before the surgical procedure (for cesarean sections, prophylaxis is usually given intraoperatively after the umbilical cord is clamped).
  - Requests order from physician for repeat dose(s) of prophylactic antibiotic if:
    - o Surgical procedure lasts longer than four hours.
    - o Major blood loss occurs.
    - o An antimicrobial with a short half-life is used.

Encourages deep breathing and coughing exercises (I33).
Encourages use of incentive spirometry (per physician order), diaphragmatic breathing, and coughing.
Preoperative phase
- Counsels patient to avoid active and passive cigarette smoking and to avoid smoke-filled rooms.
- Counsels patient to avoid exposure to persons with respiratory infections.
- Assists patient in practicing incentive spirometry, diaphragmatic breathing, and coughing as appropriate.
- Evaluates patient response:
  - Observes patient for correct demonstration of expected postoperative behaviors.
  - Asks pertinent questions to determine patient's level of understanding.
  - Reinforces information when necessary.

Postoperative phase
- Encourages and assists patient in performing incentive spirometry, diaphragmatic breathing, and coughing as appropriate.

- Encourages patient's self-use of incentive spirometer approximately 10 to 12 times per hour.
- Monitors patient's spirometer breaths, periodically increasing tidal volume as patient tolerates.
- Encourages patient to cough after deep breathing at conclusion of treatment unless contraindicated.
- Instructs patient to turn and change positions in bed to encourage deeper breathing.
- Evaluates effectiveness and patient tolerance of the treatment.
  - Auscultates chest and notes any improvement or variation.
  - Notes volume attained, effectiveness of cough, and characteristics of any secretions expectorated.

Administers care to wound sites (I4).
Examines characteristics of wound sites and provides appropriate wound care.
- Dresses wound at completion of procedure.
  - Uses sterile gloves when touching wound or dressing materials.
  - Selects dressing materials based on clinical needs so as to:
    - Cushion and protect wound from trauma and gross contamination;
    - Absorb drainage;
    - Debride wound;
    - Support, splint, or immobilize body part and incisional area;
    - Aid in hemostasis and minimize edema, as in a pressure dressing;
    - Maintain moist environment and prevent cell dehydration;
    - Apply medications; and/or
    - Accommodate specific wound characteristics (eg, site, depth, area) as well as the patient's overall condition.
  - Applies sterile dressings.
  - Secures dressings with tape. Selects tape based on:
    - Assessment of skin condition;
    - Amount of strength and elasticity required;
    - Patient allergies;
    - Anticipated frequency of dressing change:
      - Uses Montgomery straps when frequent dressing changes are anticipated.
      - Uses polyurethane dressing, elastic tape, or elastic bandages when wound compression is desired.
  - Immobilizes with soft padding, splints, elastic bandages, and/or casting materials as needed.
  - Applies ostomy bag or other appliance as needed.
- Observes characteristics of any drainage.
  - Changes dressings over closed wounds and assesses wound if patient has signs or symptoms of infection (eg, fever, unusual wound pain).
  - Evaluates drainage for signs of infection including:
    - Type of drainage,
    - Consistency of drainage,
    - Amount of drainage, and
    - Color of drainage.
- Checks casting materials for signs of circulatory impairment.
- Examines and compares characteristics of incision regularly.
  - Observes for well-approximated incision edges.
  - Observes for signs of infection (eg, heat, redness, swelling, unusual pain, odor), dehiscence, or evisceration.
- Cleans all areas of the wound.
  - Uses sterile gloves when touching incision.
  - Uses sterile supplies to prevent contamination.
  - Removes debris, pus, blood, and necrotic material.
  - Avoids disrupting sutures or irritating incision.
  - Aseptically cleans incision site with sterile normal saline.
    - Wipes only once with each sponge.
    - Moves from the top of incision site to the bottom with one sponge.
    - Continues in vertical path next to incision, moving in line parallel to incision.
    - Wipes from clean area toward less clean areas.

- o Avoids tracking wound exudate and normal body flora from the surrounding skin to clean areas.
- o Uses cotton-tipped applicators (wiping only once with each applicator) to clean tight-fitting wire sutures, deep and narrow wounds, or wounds with pockets.
- o Cleans skin around drain, if present, by wiping in half or full circles.
- o Cleans drain surface last.
  - ▪ Aseptically irrigates and packs open wounds as prescribed.
- Aseptically removes skin sutures/staples (per physician order) from the healed wound.
  - ▪ Avoids damaging newly formed tissue.
  - ▪ Cleans incision site immediately before suture/staple removal.
  - ▪ Cuts sutures portion back through the subcutaneous tissue or remove staples using a staple extractor.
  - ▪ Cleanses incision site at skin surface on one side of visible part of suture.
  - ▪ Removes suture by lifting and pulling visible end off skin.
  - ▪ Avoids drawing contaminated portion back through the subcutaneous tissue.
  - ▪ Cleanses incision site immediately following suture/staple removal.
- Covers incisions and/or wounds with appropriate dressing materials.
  - ▪ Changes dressings if patient has signs or symptoms of infection (eg, fever, unusual wound pain).
  - ▪ Changes/reinforces dressings if patient has dressings saturated with body fluids.
- Evaluates for signs of infection when dressings are removed.
- Evaluates skin condition when dressings are removed.

Administers care to invasive device sites (I3).
Examines and compares the characteristics of site, drainage, and patency of invasive devices (eg, urinary drainage systems, endotracheal tube, tracheostomy tube, drainage tube, percutaneous catheter, vascular access devices) and provides appropriate wound care.

- Examines and compares the characteristics of invasive device sites regularly.
  - ▪ Changes dressings and evaluates site for signs or symptoms of infection (eg, heat, redness, swelling, odor, drainage, unusual pain).
    - o Secures invasive devices properly.
    - o Uses sterile gloves if it becomes necessary to provide care to the invasive device insertion site, and uses sterile supplies to prevent contamination.
    - o Cleans all areas of the invasive device site to wash away debris, pus, blood, and necrotic material without disrupting sutures or irritating the site.
    - o Aseptically cleans device sites according to facility policy, wiping only once with each sponge.
    - o Moves from insertion site outward.
    - o Wipes from clean area toward less clean areas.
    - o Avoids tracking wound exudate and normal body flora from surrounding skin to clean areas.
    - o Uses cotton-tipped applicators (wiping only once with each applicator) to clean tight-fitting sutures, deep and narrow wounds, or wounds with pockets.
    - o Cleans the skin around the device by wiping in half or full circles.
    - o Cleans device surface last.
  - ▪ Applies sterile dressings following site care.
    - o Selects dressing materials based on clinical needs [see "Administers care to wound sites" (I4)].
    - o Secures dressings with tape. Selects tape based on patient need.
- Maintains patency of invasive devices (eg, tube, catheter).

<u>Drainage tube systems</u>
- ▪ Examines and compares the characteristics of drainage device sites regularly.
- ▪ Changes dressings and evaluates site for signs or symptoms of infection (eg, heat, redness, swelling, odor, unusual pain).
- ▪ Secures drainage devices.
- ▪ Uses sterile gloves to touch drainage device insertion sites.
- ▪ Uses sterile supplies to prevent contamination.
- ▪ Connects drainage tubes to be free of twists, kinks, leaks, and obstruction.
- ▪ Maintains and monitors suction devices that may be connected for drainage (eg, pleurevac, ventriculostomy).

Tracheostomy tube site care
- Provides tracheostomy care per facility policy.
- Changes tracheostomy ties daily and as needed.
- Secures ties to keep tube in stoma, but with the width of two fingers' distance between ties and neck.

Percutaneous catheter site care (eg, cystostomy, nephrostomy, ureterostomy)
- Uses sterile gloves when providing care.
- Uses sterile supplies to prevent contamination.
- Cleans site according to cleaning protocol previously identified for invasive sites.

Maintains peripheral IV sites
- Maintains sterility of IV system devices.
- Cleans around venipuncture site according to facility policy.
- Assesses and rotates IV site regularly and changes dressing, tubing, and solution according to facility policy.
    - Assesses venipuncture site for signs of infection (eg, redness, pain at puncture site).
    - Assesses site for infiltration (eg, coolness, blanching, and edema at the site).
    - Assesses site for thrombophlebitis (eg, redness, firmness, pain along the path of the vein, and edema).
    - Discontinues IV if any of above symptoms present.
    - Secures site with pressure dressing.
    - Starts IV in alternate location.

Performs percutaneous pin site care
- Cleans pin sites and removes crusts with sterile cotton-tipped applicator using solution and/or ointment as prescribed.
- Assesses wounds for signs and symptoms of infection.

Implements and maintains urinary drainage systems
- Catheterizes only when necessary.
- Maintains unobstructed urine flow.
- Aseptically empties the urinary drainage bag.
- Obtains urine samples aseptically.
- Inspects the catheter for any problems.
- Inspects the tissue around the meatus for irritation and swelling.
- Encourages patient with unrestricted fluid intake to increase fluid intake to at least 3000 mL per day to help flush the urinary system and reduce sediment formation.
    - Assesses for signs and symptoms of urinary tract infection, including cloudy urine, hematuria, fever, malaise, tenderness over the bladder, and flank pain.
- Removes indwelling catheters as soon as they are no longer needed.
    - Assesses the patient for incontinence, urgency, persistent dysuria, bladder spasm, fever, chills, or palpable bladder distention following catheter removal.

Maintains closed drainage systems (eg, bulb, vacuum, bag systems)
- Establishes vacuum in closed drainage system before closing.
- Empties reservoir frequently during periods of heavy drainage to maintain maximum suction and prevent strain on suture line from pressure due to excessive fluid buildup.
- Cleans the closed drainage system spout before and after emptying drainage.
- Secures vacuum unit to patient's bedding or gown below wound level to promote drainage.
- Avoids tension on drainage system to prevent dislodgment.

Maintains thoracic drainage system
- Checks water level in water-seal chamber.
    - Checks for fluctuation in water-seal chamber as patient breathes.
    - Checks for intermittent bubbling in water-seal chamber.

- o   Checks water level in suction-control chamber and adds sterile distilled water if necessary.
- o   Checks for gentle bubbling in suction-control chamber.
- ▪   Checks air vent in system for proper functioning.
- ▪   Secures system tubing to bed.
- ▪   Avoids kinks, dependent loops, or pressure on tubing.
- ▪   Avoids lifting drainage system above patient's chest to prevent fluid backflow into pleural space.
- ▪   Assesses patient's breath sounds.
- ▪   Avoids disrupting sutures or irritating site.
- ▪   Selects dressing materials according to patient need [see "Administers care to wound sites" (I4)].
- ▪   Secures dressings.
- ▪   Ensures suction is maintained at prescribed setting.

Administers prescribed antibiotic therapy and immunizing agents as ordered (I7).
Verifies physician orders for antibiotic therapies and immunizing agents and safely administers.
- •   Determines if physician orders for antibiotic therapy have been written.
  - ▪   Verifies physician orders and determines that orders are appropriate.
    - o   Consults with physician as needed.
    - o   Consults with pharmacist as needed.
  - ▪   Determines indications, doses, and intended effects of prescribed medications as well as interactions with other medications that the patient is receiving.
  - ▪   Confirms patient compliance with prescribed prophylactic therapies ordered to be self-administered.
  - ▪   Assesses patient before administering, delaying, or withholding medication if necessary.
  - ▪   Compares physician's order with label on medication container.
  - ▪   Confirms correct medication is administered to the right patient at the right dose via the right route at the right time.
  - ▪   Notes expiration date.
  - ▪   Safely administers antibiotic therapy as prescribed.
  - ▪   Recognizes and identifies adverse effects, toxic reactions, and medication allergies.
  - ▪   Evaluates the patient's response to medications administered.
- •   Assesses the patient's immunization history for recommended immunizations (eg, vaccines, antisera, immune globulins).
  - ▪   Obtains physician's order for any required immunizations as appropriate.
  - ▪   Follows above procedure for safely administering immunizing agents.
  - ▪   Safely administers immunization agent as prescribed.
  - ▪   Recognizes and identifies adverse effects, toxic reactions, and medication allergies.
  - ▪   Evaluates patient's response to medications administered.

Manages culture specimen collection (I83).
Collects, identifies, labels, stores, preserves, and transports specimens for microbiological testing.
- •   Collects specimen using aseptic sampling methods.
- •   Places sample(s) in sterile container with transport medium and/or an inert gas according to type of culture.

Wound cultures
- ▪   Reduces risk of contaminating specimen with skin bacteria by cleaning area around wound according to facility policy. Allows area to dry.
- ▪   Uses cotton-tipped swab to collect as much exudate as possible for aerobic culture or inserts swab deeply into wound and gently rotates it. Places swab in aerobic culture tube.
- ▪   Avoids collecting exudate from skin and then from deeper space in wound with same swab to prevent contaminating wound with skin bacteria.
- ▪   Inserts cotton-tipped swab deeply into wound and rotates it gently for anaerobic culture.
- ▪   Removes swab and immediately places swab in anaerobic culture medium or aspirates 5 to 10 mL of exudate from deep wound with sterile syringe and places aspirate into anaerobic culture medium.

Tissue cultures
- Uses sterile supplies to collect tissue for culture.
- Places tissue in sterile specimen container immediately after collection.
- Sends container to laboratory immediately to prevent deterioration and erroneous test results.

Blood cultures
- Aseptically collects venous blood sample (10 mL from adult or 2 to 6 mL from a child) and transfers sample into two sterile bottles, one containing anaerobic medium and the other aerobic medium.
- Collects three to four sets of samples at timed intervals as appropriate
- Obtains each set of samples from different site.
- Avoids using existing blood lines for cultures unless sample is drawn when line is inserted or catheter sepsis is suspected.

Urine cultures
- Obtains "clean-catch" midstream urine specimen.
  - Instructs patient regarding clean-catch midstream urine collection method.
  - Assists patient in obtaining specimen as necessary.
  - Sends specimen to laboratory immediately to prevent deterioration and altered test results.

Indwelling catheter urine specimen collection
- Aspirates urine sample with urine sampling kit or sterile syringe.
- Transfers specimen into a sterile specimen container immediately.
- Sends container to laboratory immediately to prevent deterioration and altered test results.

Maintains continuous surveillance (I128).
Acquires, interprets, and synthesizes patient data so as to detect and prevent potential adverse clinical events.
- Continually monitors physiological and psychological indicators to detect discrete changes in overall condition.
- Utilizes critical thinking.
- Recognizes patients at high risk for complications.
- Communicates information about patient's risk status to appropriate member(s) of health care team.
- Monitors and controls clinical environment for safety or infection risks and other potential hazards.
- Prioritizes nursing actions based on clinical situation and patient's condition.
- Monitors patient for changes in status that require immediate nurse attention.
- Institutes appropriate care utilizing clinical practice guidelines.
- Notes type and amounts of effluent from drainage tube and notifies appropriate member of health care team regarding significant changes.
- Troubleshoots surgical equipment and clinical systems.

WOUND/TISSUE PERFUSION

OUTCOME O11	**The patient has wound/tissue perfusion consistent with or improved from baseline levels established preoperatively.**

OUTCOME DEFINITION: Adequate surgical wound tissue perfusion is evidenced by capillary refill of less than 3 seconds and evidence of maintaining or improving circulation, sensation, and motion of wound.

INTERPRETIVE STATEMENT: Adequate wound/tissue perfusion is necessary to promote optimal healing and maintain cellular function. Preexisting conditions (eg, diabetes, vascular disease) and patient behaviors (eg, smoking) can interfere with the adequate perfusion of both oxygen and nutrients.

OUTCOME INDICATORS:

- **Skin condition (general):** conjunctiva and/or mucous membranes pink; free from cyanosis or pallor.
- **Skin condition (surgical wound):** incision edges approximated; free from ischemia (pallor, cyanosis, erythema).
- **Vital signs:** temperature, pulse, and respirations within expected ranges.
- **Cardiovascular status:** heart rate and blood pressure within expected ranges; peripheral pulses present and equal bilaterally; skin warm to touch; capillary refill less than 3 seconds.

EXAMPLES OF INTERIM OUTCOME STATEMENTS:

- The patient's surgical wound is well-approximated and covered with a sterile dressing at transfer to postoperative unit.
- The patient's vital signs are stable at time of discharge from the OR.
- The patient's surgical wound is open and covered with a sterile dressing at time of discharge from OR.

POTENTIALLY APPLICABLE NURSING DIAGNOSES:

- Decreased cardiac output (X8)
- Risk for fluid volume deficit (X18)
- Risk for infection (X28)
- Ineffective breathing pattern (X7)

NURSING INTERVENTIONS AND ACTIVITIES:

Identifies baseline tissue perfusion (I60).
Assesses tissue perfusion and identifies any impairments or risk factors prior to an operative or invasive procedure.

- Verifies procedure, recognizes and anticipates fluid loss.
- Validates nursing assessment completed preoperatively.
- Completes visual inspection and assesses peripheral tissue perfusion.
- Follows facility policies, procedures, guidelines, or protocols for skin assessment preoperatively.
- Verifies patient's preoperative hydration status, height, weight, skin turgor, and pulses.
- Verifies patient's preoperative laboratory results as appropriate (eg, hematocrit [Hct], blood urea nitrogen [BUN], urine specific gravity [SpG]).
- Validates variances from norm (eg, edema, ascites, adventitious breath sounds, elevated central venous pressure [CVP]).
- Monitors intake and output.
- Monitors physiological parameters as indicated: vital signs, CVP, mean arterial pressure (MAP), pulmonary artery pressure (PAP), pulmonary capillary wedge pressure (PCWP), ECG, arterial blood gases (ABG), SaO_2, and temperature.

- Monitors patient for changes in neurological status (eg, LOC, mentation, speech, reflexes, strength, mobility).
- Monitors patient for changes in extremities (eg, pulses, skin color, temperature, turgor, capillary refill, SaO_2 as appropriate).
- Monitors patient for changes in skin integrity (eg, cuts, abrasions, bruises, edema).
- Reports/reviews variance from norm of physiological parameters with appropriate member of health care team.

Assesses factors related to risks for ineffective tissue perfusion (I15).
Collects data to evaluate the patient's risk for ineffective tissue perfusion (eg, presence of diabetes, immunosuppression).
- Assesses nutritional status for altered nutrition.
  Increased adipose tissue
  - Maintains awareness of associated impaired circulation and respiration.
  - Maintains awareness of decreased blood flow and oxygen at wound area.
  - Maintains awareness of decreased resistance to infection.
  Decreased adipose tissue
  - Recognizes decreased cushioning over bony prominences and takes appropriate action.
  - Recognizes patient's potential inability to conserve body heat and takes appropriate action.
- Identifies patient's allergies and/or hypersensitivities to medications, tapes, iodine products, soaps, and antimicrobial solutions.
- Identifies skin reactions that occur as a result of allergy or sensitivity.
- Determines onset and associated symptoms of skin reactions, (eg, itching, burning, stinging, numbness, pain, fever, nausea and vomiting, diarrhea, sore throat, cold, stiff neck, exposure to new foods, new soaps or cosmetics, new clothing or bed linens, stressful situations).
- Identifies family history of chronic tendencies toward skin disorders.
- Identifies previous surgery sites (eg, presence of scars, degrees of keloid formation).
- Reviews chart for evidence of:
  - Diabetes—diminishes circulation to extremities and impairs the body's healing ability.
  - Cancer—previous irradiation may cause fragile and sensitive skin.
  - Immunosuppression due to corticosteroids, anti-inflammatory agents, and cytoxic medications.
  - Vascular disease—diminished circulation.
  - Hyperthermia.
  - Impaired physical immobility.
  - Urinary/bowel incontinence.
  - Abnormal lab values (eg, lower hemoglobin).
- Individualizes plan of care based on assessment.

Functions as first assistant during surgical incision, excision, and repair of pathology *(RNFA)* (I129).
Functions as first assistant during an operative or other invasive procedure.
- Implements tissue handling techniques based on assessment of tissue location, type, and health status. *(RNFA)*
- Preserves homeostasis during tissue manipulation. *(RNFA)*
- Plans approach, incises, and dissects tissue or places instrumentation for tissue dissection under the supervision of the surgeon (eg, trocar placement, saphenous vein harvesting). *(RNFA)*
- Selects suture for wound closure. *(RNFA)*
- Sutures (knot tying, ligation of vessels, and wound closure). *(RNFA)*
- Chooses appropriate suturing material and techniques based on density of tissue, support for suture line, potential tissue necrosis, everting skin edges, and cosmetic effect. *(RNFA)*
- Determines skin closure based on patient's status. *(RNFA)*
- Staples wound. *(RNFA)*
  - Assesses blood supply of tissues being stapled. *(RNFA)*
  - Inspects staple line to assess need for reinforcement. *(RNFA)*
- Removes wound closure sutures/staples when wound is healed.

Evaluates postoperative tissue perfusion (I46).
Assesses tissue perfusion throughout postoperative phase of care.
- Validates nursing assessment completed preoperatively.
- Completes visual inspection and assesses peripheral tissue perfusion.
- Follows facility policies, procedures, guidelines, or protocols for skin assessment.
- Monitors patient positioning intraoperatively.
- Ensures appropriate positioning devices are used.
- Monitors patient for changes in neurological status (eg, LOC, mentation, speech, reflexes, strength, mobility).
- Monitors patient for changes in extremities (eg, pulses, skin color, temperature, turgor, capillary refill, SaO_2 as appropriate).
- Monitors patient for changes in skin integrity (eg, cuts, abrasions, bruises, edema).
- Reports variances from norm to appropriate members of health care team.

Evaluates progress of wound healing (I130).
Assesses skin condition, tissue perfusion, and healing progress of surgical wound.
- Identifies risk factors that impair wound healing.
- Assesses wound status (approximation of skin edges, color, warmth, drainage, foul odor) regularly.
- Conducts follow-up telephone assessment of wound status in patients discharged within 24 hours of procedure.
- Reports signs and symptoms of infection to appropriate member of health care team.
- Monitors temperature for elevation.
- Provides wound care consistent with wound class.

NORMOTHERMIA

OUTCOME O12	The patient is at or returning to normothermia at the conclusion of the immediate postoperative period.

OUTCOME DEFINITION: The patient's core body temperature is within expected or therapeutic range.

INTERPRETIVE STATEMENT: The patient must be at or near normal temperature for basal metabolic processes to occur. A core temperature is preferred to assess thermoregulation. Alterations in temperature, either above or below normothermia, interfere with optimal recovery from anesthesia, thereby increasing the probability of adverse postoperative sequelae. Surgical intervention may include intentional alterations in body temperature.

OUTCOME INDICATORS:

- **Vital signs:** temperature, pulse, and respirations within expected ranges.
- **Cardiovascular status:** heart rate and blood pressure within expected ranges; peripheral pulses present and equal bilaterally; skin warm to touch; capillary refill less than 3 seconds.
- **Skin condition (general):** free from shivering; free from cyanosis or pallor.

EXAMPLES OF INTERIM OUTCOME STATEMENTS:

- The patient's temperature is greater than 36 degrees centigrade at time of discharge from the operating room.
- The patient's temperature is intentionally maintained at 33 degrees to lower cell metabolism.

POTENTIALLY APPLICABLE NURSING DIAGNOSES:

- Risk of impaired skin integrity (X51)
- Impaired skin integrity (X50)
- Hypothermia (X26)
- Risk for imbalanced body temperature (X57)
- Ineffective thermoregulation (X58)

NURSING INTERVENTIONS AND ACTIVITIES

Assesses risk for inadvertent hypothermia (I131).
Determines patients at risk for loss of body heat and plans appropriate interventions.
- Those at high risk include but are not limited to patients:
  - With preoperative baseline temperature less than or equal to 36 degrees centigrade.
  - Receiving general anesthesia (anesthetic agents impair the body's ability to control and conserve heat by inhibiting vasoconstriction and the shivering response).
  - With open exposed wound for prolonged period of time (eg trauma, long intraoperative procedure).
  - Such as infant, neonate, toddler (high body surface/kg and low subcutaneous brown fat for insulation increases rate of heat loss).
  - Including frail elderly (low basal metabolic rate, limited cardiovascular reserves, thinning of skin, and reduced muscle mass).
  - With traumatic destruction of skin (burn, industrial accidents)

Implements thermoregulation measures (I78).
Initiates thermoregulation measures and applies devices to cool or warm the patient as indicated.
- Selects temperature-monitoring and regulation devices based on identified patient needs.

- Determines that devices are readily available, clean, and functioning according to manufacturers' specifications before inserting, attaching or placing devices on patient.
- Inserts or applies temperature-monitoring and regulation devices to patient according to plan of care, facility practice guidelines, and manufacturers' documented instructions.
- Operates temperature-monitoring and regulation devices according to manufacturers' documented instructions.
- Removes temperature-monitoring and regulation devices from patient when indicated.

Monitors body temperature (I86).
Inserts, attaches, or applies temperature-monitoring devices.
- Measures core body temperature. (Sites that reflect core body temperature include esophagus, nasopharynx, tympanic membrane, bladder, rectum, pulmonary artery).
- Listens for patient verbalization of thermal comfort.
- Assesses and documents patient's body temperature at frequent intervals.
- Interprets and communicates patient temperature data to appropriate members of health care team for further evaluation and action as appropriate.
- Monitors and documents patient's pulse, respirations, blood pressure, and SaO_2 saturation.
- Assesses patient for signs of shivering.
- Monitors patient for intraoperative and immediate postoperative bleeding.
- Monitors patient for cardiac dysrhythmia and congestive heart failure.
- Reports patient's temperature to PACU nurses for determination of appropriate postoperative treatment methods.

Evaluates response to thermoregulation measures (I55).
Observes and verifies body temperature and responses to thermoregulation measures, and monitors for adverse effects.
- Measures core body temperature (sites that reflect core body temperature include esophagus, nasopharynx, tympanic membrane, bladder, rectum, pulmonary artery).
- Listens for patient verbalization of thermal comfort.
- Assesses and documents patient's body temperature at frequent intervals.
- Interprets and communicates patient temperature data to appropriate members of health care team for further evaluation and action as appropriate.
- Monitors and documents patient's pulse, respirations, blood pressure, and SaO_2.
- Assesses patient for signs of shivering.
- Monitors patient for intraoperative and immediate postoperative bleeding.
- Monitors patient for cardiac dysrhythmia and congestive heart failure.
- Reports patient's temperature to PACU nurses for determination of appropriate postoperative treatment methods.

FLUID/ELECTROLYTE/ACID-BASE BALANCES

OUTCOME O13   **The patient's fluid, electrolyte, and acid-base balances are consistent with or improved from baseline levels established preoperatively.**

OUTCOME DEFINITION: The patient's fluid, electrolyte, and acid-base balance are within expected or therapeutic range throughout the perioperative period. These parameters are continuously monitored during the perioperative period.

INTERPRETIVE STATEMENT: Continuous monitoring of fluid loss, replacement, and acid-base balance occurs during the perioperative period. Maintaining fluid electrolyte and acid-base balances is critical for optimal recovery from anesthesia and surgery.

OUTCOME INDICATORS:

- **Skin condition (general):** free from new or increasing edema in dependent areas; conjunctiva and/or mucous membranes pink; free from cyanosis or pallor.
- **Vital signs:** temperature, pulse, and respirations within expected ranges.
- **Cardiovascular status:** heart rate and blood pressure within expected ranges; peripheral pulses present and equal bilaterally; skin warm to touch; capillary refill less than 3 seconds.
- **Renal status:** output greater than 30 mL/hr; specific gravity 1.010 to 1.030.
- **Laboratory values:** arterial blood gases, serum electrolytes, and hemodynamic monitoring values (if ordered/available) within expected ranges.

EXAMPLES OF INTERIM OUTCOME STATEMENTS:

- The patient's vital signs are within expected range at discharge from the OR.
- The patient's blood pressure and pulse are within expected range and remain stable with position change at time of transfer to PACU.
- The patient's urinary output is within expected range at discharge from the OR.

POTENTIALLY APPLICABLE NURSING DIAGNOSES:

- Risk for impaired skin integrity (X51)
- Impaired skin integrity (X50)
- Risk for fluid volume deficit (X18)
- Fluid volume deficit (X17)
- Risk for fluid volume imbalance (X20)
- Impaired gas exchange (X21)

NURSING INTERVENTIONS AND ACTIVITIES:

Identifies factors associated with an increased risk for hemorrhage or fluid and electrolyte loss (I132).
Identifies individuals at risk for hemorrhage or hypovolemia including those with recent traumatic injury, abnormal bleeding or clotting time, extensive surgical procedure, complicated renal/liver disease, and major organ transplant.
Establishes and verifies nursing assessment.
- Identifies and verifies availability of blood/plasma replacement.
- Collaborates with blood bank to ensure supply of blood/plasma replacement
- Assures adequate supply of warm intravenous fluids.
- Assures adequate supply of suction containers, sponges, and hemostatic agents.

- Verifies patient's preoperative hydration status, height, weight, skin turgor, and pulses.
- Confers with physician and/or anesthesia care provider if unusual assessment data, or signs and/or symptoms of fluid, electrolyte, and/or acid-base imbalances are noted.

Recognizes and reports deviation in diagnostic study results (I111).
Identifies critical variances in fluid, electrolyte, and acid-base balances and notifies appropriate members of health care team.
- Obtains patient health data.
- Identifies patient's physiological baseline. Parameters include, but are not limited to:
  - Serum electrolyte levels;
  - Laboratory results specific to fluid balance (eg, Hct, BUN, albumin, total protein, serum osmolality, SpG);
  - Assesses patient's buccal membranes, sclera, and skin for indications of altered fluid and electrolyte balance (eg, dryness, cyanosis, jaundice);
  - ABG specific to acid-base balance (eg, pH, partial arterial oxygen [PaO_2], SaO_2, bicarbonate [HCO_3] as available);
  - Hemodynamic status, including CVP, MAP, PAP, and PCWP levels, if available;
  - Blood pressure;
  - Heart rate and rhythm;
  - Respiratory rate, method of respiration (eg, natural, spontaneous on room air; mechanical ventilation and settings);
  - Fluid and food intake, both oral and parenteral;
  - Sources of fluid loss (eg, diarrhea, draining wounds, excessive urine output);
  - Use of medications, prescribed and over-the-counter;
  - Alcohol or drug abuse;
  - Preexisting conditions and/or disease states (eg, congestive heart failure, diabetes mellitus); and
  - Inadequate oral intake and/or IV fluid flow (eg, inadequate fluid/electrolyte maintenance).
- Assesses cardiovascular status (eg, pulse, dysrhythmia, edema, ECG, hemodynamic parameters).
- Assess renal status (eg, intake and output, urinalysis, renal function studies).
- Assesses nutritional status (eg, NPO status, weight, skin turgor).
- Collaborates with other health care providers regarding laboratory or assessment findings related to fluid, electrolyte, and acid-base status.
- Plans nursing care based on physiological data.
- Communicates physical health status (eg, verbal reports, patient record).
- Implements conservative surgical techniques when hemoglobin, hematocrit, and blood availability are compromised. *(RNFA)*

Monitors physiological parameters (I89).
Monitors physiological parameters including intake and output, arterial blood gases, electrolyte levels, hemodynamic status, and SaO_2.
- Assesses and monitors neurologic status (eg, LOC, confusion).
- Auscultates breath sounds.
- Estimates blood and fluid loss by weighing sponges, measuring suctioned output, and summing fluid amounts from drainage devices (wound drains, chest tubes).
- Measures urine output.
- Monitors vital signs.
- Obtains peripheral blood specimen as ordered for monitoring of fluid and electrolyte levels (eg, hematocrit, BUN, protein, sodium, potassium, glucose levels).
- Monitors laboratory results relevant to fluid balance (eg, hematocrit, BUN, albumin, serum electrolytes, total protein, serum osmolality, specific gravity levels).
- Inserts arterial line when indicated and if within scope of practice. *(RNFA)*
- Assists with insertion of invasive hemodynamic monitoring catheters (eg, arterial line, CVP, pulmonary arterial catheter, Swan-Ganz catheter).
- Monitors hemodynamic status, including CVP, MAP, PAP, and PCWP levels, if available.
- Monitors for signs of hypervolemia/hypovolemia.

- Monitors patient's response to prescribed electrolyte/fluid therapy.
- Monitors fluid loss (eg, bleeding, vomiting, diarrhea, perspiration).
- Monitors amount of irrigation fluids administered.
- Monitors ABG, as available.
- Monitors for loss of acid (eg, vomiting, nasogastric output, diarrhea, diuresis).
- Monitors for loss of bicarbonate (eg, fistula drainage, diarrhea).
- Monitors respiratory pattern.
- Monitors for symptoms of respiratory failure (eg, PaO_2, SaO_2 and elevated $PaCO_2$ levels).
- Monitors tissue perfusion (eg, PaO_2, SaO_2, ABG, and hemoglobin levels and cardiac output), if available.

Implements hemostasis techniques (I133).
Provides supplies, instrumentation, and appropriate surgical techniques as needed to control hemorrhage.
- Provides appropriate supplies (eg, sponges, suction, electrocoagulation unit, instrumentation) to control bleeding.
- Applies pressure to bleeding sites as directed.
- Applies instrumentation to control bleeding vessels. *(RNFA)*
- Coagulates bleeding vessels with electrocautery. *(RNFA)*
- Uses hemostatic agents when appropriate for bleeding control. *(RNFA)*
- Facilitates site exposure using appropriate suctioning techniques. *(RNFA)*

Establishes IV access (I34).
Establishes and maintains peripheral IV access to administer IV fluids, medications, and blood products per physician order.
- Verifies order to establish IV access.
- Reviews chart for allergies, laboratory results, and patient history.
- Verifies barriers to communication.
- Verifies patient's ability to understand information.
- Provides information about procedure to be completed and offers emotional support.
- Reviews with patient presence of allergies, clotting disorders, or medications that would affect clotting.
- Maintains aseptic technique throughout.
- Selects and prepares all items for procedure.
- Offers emotional support.
- Requests patient hold extremity still.
- Avoids placing line in extremity with arteriovenous fistulas or shunts.
- Applies warm compresses as appropriate.
- Applies tourniquet above insertion site.
- Cleanses area with appropriate solution per facility policy or protocol.
- Inserts needle per appropriate policy or protocol.
- Observes for blood in flash chamber.
- Connects needle hub to IV tubing as appropriate.
- Applies tape and dressing per facility policy and protocol.
- Labels dressing per facility policy and protocol.
- Evaluates patient's responses to procedure.

Collaborates in fluid and electrolyte management (I23).
Collaborates with other members of health care team to monitor and implement prescribed treatments (eg, autotransfusion, IV fluids, blood products, medications).
- Verifies procedure, recognizes and anticipates fluid loss.
- Anticipates replacement requirement for large volume loss procedures.
- Verifies patient's preoperative hydration status, height, weight, skin turgor, and pulses.
- Verifies patient's preoperative laboratory results as appropriate (eg, Hct, BUN, urine SpG).

- Validates variances from norm (eg, edema, ascites, adventitious breath sounds, elevated CVP) and reports to appropriate members of health care team.
- Monitors vital signs as indicated.
- Administers or prepares for administration of IV fluid therapy.
  - Maintains patient IV access.
  - Provides [restricts] oral intake as appropriate.
  - Weighs patient and monitors trends.
  - Inserts urinary catheter when ordered.
  - Confers with appropriate health care provider if symptoms of fluid electrolyte and/or acid-base, excess/deficit persist or worsen.
  - Monitors hydration status as appropriate.
  - Monitors for infiltration of intravenous site.
  - Reports variances from norm of physiological parameters to appropriate members of health care team.
  - Evaluates patient's response to intravenous therapy.
- Monitors intake and output.
- Considers blood and fluid loss by weighing sponges, measuring suctioned output, and adding fluid amounts from drainage devices (wound drains, chest tubes).
- Inserts Foley catheter as ordered.
- Monitors physiological parameters: vital signs, CVP, MAP, PAP, PCWP, ECG, ABG, SaO_2, and temperature as appropriate.
- Reports variance from norm of physiological parameters to appropriate member of health care team.
- Retrieves additional fluids and/or supplies as indicated.
- Evaluates patient's response to fluid management.

Administers blood product therapy as prescribed (I2).
Arranges for availability and the administration of blood products or blood recovery per physician order.
- Validates order as prescribed.
- Verifies patient's consent to receive blood product therapy.
- Determines blood product has been prepared.
- Requests product delivery to area of infusion.
- Obtains supplies and prepares administration system for blood product.
- Observes standard and transmission-based precautions.
- Completes venipuncture with large bore needle.
- Follows national standards/guidelines and facility policies, procedures, or protocols for blood administration.
- Monitors patient for response to therapy.
- Monitors physiological parameters as applicable (eg, vital signs, CVP, MAP, PAP, PCWP, ECG, ABG, SaO_2, and temperature).
- Reports variances from norm of physiological parameters to appropriate member of health care team.
- Monitors for transfusion reaction, fluid shift to third space, and hypervolemia.
- Responds immediately to recognition of transfusion reaction (eg, discontinue infusion, notify physician and blood bank, treat patient's symptoms according to physician's directions and facility policies).
- Reports variances from norm to appropriate members of health care team.

Administers prescribed medications based on arterial blood gas results (I9).
Safely administers prescribed medications related to acid-base balance and monitors for complications resulting from acid-base imbalance.
- Validates nursing assessment preoperatively.
- Completes a visual inspection, physical examination, and review of laboratory data.
- Obtains specimen following facility policies, procedures, and guidelines.
- Reviews results with other members of the health care team.
- Obtains medications ordered and understands the medication actions, indications, contraindications, adverse reactions, and emergency treatment.
- Administers medication as ordered.

- Monitors patient for demonstrated sign of therapeutic effect.
- Monitors patient for signs of adverse effects.
- Monitors applicable physiological parameters (eg, vital signs, SaO_2, ABG, CVP, MAP, PAP, PCWP).
- Reports variances from norm to appropriate members of health care team.
- Retrieves emergency equipment as indicated (eg, intubation equipment, fiber-optic scope).
- Evaluates patient's response to medications administered.

Administers electrolyte therapy as prescribed (I5).

Administers medications related to electrolyte balance and monitors for complications resulting from abnormal serum electrolyte levels.
- Validates order as prescribed.
- Verifies patient's preoperative hydration status (eg, weight, height, skin turgor, pulses).
- Verifies patient's preoperative laboratory results as applicable (eg, Hct, BUN, urine specific gravity).
- Identifies nursing activities necessary for expected outcome (eg, assembles supplies to initiate IV therapy).
- Prioritizes nursing actions (eg, correct hypovolemia/hypervolemia).
- Determines availability and coordinates supplies, equipment, and personnel for fluid, electrolyte, and blood volume maintenance. This includes, but is not limited to:
  - IV catheters, infusion line, and fluids;
  - Rapid infusion systems;
  - Autotransfusion equipment;
  - Type and screen or cross-match for blood products; and
  - Personnel who manage specialty equipment (eg, perfusionist).
- Provides equipment and supplies based on patient's needs.
- Anticipates need for equipment and supplies.
- Selects equipment and supplies in an organized and timely manner.
- Determines all equipment is functioning before use.
- Administers electrolyte therapy as prescribed.
- Monitors hydration status as appropriate.
- Monitors intake and output.
- Monitors physiological parameters as appropriate (eg, vital signs, CVP, MAP, PAP, PCWP, ECG, ABG, SaO_2, temperature).
- Reports variances from norm of physiological parameters to appropriate members of health care team.
- Evaluates patient's response to electrolyte therapy.
- Confers with physician and/or anesthesia care provider concerning maintenance and/or corrective therapy (eg, IV fluids, electrolyte replacement, medications to correct acid-base balance).
- Determines that emergency equipment and supplies are available at all times (eg, defibrillator/monitor, emergency medication and supply cart).

Evaluates response to administration of fluids and electrolytes (I153).

Observes for signs and symptoms of fluid and electrolyte imbalances.
- Monitors intake and output, arterial blood gases, electrolyte levels, hemodynamic status, and SaO_2.
- Estimate blood and fluid loss.
- Monitors for signs and symptoms of fluid volume excess/deficit.
- Monitors for signs and symptoms of electrolyte imbalances.
- Monitors laboratory results relevant to fluid and electrolyte imbalance.
- Monitors patient's response to prescribed fluid/electrolyte therapy.
- Reports variances from norm to appropriate members of health care team.

RESPIRATORY	
OUTCOME O14	**The patient's respiratory function is consistent with or improved from baseline levels established preoperatively.**

OUTCOME DEFINITION: The patient's respiratory status is consistent with or improved from the baseline preoperative level. This is monitored continuously throughout the perioperative period.

INTERPRETIVE STATEMENT: Adequate respiratory status is essential to maintain oxygenation and elimination of carbon dioxide. Adequate respiratory function is critical for optimal recovery and the prevention of hypoventilation, which can lead to cardiac arrest, permanent brain injury, and death.

OUTCOME INDICATORS:

- **Cognition:** answers questions appropriately; memory intact.
- **Affective response:** awake; cooperative with plan of care
- **Vital signs:** blood pressure, temperature, and pulse within expected ranges.
- **Respiratory status:** SaO_2 within expected range; rate, depth, and symmetry of respirations unchanged or improved from preoperative assessment; breath sounds free from adventitious sounds.
- **Skin condition (general):** conjunctiva and/or mucous membranes pink; free from cyanosis or pallor.

EXAMPLES OF INTERIM OUTCOME STATEMENTS:

- The patient is breathing spontaneously on room air without assistance at discharge from the OR.
- The patient is breathing spontaneously on supplemental oxygen without assistance on transfer to postoperative unit.
- The patient is mechanically ventilated with oxygen therapy through endotracheal tube at discharge from the OR.
- The patient's SaO_2 and respiratory rate are within expected range at discharge from the postoperative unit.

POTENTIALLY APPLICABLE NURSING DIAGNOSES:

- Ineffective breathing pattern (X7)
- Ineffective airway clearance (X2)
- Impaired gas exchange (X21)
- Risk for aspiration (X5)
- Anxiety (X4)

NURSING INTERVENTIONS AND ACTIVITIES:

Monitors changes in respiratory status (I87).
Assesses respiratory status and monitors for changes in respiratory status.
- Validates nursing assessment completed preoperatively.
- Anticipates and assists in maintaining or establishing patent airway.
- Monitors rate, rhythm, and depth of respirations.
- Monitors chest movement for symmetry and/or any use of accessory muscles.
- Monitors for sound of respirations (eg, noisy, wheezy, snoring, crowing).
- Auscultates breath sounds for depth and quality and presence of adventitious sounds.
- Provides airway maintenance as applicable (eg, suctioning and/or repositioning, chin lift, oral or nasal pharyngeal airway for ineffective airway).
- Administers oxygen as needed.
- Monitors physiological parameters as applicable (eg, vital signs, ABG, SaO_2).

- Monitors for restlessness, agitation, apprehension, or lethargy.
- Monitors for airway compromise (ie, laryngospasms unresolved with routine protocols).
- Reports variances from norms to appropriate members of health care team.
- Has emergency medications and equipment available.
- Maintains pharyngeal airway until patient demonstrates return of protective reflexes, then removes assistive airway device to minimize gag reflex.
- Extubates patient per facility extubation protocol.
- Monitors tidal volume to evaluate patient readiness for extubation.
- Positions patient for maximum lung expansion unless contraindicated.
- Monitors for pain and anxiety.
- Provides pain relief as applicable.
- Evaluates patient's responses to respiratory interventions.

Uses monitoring equipment to assess respiratory status (I121).

Assesses respiratory status and SaO_2.

- Reads and understands manufacturers' documented instructions for all monitoring equipment used by the perioperative nurse.
- Recognizes normal and abnormal blood pressure, interprets monitoring device readings, and recognizes abnormal readings.
- Validates nursing assessment completed preoperatively.
- Completes visual inspection of respiratory functions.
- Monitors rate, rhythm, depth, symmetry of chest muscle movement, and use of accessory muscles.
- Monitors for audible sounds (eg, noisy, wheezy, snoring, crowing) and auscultates breath sounds.
- Applies and operates pulse oximeter according to manufacturers' documented instructions.
- Applies, attaches, or inserts a conventional, electronic, or temperature-sensitive patch or tape thermometer according to manufacturer's documented instructions.
- Attaches ECG leads and operates ECG monitor.
- Attaches blood pressure monitoring equipment and operates equipment.
- Interprets SaO_2.
- Interprets temperature readings done with a conventional, electronic, or temperature-sensitive patch or tape thermometer.
- Interprets ECG tracings.
- Monitors assisted ventilation parameters as appropriate (ie, ventilator settings and alarms).
- Maintains pharyngeal airway until patient demonstrates return of protective reflexes, then removes assistive airway device.
- Monitors for airway compromise (ie, laryngospasm unresolved with routine protocols).
- Positions patient for maximal lung expansion unless contraindicated.
- Provides pain relief as applicable.
- Has emergency equipment and medications available.
- Administers oxygen as needed.
- Evaluates patient's response to respiratory-related interventions.

Recognizes and reports deviation in arterial blood gas studies (I110).

Identifies critical variances in acid-base balance and notifies appropriate members of health care team.

- Validates nursing assessment completed preoperatively.
- Reviews preoperative laboratory values.
- Monitors physiological parameters as applicable (eg, vital signs, SaO_2, ABG).
- Repeats tests whenever indicated.
- Reports variances from norms to appropriate members of health care team.
- Provides medications or equipment as requested.
- Evaluates patient's responses to interventions.

Evaluates postoperative respiratory status (I45).
Observes and monitors respiratory status throughout postoperative phase of care.

- Continually reassesses respiratory status;
- Completes visual inspection of respiratory function;
- Monitors rate, rhythm, and depth of respirations;
- Monitors chest movement for symmetry and/or any use of accessory muscles;
- Monitors sounds of respirations (eg, normal, noisy, wheezing, snoring, crowing);
- Auscultates breath sounds for depth and quality and presence of adventitious sounds;
- Monitors airway for patency and secretions;
- Provides airway maintenance as indicated;
- Monitors physiological parameters as indicated (eg, vital signs, SaO_2, ABG); and
- Reports variances from norm to the appropriate members of health care team.

CARDIAC	
OUTCOME O15	**The patient's cardiovascular status is consistent with or improved from baseline levels established preoperatively.**

OUTCOME DEFINITION: The patient's cardiac status is consistent with or improved from baseline levels established preoperatively. Cardiac status is monitored continuously throughout perioperative period.

INTERPRETIVE STATEMENT: Adequate cardiac output is essential to maintain perfusion of tissues. Cardiovascular status contributes to tissue perfusion of oxygen and nutrients, removal of cellular waste, and temperature regulation. Cardiac monitoring can be invasive or noninvasive depending on the type of procedure.

OUTCOME INDICATORS:

- **Cardiovascular status:** heart rate and blood pressure within expected ranges; peripheral pulses present and equal bilaterally; skin warm to touch; capillary refill less than 3 seconds.
- **Respiratory status:** SaO_2 within expected range; rate, depth, and symmetry of respirations unchanged or improved from preoperative assessment; free from adventitious breath sounds.
- **Skin condition (general):** conjunctiva and/or mucous membranes pink; free from cyanosis or pallor.
- **Renal status:** output greater than 30 mL/hr; specific gravity 1.010 to 1.030.

EXAMPLES OF INTERIM OUTCOME STATEMENTS:

- The patient's vital signs are within expected range at discharge from OR.
- The patient's hemodynamic status within expected range at transfer to postoperative unit.
- The warmth of the patient's skin is consistent with adequate perfusion at discharge from the OR.

POTENTIALLY APPLICABLE NURSING DIAGNOSES:

- Decreased cardiac output (X8)
- Fluid volume deficit (X17)
- Fluid volume excess (X19)
- Risk for fluid volume imbalance (X20)
- Risk for peripheral neurovascular dysfunction (X41)

NURSING INTERVENTIONS AND ACTIVITIES:

Identifies baseline cardiac status (I59).
Assesses blood pressure, heart rate and rhythm, SaO_2, and other parameters as appropriate.
- Validates nursing assessment completed preoperatively.
- Completes assessment of tissue perfusion, respiratory function, and cardiac status.
- Assesses cognition to include LOC; orientation to person, place and time; and presence of restlessness or agitation.
- Assesses respiratory function:
  - Inspects for symmetry of movement and any use of accessory muscles;
  - Notes noisy, wheezy, snoring, or crowing respirations and depth and quality of respirations; and
  - Auscultates breath sounds.
- Assesses cardiac function:
  - Reviews physiological parameters (eg, vital signs; CVP, SaO_2, MAP, PAP, PCWP, and ECG; regular rhythm, dysrhythmias or changes);
  - Auscultates for quality and regularity of rhythm; and
  - Palpates for equality, volume, and rate of pulses.

- Assesses extremities:
  - Inspects color, size, and shape;
  - Palpates for warmth, dryness, and capillary refill; and
  - Palpates for quality and volume of pulses.
- Assesses and reviews all pertinent laboratory studies.
- Reports variances from norms to appropriate members of health care team.

Uses monitoring equipment to assess cardiac status (I120).
Assesses blood pressure, heart rate and rhythm, SaO_2, and other parameters as appropriate.
- Reads and understands manufacturers' documented instructions for all monitoring equipment used by the perioperative nurse.
- Recognizes normal and abnormal blood pressure, interprets monitoring device readings, and recognizes and reports abnormal readings.
- Applies and operates the pulse oximeter according to manufacturer's documented instructions.
- Monitors and interprets SaO_2.
- Applies, attaches, or inserts a conventional, electronic, or temperature-sensitive patch or tape thermometer according to manufacturer's documented instructions.
- Interprets temperature readings obtained with a conventional, electronic, or temperature-sensitive patch or tape thermometer.
- Attaches ECG leads and operates ECG monitor.
- Interprets ECG tracings.
- Attaches blood pressure monitoring equipment and operates equipment.
- Validates nursing assessment completed preoperatively.
- Completes assessment of peripheral tissue perfusion.
- Monitors heart rate, rhythm, and quality.
- Monitors respiratory status visually, audibly, and through monitoring indices (eg, SaO_2, ABG).
- Monitors physiological parameters as appropriate (eg, vital signs, CVP, MAP, PAP, PCWP, ECG, laboratory studies).
- Monitors fluid volume status: initial baseline, estimated blood loss, and fluid replacement therapy.
- Monitors mentation and assesses LOC, orientation, presence of restlessness or agitation.
- Monitors extremities for warmth, color, dryness, pulse quality, and capillary refill.
- Monitors incision site for drainage type and amount.
- Recognizes early signs of cardiac complications.
- Recognizes the cardiac effect of intra-abdominal or intrathoracic pressure causing vagal stimulation or surgical manipulation. *(RNFA)*
- Monitors cardiac rate and rhythm when activating electrocautery. *(RNFA)*
- Reports variances from norms to appropriate members of health care team.
- Evaluates patient's responses.

Identifies and reports the presence of implantable cardiac devices (I58).
Verifies presence of pacemaker and/or automatic implantable cardioverter-defibrillator and notifies the appropriate members of the health care team.
- Validates nursing assessment completed preoperatively.
- Validates medical history and physical.
- Completes baseline cardiac assessment.
- Prepares for unplanned cardiac dysfunction due to device (eg, pacemaker magnet, bipolar or battery operated electrocautery).
- Notes any variances from norms (eg, scar tissues).
- Requests additional information from patient regarding any variances.
- Shares information with appropriate members of health care team.

Evaluates postoperative cardiac status (I44).

Observes and monitors cardiac status throughout postoperative phase of care.

- Validates nursing assessment completed preoperatively.
- Monitors mentation and assesses LOC; orientation to person, place and time; and presence of restlessness or agitation.
- Completes visual inspection of tissue perfusion, respiratory function, and cardiac status.
- Assesses respiratory function visibly, audibly, and ausculatory.
- Assesses cardiac status visibly, ausculatory, and by palpation.
- Assesses extremities visually, by palpation, and ausculatory as indicated.
- Assesses fluid volume status preoperatively and intraoperatively with estimated blood loss and replacement therapy.
- Monitors physiological parameters (eg, vital signs, CVP, SaO_2, MAP, PAP, PCWP, ECG, pertinent laboratory studies).
- Reports variances from norms to appropriate members of the health care team.

NEUROLOGIC

OUTCOME O30

The patient's neurological status is consistent with or improved from baseline levels established preoperatively.

OUTCOME DEFINITION: The patient's neurological status is consistent with or improved from the preoperative level. Neurologic parameters are monitored continuously throughout the perioperative period.

INTERPRETIVE STATEMENT: Adequate neurologic output is essential to maintain affective, cognitive, and neuromuscular function. Neurologic procedures are classified as cranial (brain and accessory structures), spinal (cord and nerves), and peripheral (all other neural tissue). Neurologic status can be measured by noninvasive or invasive methods depending on the type of procedure.

OUTCOME INDICATORS:

- **Cognition:** responds appropriately to questioning; memory intact
- **Affective response:** awake; cooperative with plan of care.
- **Psychomotor response:** verbal and motor responses equal to or improved from baseline levels; free of abnormal posturing; follows commands appropriately.
- **Neuromuscular status:** independently flexes and extends extremities; denies numbness or tingling of extremities; pupils equal and reactive to light; swallows without difficulty; reports vision unchanged; tremors decreased from baseline.
- **Cardiovascular status:** heart rate and blood pressure within expected ranges; peripheral/intracranial pulses present and equal by Doppler; skin warm to touch; capillary refill less than 3 seconds.
- **Skin condition (general):** smooth, intact, and free of ecchymosis, cuts, abrasions, shear injury, rash, or blistering.

EXAMPLES OF INTERIM OUTCOME STATEMENTS:

- The patient's vital signs are within expected range at the time of transfer to the PACU.
- The patient is awake and verbally responds appropriately to questioning at discharge from OR.
- The patient flexes and extends all extremities at discharge from the OR.
- The patient's sensory responses are within expected ranges at discharge from OR.
- The patient's peripheral pulses and Doppler readings are present, equal bilaterally at discharge from OR.

POTENTIALLY APPLICABLE NURSING DIAGNOSES:

- Acute confusion (X11)
- Decisional conflict (X12)
- Ineffective protection (X44)
- Risk for infection (X28)

NURSING INTERVENTIONS AND ACTIVITIES:

Identifies physiological status (I66).
Assesses current physiological status and reports variances to appropriate members of health care team.
- Establishes/reviews assessment of peripheral tissue perfusion. Assessment includes but is not limited to:
  - Blood pressure.
  - Peripheral pulse—equal bilaterally, quality.
  - Doppler readings.
  - Cardiac output.
  - Presence/absence of deep vein thrombosis.

- Evaluates laboratory values:
    - Monitors physiological parameters (eg, CBC, PT, and PTT).
    - Monitors drug and alcohol levels.
- Establishes/reviews assessment of respiratory status. Assessment includes but is not limited to:
    - Rate and depth of respirations.
    - Use of ventilatory support/oxygen.
    - Airway patency.
    - ABG.
- Assesses temperature.
- Monitors urinary output.
- Reviews pertinent laboratory test results (eg, electrolytes, hormone levels, basal metabolic rate, tissue pathology, culture sensitivities, CSF analyses, drug/alcohol levels).
- Notes presence of neurological implants (eg, VP/VA/LP shunts, stimulators, aneurysm clips).

Assesses baseline neurological status (I144).
Collects data to evaluate patient's current neurological status.
- Assesses patient by scoring the Glasgow coma scale (includes eye response, verbal response, and motor response).
- Assesses while awake preoperatively for:
    - Presence of nausea and vomiting.
    - Ability to flex and extend extremities.
    - Presence of numbness, tingling, or paresthesia in nontargeted areas.
    - Grip strength and ensures equality bilaterally.
- Validates skin integrity and the presence of any muscle wasting.
- Reviews chart for current neurological status. Review should include:
    - Latex allergy in patients with spina bifida history including number of previous surgical procedures.
    - History of seizure activity – occurrence, variety, frequency, stimulus, medications.
    - Cranial nerve assessment, including swallowing ability, speech, vision, pupil response.
    - EEG activity.
    - Diagnostic test results (eg, x-rays, CT scans, MRI, angiograms).
- Notes presence of tremors, plegia, palsy.
- Reviews history and physical for indications of Creutzfeldt-Jakob disease.
- Evaluates current headache/pain/discomfort level using a recognized pain scale (eg, patient with loss of cognition may need the "faces" scale).
- Identifies triggers for patients with seizures or tic Douloureux.
- Notes presence of decerebrate rigidity in patient posturing.
- Notes presence of intracranial pressure monitoring and values prior to surgery.
- Notes presence of neurological implants (eg, VP/VA/LP shunts, stimulators, aneurysm clip).
- Assesses psychosocial status.

Implements protective measures during neurosurgical procedures (I145).
Protects patient from harm caused by equipment, supplies, or positioning specific to neurosurgical procedures.
- Reviews/establishes neurological nursing assessment.
- Obtains previous diagnostic tests for comparison during the surgical procedure (eg, x-rays, CT scans, MRI, angiograms).
- Prevents potential cross-contamination by prion infection.
    - Informs health care team when diagnosis is probable or known.
    - Collects supplies and equipment required for care.
    - Implements precautions according to facility policy.
    - Provides health care team with education regarding special handling of instruments/equipment/supplies.
    - Arranges for appropriate postoperative care.
- Implements latex allergy precautions as necessary (spina bifida cases are high risk patients).

- Implements spine precautions in patients with known or suspected spinal injury.
- Implements aneurysm precautions as needed (eg, decrease light stimulus, decrease noise stimulus, maintain medications to lower blood pressure).
- Preserves patient dignity by providing privacy for head shave.
  - Stores hair in labeled container according to facility policy.
- Considers safety and surgical visibility when positioning for neurosurgical procedure.
  - Uses adequate personnel to move patient into sitting, side-lying, or prone position.
  - Positions patient with head slightly higher than heart to improve venous drainage and prevent an air embolus.
  - Assists with placement of positioning tongs and attempts to avoid placement in highly visible locations such as the forehead.
- Ensures that drills and perforators used to penetrate the skull are functioning and readily available to relieve intracranial pressure.
  - Has alternative measures available (manual cranial drill).
- Ensures availability of medications to decrease intracranial volume as needed (eg, mannitol, dexamethasone).
- Provides suction and warm irrigation continuously to prevent accumulation of fluids/debris in cranium.
- Monitors cognition, LOC, orientation to person, place, and time, and the presence of restlessness or agitation during awake procedures.
- Implements safety precautions when intended hypothermia is required during procedure.
- Maintains tissue hydration by covering with wet material or moistening with warm saline.
  - Ensures all sponges, cotton, and cottonoids utilized have x-ray detectable strings attached.
  - Ensures sponges, cotton, and cottonoids are not cut or torn.
  - Ensures all sponges and cottonoids remain in units of 5 or 10 according to packaging.
  - Avoids use of water for irrigation.
- Provides hemostatic agents to minimize cranial bleeding (eg, local anesthesia for skin edges, skin (Raney) clips, bone wax or equivalent, hemostatic chemical agents).
- Observes for signs and symptoms of venous air embolus (eg, end-tidal PCO_2 decline, decreased blood pressure, bradycardia, and convulsions) when patient is placed in the sitting position.
- Ensures micro-Doppler is available and functioning.
- Administers care to invasive device sites (eg, ventriculostomy, ICP monitor).

Evaluates postoperative neurological status (I146).
Assesses and monitors neurological status throughout postoperative phase of care.
Validates nursing assessment completed preoperatively.
- Completes a Glasgow coma evaluation post-procedure and compares to preoperative values.
- Observes for seizure occurrence, variety, frequency, and duration.
- Monitors for changes between preoperative and postoperative cranial nerves function.
- Assesses pain/headache/discomfort level using a recognized pain scale.
- Evaluates changes in intracranial pressure, levels in skin sensation, and neurological rigidity posturing.
- Evaluates physiological parameters (eg, vital signs, ICP, CPP, MAP, SaO_2, ECG, ABGs, evoked potentials (BAEP and SSEP) and pertinent laboratory studies.
- Reports variances from norms to appropriate members of the health care team.
- Inspects location of tong placement and applies ointment and dressing postoperatively.
- Evaluates for foreign body/implant function and response – biologic (dura grafts, bone grafts) vs. non biologic (hardware, aneurysm clips). *(RNFA)*
- Considers long term neurological follow-up of: *(RNFA)*
  - Devices implanted during surgery (eg, functionality of VP shunt).
  - Social relationships.
  - Leisure activities.
  - Activities of daily living.
  - Neuropsychological tests.
  - Quality of life.
  - Family burden.

PAIN CONTROL	
OUTCOME O29	**The patient demonstrates and/or reports adequate pain control throughout the perioperative period.**

OUTCOME DEFINITION: Adequate pain control/management is the alleviation or reduction in pain to a level of comfort that is acceptable to the patient.

INTERPRETIVE STATEMENT: Patient comfort and pain relief is critical to recovery from anesthesia and surgery. Methods to alleviate or reduce pain and/or discomfort may include pharmacologic and/or nonpharmacologic means.

OUTCOME INDICATORS:

- **Pain perception:** patient reports pain controlled based on a recognized pain scale (eg, less than 4 on a 1-10 scale); facial expression relaxed; rests comfortably; denies discomfort in nontargeted areas.
- **Cognition:** uses pain scale appropriately to describe level of discomfort.
- **Affective response:** cooperative with plan of care; relaxed body position; verbalizes ability to cope.
- **Vital signs:** blood pressure, pulse, and respiration within expected ranges.
- **Patient satisfaction:** reports satisfaction with level of pain control.

EXAMPLES OF INTERIM OUTCOME STATEMENTS:

- The patient cooperates by lying quietly during intraoperative procedure utilizing block/local anesthesia.
- The patient's vital signs at discharge from the OR are equal to or improved from preoperative values.
- The patient verbalizes control of pain.

POTENTIALLY APPLICABLE NURSING DIAGNOSES:

- Acute pain (X38)
- Chronic pain (X74)
- Fear (X16)
- Anxiety (X4)

NURSING INTERVENTIONS AND ACTIVITIES:

Assesses pain control (I16).
Uses validated pain scale to assess pain control.
- Reviews patient assessment for type of pain being treated and medical condition.
- Reviews current treatment protocol.
- Reviews potential interactions of pain medication(s) with other medications or food.
- Requests patient verbalize effectiveness of treatment with recognized assessment tool (eg, numerical scale, face scale).
- Requests verbalization of patient's expectation of acceptable pain score.
- Encourages questions related to pain management.
- Offers information to patient, family members about pain, pain relief measures, rating scales, and other assessment data to report.
- Monitors patient for congruence of verbal and nonverbal cues.
- Evaluates patient's responses to pain regimen.

Implements pain guidelines (I71).
Provides care consistent with clinical practice guidelines related to pain assessment and management.
- Reviews patient assessment for type of pain being treated, medical condition, and health status.
- Reviews facility pain guidelines.
- Initiates protocols identified in guidelines.
- Positions for comfort unless contraindicated.
- Determines regimen meets identified need.
- Monitors relationship of patient progress to pain control.
- Monitors pain guideline effectiveness.
- Administers medications as prescribed.
- Prescribes analgesics according to protocol and state regulations. *(RNFA)*

Collaborates in initiating patient-controlled analgesia (I24).
Identifies and collaborates in identifying patients who will benefit from patient-controlled analgesia.
- Review assessment for type of pain being treated and patient medical condition.
- Reviews with patient goals of pain management therapy.
- Reviews treatment protocol for administration.
- Encourages titration to effective relief levels.
- Monitors administration process.
- Provides teaching related to patient-controlled analgesia.
- Evaluates patient's response to medication administration.

Implements alternative methods of pain control (I69).
Uses diversified activities, therapeutic touch, meditation, breathing, and positioning to augment pain control methods.
- Reviews patient assessment for type of pain being treated and medical condition.
- Reviews current treatment protocol.
- Asks patient to verbalize effectiveness of treatment regimen.
- Reviews non-medication pain treatments (eg, cold therapy, heat therapy, music distraction, relaxation therapy, physical rehabilitation, visualization, pacing, and transcutaneous electrical nerve stimulation).
- Identifies patient's coping style and cultural influences regarding pain management.
- Assesses patient's level of fatigue, cognition, and ability to follow instruction.
- Offers information about methods that will assist in pain control.
- Includes family/significant other in educational process.
- Initiates alternative method following institutional guidelines.
- Monitors progress.
- Evaluates patient's responses.

Evaluates response to pain management interventions (I54).
Assesses patient's responses to pain management interventions, including physiological parameters and subjective and objective findings.
- Identifies and documents how the patient expresses pain (eg, facial expressions, irritability, restlessness, verbalization).
- Observes for clues indicating the patient is in pain (eg, restlessness, increased or decreased blood pressure, pallor, sweating, increased heart rate, nausea, irregular shallow breathing patterns, agitation, crying).
- Assesses the nature of the pain and any changes in pain level after pain management interventions.
- Uses recognized pain scale to quantify and measure adult patient's pain level in response to pain management interventions.
- Uses recognized pain observational scale to quantify and measure change in pediatric/neonate patient's pain level.

KNOWLEDGE OF EXPECTED RESPONSES

OUTCOME O31	The patient demonstrates knowledge of the expected responses to the operative or invasive procedure.

OUTCOME DEFINITION: The patient/family members communicate an understanding of the operative or other invasive procedure and effects they can expect. This is evidenced by their consent for the procedure and description of the perioperative sequence of events and outcomes.

INTERPRETIVE STATEMENT: The patient needs information regarding the expected outcomes, benefits, risks, surgical experience, and recovery process related to the planned operative or other invasive procedure. The information is shared with the patient's family members according to the patient's preference.

OUTCOME INDICATORS:

- **Cognition:** describes sequence of planned procedure; repeats instructions correctly; asks questions based on information provided; participates in plan of care.
- **Affective response:** calm; cooperates with plan of care; relaxed facial expression; verbalizes ability to cope.
- **Psychomotor skills:** correctly demonstrates deep breathing, coughing, leg exercises, wound care.
- **Supportive resources:** family demonstrates willingness to be actively involved in rehabilitation.
- **Patient satisfaction**: verbalizes satisfaction with content and process of teaching.

EXAMPLES OF INTERIM OUTCOME STATEMENTS:

- The patient verbalizes the sequence of events to expect before and immediately after surgery.
- The patient states realistic expectations regarding recovery from procedure.
- The patient and family members identify signs and symptoms to report to the surgeon/health care provider.
- The patient and family describe the prescribed postoperative regimen accurately.

POTENTIALLY APPLICABLE NURSING DIAGNOSES:

- Deficient knowledge (X30)
- Anxiety (X4)
- Impaired home maintenance (X23)
- Ineffective coping (X68)
- Compromised family coping (X14)
- Decisional conflict (X12)
- Body image disturbance (X6)

NURSING INTERVENTION AND ACTIVITIES:

Notes sensory impairments (I90).
Determines the patient's ability to see and hear without corrective devices.
- Identifies presence of the following:
    - Visual impairment,
    - Auditory impairment, or
    - Speech impairment.
- Modifies plan of care to accommodate sensory impairments.

Identifies barriers to communication (I134).
Assesses factors that could affect ability to communicate, comprehend, and demonstrate understanding of new information.

- Evaluates patient's communication skills.
- Observes and identifies the patient's:
  - Age and developmental needs;
  - Understanding of spoken words and ability to hear (presence of hearing aid);
  - Presence of airway adjuncts (eg, tracheotomy, laryngectomy, endotracheal tube);
  - Presence of alternative methods of speech (eg, sign language, voice box, keyboard, writing tools);
  - Nonverbal cues;
  - Need for interpreter or provides alternative to direct interpretation (written literature, telephone service) if needed.
- Listens to patient's speech pattern to identify:
  - Age and developmental needs,
  - Speech patterns,
  - Clarity of speech,
  - Complete thoughts,
  - Grammar and vocabulary patterns,
  - Discrepancies between words spoken and tone of voice, and
  - Patient comprehension from simple to complex.
- Provides the privacy necessary for patient to share confidential information.
- Provides environment that facilitates understanding:
  - Ensures room is quiet and has adequate lighting with minimal distractions;
  - Attracts patient's attention before speaking;
  - Looks at patient while speaking;
  - Speaks clearly and slowly in moderate tone;
  - Uses facial expressions, touch, and nonverbal cues appropriately to enhance communication; and
  - Uses visual aids as appropriate to assist with explanations.
- Evaluates patient's responses to teaching.

Determines knowledge level (I135).
Assesses knowledge and comprehension of new information and ability to apply in self-care activities.

- Establishes rapport.
- Evaluates language and cognitive skills relative to age and developmental stage of growth.
- Identifies barriers to communication.
- Identifies presence of altered thought processes.
- Verifies understanding of procedure and perioperative events.
- Identifies physiological variables that may interfere with learning such as central nervous system impairment, confusion, poor cognition, or medicated state.
- Assesses behaviors for appropriateness to situation (eg, calm, quiet, attentive, nervous, tense, agitated, apathetic).
- Observes for behaviors that demonstrate compliance with an understanding of previous instruction or therapeutic regimens.
- Evaluates patient's responses to identify level of knowledge and understanding.

Assesses readiness to learn (I136).
Evaluates factors that may affect abilities to learn or demonstrate knowledge.

- Identifies barriers to communication.
- Determines knowledge level.
- Identifies deviations from cognitive and psychomotor norms of age group.
- Identifies philosophical, cultural, and spiritual beliefs and values.
- Assesses coping mechanisms.
- Assesses patient's self-perception and self-concept patterns considering self-image, self-worth, and emotional responses.

- Identifies barriers to readiness to learn, including:
  - Anxiety,
  - Ineffective coping,
  - Ineffective denial,
  - Fatigue,
  - Anticipatory grieving,
  - Hopelessness,
  - Pain,
  - Powerlessness,
  - Ineffective role performance,
  - Spiritual distress, and
  - Disturbed thought process.
- Evaluates patient's responses to teaching.

Identifies psychosocial status (I68).
Assesses the psychosocial factors that influence that patient's care and develops and implements plan of care to address those needs.
- Evaluates psychosocial status relative to age and stage of development.
- Verifies psychosocial status.
- Identifies barriers to communication.
- Determines knowledge level.
- Determines patient's ability to understand information offered.
- Assesses coping mechanisms.
- Identifies patient home profile: household composition, ages, gender, and occupations; and family coping skills, limitations, and roles.
- Identifies patient's resources (eg, insurance, home environment, extended family, community).
- Identifies patient's religious practices.
- Identifies cultural practices and their affect on health behaviors and impending surgical event.
- Elicits perceptions of surgery.
- Evaluates patient's responses to psychosocial status.

Assesses coping mechanisms (I137).
Assesses the influence of coping practices and availability of support from family members.
- Reviews patient's coping pattern and its effectiveness.
- Identifies barriers to communication.
- Determines knowledge level.
- Identifies psychosocial status.
- Identifies philosophical, cultural, and spiritual beliefs and related practices.
- Asks patient to describe current methods of dealing with stress.
- Observes for behavior that may indicate ineffective coping (eg, verbalization of anger, depression, ineffective coping, alterations in diet, disruption of sleep pattern; restlessness; absence of eye contact; absence of or reduced participation in plan of care; withdrawal from family or staff; hostility toward family or staff).
- Determines when these behaviors became first apparent.
- Evaluates patient's potential for harming/injuring self or others.
- Encourages patient to express feelings.
- Determines the most effective methods of communication and support.
- Evaluates patient's previous and current coping patterns.
- Evaluates availability and effectiveness of support system.

Implements measures to provide psychological support (I147).
Offers assistance, advocates for patient, and provides psychological support during perioperative phases of care.
- Assesses for signs and symptoms of anxiety/fear (eg, fears and concerns, preoperative insomnia, muscle tenseness, tremors, irritability, change in appetite, restlessness, diaphoresis, tachypnea, tachycardia, elevated blood pressure, facial pallor or flushing, withdrawn behavior).

- Orients patient to environment and care routines/practices.
- Introduces staff members.
- Assures patient that a member of the staff is nearby.
- Provides information and answers questions honestly.
- Maintains a calm, supportive, confident manner.
- Provides an atmosphere of care and concern (privacy, nonjudgmental approach, empathy, and respect).
- Identifies sociocultural variables such as cultural or religious beliefs, values, and attitudes toward health and health practices.
- Observes for increased anxiety demonstrated through behavior (eg, hand tremor, shakiness, restlessness, facial tension, voice quivering, increased perspiration).
- Offers alternative methods to minimize anxiety (music, humor).
- Reinforces physician's explanations and clarifies any misconceptions.
- Explains purpose of preoperative preparations prior to implementation.
- Encourages patient participation in decision making and planning for postoperative care.

Evaluates psychosocial response to plan of care (I47).
Determines effectiveness of plan and psychosocial responses of patient/family members and modifies plan as indicated.
- Identifies barriers to communication.
- Determines knowledge level.
- Verifies patient's ability to understand information.
- Provides necessary time to process information.
- Appears relaxed and unhurried in interactions with patient.
- Obtains interpreter as appropriate.
- Provides culturally sensitive nursing care.
- Reviews nursing care plan with patient/family members.
- Discusses specific cultural influences (eg, folk medicine/home remedies; religious or spiritual aspects; food preferences or avoidance aspects; socioeconomic aspects; family structure).
- Provides for continuation of cultural practices and beliefs.
- Encourages use of family members as support as appropriate.
- Collaborates with patient/family member regarding expectations of care.
- Verifies patient's/family member's understanding of plan of care.
- Evaluates patient's/family member's response to plan of care.

Elicits perceptions of surgery (I32).
Assesses responses to the procedure and ensures access to correct information.
- Identifies barriers to communication.
- Verifies surgical procedure.
- Encourages patient to verbalize understanding of procedure.
- Observes behavior for nonverbal cues.
- Listens for verbalization of apprehension, uncertainty, fear, distress, or worry.
- Encourages patient to verbalize possible outcomes of surgery.
- Encourages patient's expression of fear or anxiety related to surgery and the outcomes of surgery.
- Evaluates patient's responses.

Explains expected sequence of events (I56).
Describes routines and protocols related to perioperative care.
- Provides preoperative instruction based on age and identified needs.
- Reviews environmental aspects of expected times and location:
  - Expected time of arrival and location,
  - Expected time of procedure,
  - Waiting time and location,
  - Directions to facility,
  - Location of postoperative discussion with physician, and
  - Anticipated time to see family/family member.

- Reviews preoperative instructions as indicated discussing importance of:
  - Diet,
  - Fluids intake (clear liquids allowed or NPO preoperatively and time frame),
  - Preoperative medications to take/hold and time frame,
  - Bowel prep if ordered,
  - Voiding,
  - Skin prep,
  - Clothing, and
  - Any anticipated transportation/discharge needs and home care.
- Reviews postoperative routines, procedures, and equipment.
- Communicates detailed procedural process and answers questions about postoperative medical regimen. (RNFA)
- Describes potential alterations in comfort levels to be expected postoperatively.
- Offers information on how to most effectively minimize postoperative discomfort.
- Evaluates patient's responses to teaching.

Screens for substance abuse (I114).
Assesses for past or present substance abuse, monitors for and reports defining characteristics of substance abuse or withdrawal, and makes appropriate referrals.
- Assesses for history of or current substance abuse.
- Listens for statements from the patient about how often substance is used and duration and quantity of use.
- Determines blood drug/alcohol levels.
- Observes behavior for signs and symptoms of substance abuse or withdrawal.
- Monitors vital signs.
- Offers appropriate referrals.
- Notifies appropriate members of healthcare team regarding history of or present abuse of drugs/alcohol.

Screens for physical abuse (I113).
Identifies defining characteristics for actual or risks for physical abuse and offers appropriate referrals.
- Assesses the patient for impaired skin or tissue integrity such as bruising, cuts, burns, and neuromuscular or skeletal impairment.
- Recognizes patient statements indicative of abuse.
- Protects the patient from and prevents further abuse.
- Provides information related to available resources (eg, social services, case management).
- Reports suspected abuse in accordance with facility policy and state reporting laws.

Provides status reports to family members. (I109).
Reports progress to family members by telephone or in person.
- Offers instruction to family members as indicated.
- Reviews expected protocols and patient progress through surgical day.
- Addresses family members' questions, concerns, and feelings.
- Identifies family members' emotional reaction to condition.
- Offers messages of assurance to family members.
- Provides answers to questions or assists in obtaining answers.
- Provides status reports to family members frequently or per facility/physician practice.
- Evaluates family members' response to information provided.

Evaluates response to instructions (I50).
Evaluates patient's/family member's understanding of instructions regarding perioperative experience and ongoing care.
- Observes patient's responses to instructions.
- Encourages patient to verbalize understanding of instructions.

- Requests patient family members to describe in their own words the anticipated physical and psychological effects of surgery, their feelings regarding surgery, and expected outcomes.
- Observes patient demonstration of sequential progressive steps of the following appropriate skills:
  - Deep breathing,
  - Use of incentive spirometer
  - Wound splinting,
  - Passive leg exercises,
  - Progression to ambulation, and
  - Wound and dressing care.
- Assesses the patient's and family member's ability to demonstrate understanding of:
  - Medication schedule;
  - Activity limitations and exercise regimen;
  - Dietary restrictions or supplements;
  - Wound care;
  - Prescribed treatments;
  - Follow-up appointments, including signs and symptoms to report; and
  - Emergency protocols.
- Observes return demonstrations of perioperative instruction.
- Provides patient/family member with written discharge and at-home instructions.
- Reinforces information provided by other members of health care team.
- Observes patient's responses to instructions.
- Clarifies information.
- Encourages patient/family member to describe in their own words their understanding of instructions.
- Encourages patient/family member communicate feelings regarding surgery and expected outcomes.
- Provides time for patient/family member to ask questions.
- Evaluates patient/family member responses to perioperative instruction.

	KNOWLEDGE OF NUTRITION MANAGEMENT
OUTCOME O18	**The patient demonstrates knowledge of nutritional management related to the operative or other invasive procedure.**

OUTCOME DEFINITION: Patient/family member communicates understanding of nutritional management and requirements related to the operative or other invasive procedure.

INTERPRETIVE STATEMENT: The patient needs information regarding nutritional management and requirements related to the operative or other invasive procedure. The information is shared with the patient's family members according to the patient's preference.

OUTCOME INDICATORS:

- **Cognition:** repeats instructions correctly; asks questions based on information provided; verbalizes ability to manage dietary requirements; describes preferred foods/fluids consistent with dietary requirements.
- **Affective response:** verbalizes understanding of the importance of balanced diet to facilitate healing.
- **Supportive resources:** family demonstrates willingness to obtain appropriate food and assist with meal preparation.
- **Patient satisfaction:** verbalizes satisfaction with content and process of teaching.

EXAMPLES OF INTERIM OUTCOME STATEMENTS:

- The patient verbalizes compliance with food and fluid restrictions prior to surgery.
- The patient describes appropriate home management of sore throat, nausea, and vomiting at time of discharge.
- The patient describes recommended postoperative nutritional intake regimen for the recovery period at time of discharge.

POTENTIALLY APPLICABLE NURSING DIAGNOSES:

- Imbalanced nutrition: less than body requirements (X36)
- Imbalanced nutrition: more than body requirements (X37)
- Nausea (X73)
- Ineffective health maintenance (X71)

NURSING INTERVENTIONS AND ACTIVITIES:

Assesses nutritional habits and patterns (I148).
Identifies usual dietary intake, habits, and patterns.
- Validates preoperative nutritional assessment including nutritional history and physical examination (eg, 24 hour recall, food record) and laboratory data.
- Verifies patient's ability to understand information.
- Provides necessary time to process information.
- Obtains interpreter if needed.
- Identifies food allergies.
- Identifies food preferences, cultural practices, and routine habits.
- Identifies cultural dietary preferences and practices.
- Compares usual dietary intake to prescribed postoperative diet.
- Individualizes postoperative dietary plan.
- Evaluates nutritional status.

Assesses psychosocial issues specific to the patient's nutritional status (I18).
Identifies any variances in nutritional plan related to psychosocial status.
- Identifies barriers to communication.
- Determines knowledge level.
- Obtains interpreter if needed.
- Verifies food preferences and routine practices.
- Involves patient when planning and providing care.
- Encourages family member participation in discussions and care processes.
- Evaluates effects of psychosocial issues on nutritional state.

Provides instruction regarding dietary needs (I107).
Explains dietary needs or restrictions.
- Obtains nutritional assessment.
- Reviews food preferences and routine practices.
- Obtains interpreter if needed.
- Provides alternatives to interpreter when appropriate (written material, video, tape recording in primary language).
- Verifies any food allergies.
- Explains purpose of dietary regimen.
- Provides age-specific, culturally-sensitive information about prescribed dietary regimen.
- Prepares patient for parenteral/enteral feedings when ordered.
- Instructs patient on appropriate food for the regimen and those prohibited.
- Reviews applicable food/medication interactions.
- Answers questions.
- Provides written instructions.
- Encourages participation of family members in process.

Evaluates response to nutritional instruction (I52).
Evaluates understanding of nutritional instruction by listening to explanations and observing return demonstrations.
- Requests patient/family member verbalize dietary regimen prescribed and review its purpose.
- Reviews cultural dietary practices.
- Requests patient/family member verbalize foods allowed and prohibited on prescribed regimen.
- Requests patient/family member verbalize specific medication/food interactions known from current medical regimen.
- Encourages and answers questions.
- Requests patient/family member verbalize understanding of dietary plan.

KNOWLEDGE OF MEDICATION MANAGEMENT

OUTCOME O19   **The patient demonstrates knowledge of medication management.**

OUTCOME DEFINITION: The patient communicates understanding of medication management. Communication includes knowledge of medications to be used, to include dose, purpose, frequency, route, and desired, side, and adverse effects.

INTERPRETIVE STATEMENT: The patient needs information regarding administration and management of medication. The information is shared with the patient's family according to the patient's preference.

OUTCOME INDICATORS:

- **Cognition:** repeats instructions correctly; asks questions based on information provided; states dose, purpose, frequency, route, side effects, and symptoms to report for each medication.
- **Affective response:** verbalizes acceptance of medication administration responsibility.
- **Psychomotor skills:** demonstrates how to care for surgical wound; prepares and self-administers injectable medication safely and correctly; demonstrates procedure required prior to medication administration (eg, pulse check).
- **Supportive resources:** family demonstrates willingness to be actively involved in medication management including medication acquisition.
- **Patient satisfaction:** verbalizes satisfaction with medication teaching and information provided.

EXAMPLES OF INTERIM OUTCOME STATEMENTS:

- The patient and family members verbalize realistic expectations regarding the effect of medications on postoperative recovery prior to discharge.
- The patient describes medication side effects to report at time of discharge.
- The patient and family members can state the correct dose, frequency of administration, and purpose of each prescribed medication at time of discharge.

POTENTIALLY APPLICABLE NURSING DIAGNOSES:

- Ineffective health maintenance (X71)
- Ineffective therapeutic regimen management (X33)
- Acute confusion (X11)
- Risk for caregiver role strain (X10)

NURSING INTERVENTIONS AND ACTIVITIES:

Verifies allergies (I123).
Identifies allergies, idiosyncrasies, and sensitivities to medications, latex, chemical agents, foods, and/or adhesives.
- Queries patient about allergies or hypersensitivity reaction to adhesives, egg products or iodine products.
- Queries patient about medications and foreign proteins that cause anaphylaxis (eg, antibiotics, opiates, vasopressin, protamine, allergen extracts, muscle relaxants, vaccines, local anesthetics, whole blood, cryoprecipitate, immune globulin, and radiocontrast media).
- Determines type of food or substance and type of reaction experienced, if any, as reported by the patient.
- Records and communicates to the anesthesia care provider a patient history of anaphylaxis, asthma, or other respiratory difficulties related to the presence of allergens, toxins, or antigens.

Assesses psychosocial issues specific to the patient's medication management (I17).
Identifies any variances in medication plan related to psychosocial status.
- Identifies barriers to communication.
- Determines knowledge level.
- Verifies patient's ability to understand information.
- Approaches patient in a calm and unhurried manner.
- Obtains interpreter if needed.
- Identifies influence of health beliefs and folk practices.

- Provides culturally sensitive nursing care.
- Reviews current medication regimens in detail with patient and family members.
- Reviews factors that may prevent the patient from taking medications as prescribed.
- Identifies effects of medication use on patient's lifestyle.
- Evaluates psychosocial issues specific to patient's medication administration.

Provides instruction about prescribed medications (I104)
Provides information about prescribed medications, such as purpose; administration; and desired, side, and adverse effects.
- Verifies any allergies and sensitivity reactions.
- States names and purpose of medications.
- Identifies dose, route, and appropriate times of administration.
- Instructs patient/family member of specific procedures necessary before medication administration (eg, checking pulse).
- Provides clear, understandable explanations about procedures.
- Communicates discharge instructions verbally and in writing.
- Communicates instructions that reinforce information provided in the preoperative period.
- Assesses patient's/family member's ability to understand information.
- Encourages family member participation in the instructional process.
- Offers teaching methods relevant to the patient's ability to comprehend information. This could include handouts, audio or video presentations, lecture, discussions, return demonstration, and class/group discussion.
- Evaluates the patient's ability to safely and correctly self-administer medications.
- Provides instruction about prescribed medications to include:
  - How to obtain and store medications,
  - The purpose and action of medication,
  - Differences in name and appearance of generic and brand names of medications,
  - Dose and times,
  - How medication should given,
  - Side effects/adverse reactions that may occur,
  - Side effects/adverse reactions to be reported immediately,
  - Symptoms indicating medication is not effective,
  - Any dietary or fluid restrictions that accompany prescribed medication,
  - Activity restrictions when taking medications,
  - Signs and symptoms of over- and under-dose,
  - Consequences of not taking or abruptly discontinuing medications,
  - Risks of taking expired medication,
  - Proper disposal of needles and syringes and where to dispose of sharps in the community,
  - Action to be taken if a dose is missed,
  - Applicable food/medication interactions, and
  - Appropriate storage practices and care of devices required for medication administration.
- Provides written instructions.
- Instructs to take a list of all medications to doctor's office appointment
- Evaluates patient's responses to instruction.

Evaluates response to instruction about prescribed medications (I48).
Evaluates understanding of medication instruction by listening to explanations and observing return demonstrations of activities related to the administration and management of medications.
- Requests patient/family member verbalize name of medication prescribed and its purpose.
- Reviews any cultural practices related to medication administration.
- Requests patient/family member verbalize dose, route, and frequency of medication administration.
- Requests patient/family member verbalize action to be taken when a dose is missed.
- Requests patient/family member identify where written instructions will be kept for reference.
- Requests patient/family member demonstrate specific procedures required prior to medication administration (eg, check pulse).
- Encourages and answers questions.

KNOWLEDGE OF PAIN MANAGEMENT

OUTCOME O20   **The patient demonstrates knowledge of pain management.**

OUTCOME DEFINITION: Patient/family members communicate/demonstrate knowledge of pain management as evidenced by an understanding of the plan for pain assessment and management, including knowledge of pharmacologic and nonpharmacologic methods of pain management, and the need to report pain in a timely manner.

INTERPRETIVE STATEMENT: The patient needs information regarding pain assessment and management plan, realistic outcomes, and pharmacologic and nonpharmacologic methods of pain management. The pain management plan reflects the patient's age, cultural background, and previous experiences with pain and surgery.

OUTCOME INDICATORS:

- **Cognition:** repeats instructions correctly; asks questions based on information provided; states dose, purpose, frequency, route, and which side effects from pain medication(s) to report; evaluates effect of pain medication using a recognized pain scale; recognizes the importance of timing of administration.
- **Affective response:** verbalizes willingness to accept responsibility for medication administration; agrees to notify health care provider with worsening or uncontrolled pain.
- **Psychomotor skills:** prepares and self-administers injectable medication appropriately; demonstrates ability to use patient controlled analgesic device.
- **Supportive resources:** family member demonstrates willingness to be actively involved in pain management plan including medication acquisition.
- **Patient satisfaction:** verbalizes satisfaction with pain management teaching and information provided.

EXAMPLES OF INTERIM OUTCOME STATEMENTS:

- The patient participates in management of pain control before and immediately after surgery.
- The patient and family member verbalize realistic expectations regarding discomfort after surgery.
- The patient verbalizes side effects of analgesic to report to the health care provider at time of discharge.
- The patient accurately describes the prescribed regimen for postoperative pain control at time of discharge.

POTENTIALLY APPLICABLE NURSING DIAGNOSES:

- Acute pain (X38)
- Ineffective coping (X68)
- Caregiver role strain (X9)
- Nausea (X73)
- Nutrition imbalance: less than body requirements (X36)

NURSING INTERVENTIONS AND ACTIVITIES:

Identifies cultural and value components related to pain (I61).
Provides pain control considering cultural factors and manifestations of values (eg, stoicism, alternative therapy, verbalization, meditation).
- Reviews records for type of pain being treated, medical condition, demographics, and cultural cues.
- Establishes rapport.
- Evaluates language and cognitive skills relative to age and developmental stage.

- Identifies barriers to communication.
- Identifies presence of altered thought processes.
- Determines educational background.
- Obtains interpreter if needed.
- Requests patient verbalize pain management protocol and its purpose.
- Identifies patient's preference of pain therapy and coping methods.
- Asks patient to describe pain and intensity of pain.
- Offers assessment tool most appropriate to patient need (ie, numerical scale, color scale, face scale).
- Verifies assessment tool is clearly understood.
- Provides culturally sensitive nursing care.
- Identifies mutual goals of care that consider different preferences (eg, alert versus pain free).

Provides pain management instruction (I108).
Provides information about the purpose; administration; and desired, side, and adverse effects of prescribed medications and nonpharmacological techniques for managing pain.
- Validates orders for prescribed medication.
- Verifies patient's ability to understand information.
- Provides necessary time to process information.
- Identifies patient's cultural practices.
- Obtains interpreter if needed.
- Verifies allergies and any sensitivity reactions.
- Explains names and purposes of medications.
- Identifies dose, route, and appropriate times of administration.
- Instructs patient/family member of specific protocols for medication administration (eg, use of patient-controlled analgesia pump).
- Reviews action to be taken if a dose is missed.
- Encourages notification of health care provider when discomfort after pain medication is unrelieved by ordered medications or is worsening.
- Reviews desired, side, and adverse effects.
- Reviews applicable food/medication interactions.
- Reviews appropriate storage practices and care of equipment.
- Provides written instructions.
- Encourages family member participation in the instruction process.
- Evaluates patient's understanding of medication administration, purpose, and effects.

Evaluates response to pain management instruction (I53).
Evaluates understanding of pain management instruction by listening to explanations and observing return demonstrations.
- Requests patient/family member to verbalize understanding of pain medication and its purpose.
- Requests feedback on level of pain management achieved using a recognized pain measurement tool (numbers, faces).
- Observes patient for nonverbal cues regarding pain (ie, grimacing movement, splinting).
- Reviews cultural influences on pain assessment and management.
- Requests patient/family member verbalize dose, route, and frequency of medication.
- Requests patient/family member verbalize action to be taken when dose missed.
- Requests patient/family member identify where written instructions will be kept for reference.
- Determines patient's understanding to notify health care provider if pain is not controlled or is worsening.
- Encourages questions and clarifies information.

KNOWLEDGE OF REHABILITATION PROCESS

OUTCOME O21   **The patient participates in the rehabilitation process.**

OUTCOME DEFINITION: The patient/family participates in decision making, discharge planning, and goal identification throughout the rehabilitation process as evidenced by communication of concerns related to care.

INTERPRETIVE STATEMENT: The patient can expect continuity of care. The rehabilitation process begins with the initial patient contact. Appropriate resources are identified and referrals are initiated to support continuity of care throughout the perioperative experience.

OUTCOME INDICATORS:

- **Cognition:** repeats instructions correctly; asks questions based on information provided; verbalizes expected sequence of events for rehabilitation plan; states activities to avoid/limit during recovery process.
- **Affective response:** cooperates with plan of care; verbalizes willingness to participate in rehabilitation plan and ability to cope.
- **Psychomotor skills:** correctly demonstrates techniques required for postoperative recovery (eg, deep breathing, coughing, leg exercises, wound care).
- **Supportive resources:** family demonstrates willingness to be actively involved in rehabilitation; transportation is available for follow-up visits; states date and time for follow-up appointments.
- **Patient satisfaction:** verbalizes satisfaction with content and process of teaching.

EXAMPLES OF INTERIM OUTCOME STATEMENTS:

- The patient voices concerns related to postoperative recovery and rehabilitation.
- The patient and family verbalize realistic expectations regarding rehabilitation after surgery.
- The patient verbalizes signs and symptoms to report immediately to the surgeon.
- The patient describes the prescribed rehabilitation regimen to follow immediately after discharge from the facility.

POTENTIALLY APPLICABLE NURSING DIAGNOSES:

- Impaired physical mobility (X34)
- Fatigue (X70)
- Ineffective therapeutic regimen management (X33)

NURSING INTERVENTIONS AND ACTIVITIES:

Provides instruction based on age and identified needs (I106).
Provides perioperative instructional activities that promote rehabilitation based on age and developmental and situation-specific needs.
- Identifies barriers to communication.
- Determines knowledge level and psychosocial status.
- Assesses readiness to learn.
- Assesses coping mechanisms.
- Identifies teaching strategies appropriate to age and developmental stage.
- Encourages family member participation in process.
- Formulates plan to offer instruction to meet individual need.
- Provides environment conducive to teaching and learning (ie, room is quiet, with adequate lighting and minimal distraction).
- Uses learning theory and communication skills to facilitate understanding:
  - Attracts patient's attention before speaking;
  - Maintains eye contact;

- Speaks clearly and slowly in a moderate tone;
- Uses facial expressions, touch, and nonverbal cues as appropriate to enhance communication;
- Uses visual aids as appropriate to assist in teaching method; and
- Offers age-appropriate materials as indicated (ie, toys, pictures, written materials).
- Establishes priorities offering age-appropriate instruction to patient/family focusing on individual need.
- Describes preoperative preparation activities and behaviors expected:
  - Diet,
  - NPO,
  - Bowel prep,
  - Voiding,
  - Skin prep
  - Clothing,
  - Transportation, and
  - Discharge planning to include:
    o Need for responsible adult to assist with home care.
    o Availability of safe transport.
    o Preparation of the home.
    o Postoperative/postprocedural physical limitations.
    o Methods of obtaining referrals for assistance
    o Procurement of supplies/equipment as needed.
- Describes equipment that may be potentially frightening. Offers child opportunity to hold and explore items (eg, toys, hats, masks, blood pressure cuff, stethoscope).
- Describes how surgical suite environment and surgical experience may affect all senses (eg, noise, coolness, hardness of bed, attire of health care workers, lights, medication taste).
- Describes potential alterations in comfort level to be expected postoperatively (eg, wound pain, soreness, achiness, nausea, bloating, referred pain).
- Offers information regarding how to best minimize discomfort (eg, request pain medication for pain).
- Describes routine activities and equipment.
- Identifies resource contact for home care needs (eg, visiting nurse, medical equipment).
- Identifies potential limitations to normal routines and explores solutions to minimize those limitations (eg, may fatigue easily—plan to gradually increase activities).
- Describes postoperative home care instructions to allow for advance preparation (eg, general anesthesia, and securing a responsible person to provide transportation from the facility and to provide supportive care for 24 hours postoperatively).
- Uses instruction method that facilitates learning.
  - Offers information in basic elements, one aspect at a time, each component part of the task (eg, sit upright, take a deep breath through open mouth).
  - Offers rationale and benefits to facilitate understanding.
  - Modifies methods as needed for individual patients with ineffective coping (eg, repeat process steps to encourage gradual mastery of skills; assist patient in identifying appropriate short- and long-term goals).
- Provides adequate time for patient or family member to review information and ask questions.
- Offers demonstrations for the following skills:
  - Deep breathing,
  - Coughing and wound splinting,
  - Passive leg exercises,
  - Progression of diet postoperatively, and
  - Wound and dressing care.
- Clarifies information.
- Selects an alternate teaching method if indicated.
- Conducts patient/family learning conferences specific to rehabilitation process.
- Provides follow-up rehabilitation instructions as needed.
- Modifies postoperative rehabilitation instructions based on individual findings at the time of surgery. *(RNFA)*

Identifies expectations of home care (I62).

Identifies home care needs relative to performing the activities of daily living, managing self-care, and returning to usual activities.

- Assesses the patient's/family members ability to verbalize feelings about:
  - Physical changes that occur as a result of surgical intervention and how life will be affected;
  - Psychological changes that occur as a result of surgical intervention and how life will be affected; and
  - Concerns about the surgical experience, desired outcomes, or involvement in the recovery process.
- Identifies nursing diagnoses that describe the patient's needs for postoperative home care.
- Identifies expected outcomes for patient for home care following a surgical or invasive procedure.
- Assists patient/family member to identify and achieve realistic, measurable goals to attain desired outcomes.
- Encourages patient to identify own strengths and weaknesses.
- Assists patient/family member develop realistic expectations of themselves in performance of roles.
- Assists patient in breaking down complex goals into small, manageable steps and in prioritizing activities leading toward goal achievement.
- Assists patient/family member in setting definitive activity targets to achieve goals.
- Helps patient with methods to measure progress toward goals.
- Explains safety and comfort home care measures appropriate for procedure. Examples of these measures include, but are not limited to:
  - Rest frequently for limited periods during early recovery.
  - Have family member in the home when taking first shower.
  - When getting out of bed the first few times, roll to side of bed, then use arms to elevate to sitting position.
  - Sit in car seat, then rotate legs into vehicle.
  - Take pain medication as ordered with food/fluids. Notify health care provider if pain persists or worsens.
  - Remove throw rugs from walking pathway.
  - Use handrail when descending stairs.
  - Do not drive a mechanized vehicle (car, motorcycle, scooter) after general anesthesia until released by surgeon.
- Arranges for home health care and support in the community if indicated.
- Provides time for patient to ask questions and discuss concerns.
- Explains alternatives for home care rehabilitation. *(RNFA)*

Evaluates environment for home care (I35).

Identifies needs after discharge by identifying those at risk and the presence of any physical barriers and potential hazards in the home and by collaborating with the patient, family members, and discharge coordinators about home care needs.

- Identifies patients who live alone.
- Identifies patients who may not be able to independently perform activities of daily living.
- Identifies patients who live in nursing homes or residential facilities.
- Identifies homeless patients.
- Identifies patients with special equipment needs.
- Identifies patients with financial needs.
- Identifies patients with transportation needs.
- Identifies physical barriers in the home that may interfere with the patient's ability to care for self (eg, stairs, accessibility of bathroom, presence of safety rails in bathroom, potential safety hazards).
- Identifies potential safety hazards and risks for injury in the home.

Evaluates response to instructions (I50).

Evaluates patient's/family member's understanding of instructions regarding perioperative experience and ongoing care.

- Observes patient demonstration of sequential progressive steps of the following appropriate skills:
  - Deep breathing,
  - Coughing and wound splinting,
  - Passive leg exercises,
  - Progression to ambulation, and
  - Wound and dressing care.
- Assesses the patient's and family members' management skills of:
  - Medication schedule;
  - Activity limitations and exercise regimen;
  - Dietary restrictions or supplements;
  - Wound care;
  - Prescribed treatments;
  - Follow-up appointments, which may include signs and symptoms to report; and
  - Emergency protocols.
- Observes return demonstrations of self-care instruction.
- Provides patient/family member with written discharge and at-home instructions.
- Reinforces information provided by other members of health care team.
- Observes patient's responses to instructions.
- Requests verbalization of instructions.
- Clarifies information.
- Encourages patient/family member to describe in their own words the anticipated physical and psychological effects of surgery, feelings regarding surgery, and expected outcomes.
- Encourages patient/family member communicate feelings regarding surgery and expected outcomes.
- Requests patient/family member communicate understanding of preoperative instructions.
- Provides time for patient/family member to ask questions.
- Evaluates patient/family responses to perioperative instruction.

KNOWLEDGE OF WOUND MANAGEMENT

OUTCOME O22   **The patient demonstrates knowledge of wound management.**

OUTCOME DEFINITION: The patient/family member demonstrates knowledge of wound management by verbalizing phases of wound healing relative to operative or other invasive procedure, and demonstrating dressing and wound care.

INTERPRETIVE STATEMENT: The patient needs information regarding wound healing and management. Wound healing is a complex and highly organized physiological response caused by intentional or accidental injury to tissue. The information is shared with the patient's family members according to the patient's preference.

OUTCOME INDICATORS:

- **Cognition:** repeats instructions correctly; asks questions based on information provided; verbalizes expected sequence for wound healing; describes plan for wound care correctly.
- **Affective response:** cooperates with plan of care; verbalizes ability to manage and cope with wound care.
- **Psychomotor skills:** correctly demonstrates postoperative wound care.
- **Supportive resources:** family member demonstrates willingness to be actively involved in wound care.
- **Patient satisfaction:** verbalizes satisfaction with content and process of teaching.

EXAMPLES OF INTERIM OUTCOME STATEMENTS:

- The patient verbalizes the expected sequence of events for wound healing at time of discharge.
- The patient and family member voice realistic expectations for wound healing at time of discharge.
- The patient verbalizes signs and symptoms of wound infection to report immediately to the surgeon at time of discharge.
- The patient and family member demonstrate correct technique for applying a wound dressing at time of discharge.

POTENTIALLY APPLICABLE NURSING DIAGNOSES:

- Knowledge deficit (X30)
- Delayed surgical recovery (X56)
- Ineffective therapeutic regimen management (X33)
- Risk for infection (X28)
- Disturbed body image (X6)

NURSING INTERVENTIONS AND ACTIVITIES:
Assesses knowledge regarding wound care and phases of wound healing (I149).
Determines knowledge level about wound care and wound healing process.
- Establishes/reviews preoperative assessment and risk for surgical site infection:
  - Wound classification,
  - Age,
  - Cardiovascular status,
  - Nutritional status,
  - Metabolic or systemic disease,
  - History of smoking, and
  - Other immune system disorders.
- Verifies patient's ability to understand information.

- Obtains interpreter if needed.
- Provides necessary time to process information.
- Identifies patient's cultural practices.
- Individualizes postoperative wound care plan to accommodate patient's lifestyle.

Provides instruction about wound care and phases of wound healing (I105).
Provides necessary information about the phases of wound healing, techniques of wound care, and signs and symptoms to report.
- Reviews preoperative nursing assessment data.
- Reviews procedure for incision site care and dressing application.
- Discusses phases of wound healing.
- Discusses protocol for drain care as appropriate.
- Discusses potential untoward changes in wound and signs and symptoms to monitor/report.
- Demonstrates prescribed procedure for wound care.
- Encourages family/member participation in instruction process.
- Provides written instruction.

Evaluates response to instruction about wound care and phases of wound healing (I49).
Evaluates understanding of instruction about wound healing and wound care by listening to explanations and observing return demonstrations.
- Requests verbalization of procedure for incision site care.
- Requests verbalization of procedure for dressing application.
- Requests verbalization of wound progress through healing.
- Requests verbalization of procedure for drain care as appropriate.
- Requests verbalization of untoward changes in wound.
- Encourages questions and offers clarification.
- Encourages family/member participation in instruction process.
- Observes return demonstration of incision care and dressing application if indicated.

PARTICIPATES IN DECISIONS

OUTCOME O23	**The patient participates in decisions affecting his or her perioperative plan of care.**

OUTCOME DEFINITION: Patient/family member participates in decisions affecting the perioperative plan of care. The patient receives accurate and timely information to support informed decision making.

INTERPRETIVE STATEMENT: Clinical processes support the patient's informed decision-making process in accordance with facility and regulatory standards. The patient receives timely and accurate information regarding diagnosis, surgery and treatment options, and has his or her questions answered. Care is individualized, and the perioperative plan of care addresses the unique needs of each patient related to

- informed surgical consent,
- informed consent for research/clinical trials, and
- decisions related to self-determination including resuscitative measures, life-sustaining treatment, and end-of-life decisions.

OUTCOME INDICATORS:

- **Cognition:** verbalizes understanding of treatment options; describes sequence of planned procedure; repeats provided information correctly; asks questions based on information provided; participates in plan of care.
- **Affective response:** verbalizes concerns about decisions.
- **Clinical documentation:** surgical consent for procedure is signed according to facility policy; Self-Determination Act is implemented according to patient wishes.
- **Supportive resources:** family member participates in perioperative plan of care according to patient's preference.
- **Patient satisfaction:** expresses satisfaction with level of involvement in plan of care and decision-making process.

EXAMPLES OF INTERIM OUTCOME STATEMENTS:

- The patient verbalizes satisfaction with decision-making process and level of involvement concerning perioperative plan throughout the perioperative experience.
- The patient and family members ask questions regarding care options throughout the perioperative experience.
- The patient and family members voice preferences in care throughout the perioperative experience.

POTENTIALLY APPLICABLE NURSING DIAGNOSES:

- Decisional conflict (X12)
- Ineffective denial (X13)
- Caregiver role strain (X9)
- Fear (X16)
- Anxiety (X4)

NURSING INTERVENTIONS AND ACTIVITIES:

Verifies consent for planned procedure (I124).
Determines that informed consent has been granted for planned operative or invasive procedure and any related activities (eg, photographs, investigational studies).
- If consent is present:
  - Establishes rapport.
  - Identifies barriers to communication.
  - Obtains interpreter if needed.

- Determines knowledge level.
- Identifies psychosocial status.
- Elicits perceptions of surgery.
- Verifies surgical procedure.
- Encourages questions by patient/family members
- Answers patient's/family member's questions.
- Refers questions regarding surgical risks, benefits, alternatives, or adverse reactions to physician.
- Ensures documents are filed in appropriate section of medical record.
- If consent is not present for alert and oriented patient:
  - Establishes rapport.
  - Identifies barriers to communication.
  - Obtains interpreter is needed.
  - Determines knowledge level.
  - Identifies psychosocial status.
  - Elicits perceptions of surgery.
  - Verifies surgical procedure.
  - Contacts surgeon to answer questions regarding surgical risks, benefits, alternatives, or adverse reactions.
  - Completes consent forms per facility policy and procedure.
  - Witnesses patient's/parent's/family member's signature on consent form.
  - Answers patient's/parent's/ family member's questions as appropriate.
  - Files documents in appropriate section of medical record.
- If surgery is emergent:
  - Attempts to establish rapport.
  - Identifies barriers to communication.
  - Obtains interpreter is needed.
  - Determines availability of family members or legal guardian.
  - Verifies procedure to be completed with physician.
  - Delegates to another member of health care team notification of appropriate family members.
  - Obtains telephone consent from next of kin with witnesses listening to and documenting telephone consent.
- If the patient is incompetent:
  - Attempts to establish rapport.
  - Identifies barriers to communication.
  - Determines knowledge level.
  - Identifies psychosocial status.
  - Attempts to elicit patient's perceptions of surgery.
  - Attempts to verify surgical procedure.
  - Completes consent forms per facility policy and procedure.
  - Witnesses next of kin signature on consent form or verifies legal guardianship documents are present and completed.
  - Encourages questions by next of kin/legal guardian.
  - Determines that person present is individual identified on consent.

Identifies individual values and wishes concerning care (I63).
Assesses values, beliefs, and preferences and includes in plan of care.
- Identifies barriers to communication.
- Determines knowledge level.
- Verifies patient's ability to understand information.
- Provides sufficient time to process the information.
- Appears relaxed and unhurried in interactions with patient.
- Identifies influences of beliefs and values.
- Uses interpreter/family member in a manner that is sensitive to cultural values.
- Obtains information regarding current philosophical, cultural, and spiritual beliefs and values towards health and health practices.

- Recognizes patient's philosophical, cultural, and spiritual beliefs and values and their influence on health and health practices.
- Encourages family member participation in discussions as appropriate.
- Encourages family member to remain in attendance preoperatively and postoperatively.
- Provides culturally sensitive nursing care.

Includes family members in preoperative teaching (I79).
Identifies family members' knowledge and provides education and support.
- Establishes rapport with patient/family members.
- Identifies self and role as perioperative registered nurse.
- Identifies barriers to communication.
- Determines knowledge level.
- Assesses coping mechanisms.
- Assesses readiness to learn.
- Encourages verbalization of questions.
- Encourages verbalization of feelings and expectations.
- Communicates potential treatment options/choices in perioperative plan. *(RNFA)*
- Requests family members verbalize understanding of and return demonstration of preoperative instruction.

Includes patient and family members in discharge planning (I80).
Reviews with patient/family members the patient's capabilities, anticipated plan for care, and resources available to facilitate the rehabilitation process.
- Identifies availability of family member and encourages their involvement in care.
- Assesses physical, emotional, and educational resources of family member.
- Assists family member to understand patient's condition.
- Provides information to family members in accordance with the patient's preferences.
- Encourages patient and family members to participate in rehabilitative process.
- Assesses patient's capabilities, strengths, and limitations.
- Assesses family members' capabilities, strengths, limitations, perception of situation, and understanding about patient's recovery from surgery.
- Identifies family member's expectations for patient.
- Determines patient's level of dependency on family members, considering age and health status.
- Identifies realistic outcomes.
- Provides support to patient/family members.
- Evaluates response to discharge planning.

Provides information and explains Patient Self-Determination Act (I103).
Assesses current knowledge of the Patient Self-Determination Act (eg, the living will, power of attorney for health care, do not resuscitate, informed consent, organ procurement) and provides copy of resources/referral related to the Patient Self-Determination Act.
- Verifies presence of advance directive documents in current medical records. If documents are present:
  - Establishes rapport.
  - Identifies barriers to communication.
  - Obtains interpreter if needed.
  - Determines knowledge level.
  - Identifies psychosocial status.
  - Inquires if patient has considered or desires any changes to current advance directive document.
  - Reassures patient no discrimination in provision of care will occur based on whether patient has provided an advance directive.
  - Encourages questions regarding the Patient Self-Determination Act.
  - Clarifies information or misinterpretations as requested.
  - Seeks consultation with designated facility resource person for those patients requesting assistance in completion of advance directive documents.

- Completes proper placement of documentation/forms in patient's records as designated by facility policy and procedure.
- If documents are not present:
  - Establishes rapport.
  - Identifies barriers to communication.
  - Determines knowledge level.
  - Identifies psychosocial status.
  - Verifies patient has received written information regarding Patient Self-Determination Act.
  - Encourages questions regarding Patient Self-Determination Act.
  - Clarifies information as requested.
  - Reassures patient no discrimination in provision of care will occur based on whether patient has provided an advance directive.
  - Offers assistance in the completion of the documents per facility policy and procedure.
  - Seeks consultation with designated resource person within facility as requested by patient.
  - Places documentation/forms in patient's records as designated by facility policy and procedure.
  - Evaluates patient's knowledge of the Patient Self-Determination Act.

INDIVIDUALIZED CARE

OUTCOME O24   **The patient's care is consistent with the individualized perioperative plan of care.**

OUTCOME DEFINITION: The treatment and care received is consistent with an individualized perioperative plan of care.

INTERPRETIVE STATEMENT: The patient receives quality health services and continuity of care consistent with the planned intervention that addresses and meets the patient's unique needs throughout the perioperative continuum of care.

OUTCOME INDICATORS:

- **Cognition:** describes sequence of planned procedure; repeats instructions correctly; asks questions based on information provided; participates in plan of care.
- **Clinical documentation:** plan of care is documented and reflects individual preferences.
- **Supportive resources:** family member demonstrates willingness to participant in plan of care.
- **Patient satisfaction:** expresses satisfaction with delivered care.

EXAMPLES OF INTERIM OUTCOME STATEMENTS:

- The patient's actual procedure is consistent with signed consent form.
- The patient reports that individual choices were honored before and after surgery.

POTENTIALLY APPLICABLE NURSING DIAGNOSES:

- Ineffective therapeutic regimen management (X33)
- Decisional conflict (X12)

NURSING INTERVENTIONS AND ACTIVITIES:

Develops individualized plan of care (I30).
Considers all assessment information including patient's preferences and unique needs when developing an individualized nursing care plan.
- Introduces self and explains role
- Establishes/reviews nursing assessment data, preferences individual values, and cultural patterns.
- Organizes information into concise problem statements/nursing diagnoses.
- Identifies goals clearly as statements of outcome and congruent with patient's wishes and health status.
- Provides opportunity for mutual goal setting with patient, family member, and members of health care team as appropriate.
- Identifies measurable outcome indicators related to goal attainment.
- Identifies actions to achieve outcomes.
- Prioritizes nursing actions.
- Compares individualized plan with standards of care.
- Reviews plan of care with patient and revises as necessary.
- Evaluates patient's participation in plan of care.
- Communicates and coordinates patient's needs.
- Collaborates with surgeon to achieve consensus regarding delegated medical functions and prescribed interventions. *(RNFA)*
- Makes patient care assignments.
- Identifies and prepares for potential emergency situations.

- Prepares to implement perioperative plan.
  - Selects and gathers appropriate and properly functioning instruments, equipment, and supplies required for patient care.
  - Prepares OR or invasive procedure room for patient care.
- Plans for patient's discharge.

Obtains consultation from appropriate health care providers to initiate new treatments or change existing treatments (I92).
Involves and/or consults other members of health care team if the patient's condition or planned procedure changes.
- Validates nursing assessment completed preoperatively.
- Continually reassesses physiological parameters as applicable.
- Validates variances from norms that are identifiable from the assessment and monitoring indices.
- Reports variances from norm to appropriate members of health care team.
- Revises treatment regimen at direction of appropriate members of health care team.
- Monitors emerging treatment modalities potentially applicable to perioperative environment.
- Evaluates new products to determine risk/benefit for patient/facility.
- Initiates new treatment regimen at the direction of appropriate members of health care team.
- Evaluates response to new treatment or change in existing therapy.
- Documents operative procedure and postoperative orders according to practice guidelines and within institutional policy. *(RNFA)*
- Communicates modification in plan of care through postoperative progress notes. *(RNFA)*
- Makes postoperative visits to evaluate recovery progress.

Uses a clinical pathway (I119).
Actions performed are consistent with predetermined clinical pathway.
- Identifies clinical pathway which best correlates with planned procedure and individualized care.
- Shares clinical pathway with all members of the perioperative team.
- Implements actions according to prescribed pathway.
- Evaluates outcomes of actions taken.
- Recognizes variances from prescribed plan.
- Modifies actions based on evaluation.

Ensures continuity of care (I27).
Provides for a continuum of care throughout the perioperative phases of care.
- Reviews medical records for history and physical and nursing assessment.
- Identifies barriers to communication.
- Determines knowledge level.
- Verifies patient's ability to understand information.
- Obtains interpreter as appropriate.
- Validates completed nursing assessment or completes nursing assessment.
- Identifies potential risk factors.
- Identifies plan of care to meet individual patient needs.
- Includes patient and family members in establishment of plan of care.
- Shares plan of care with other members of health care team if appropriate.
- Implements perioperative plan of nursing care.
- Monitors patient status throughout perioperative experience.
- Reports any variances from norm to appropriate members of health care team.
- Performs actions or treatments as prescribed.
- Prioritizes actions based on patient's needs.
- Evaluates patient's responses to actions and treatments.
- Evaluates patient's responses to the plan of care.
- Shares evaluation of plan with appropriate members of the health care team.

PRIVACY RIGHTS

OUTCOME O25	**The patient's right to privacy is maintained.**

OUTCOME DEFINITION: The patient's personal privacy, confidentiality, and security within the perioperative environment are maintained. This includes maintaining the patient's privacy; securing patient records, personal belongings, and valuables; entering appropriate and accurate information into the patient record; and maintaining confidentiality of patient information.

INTERPRETIVE STATEMENT: Confidentiality of patient information is an integral component of patient privacy. Caregivers protect patients from undue physical exposure or unwarranted breaches of privacy or confidentiality.

OUTCOME INDICATORS:

- **Affective response:** verbalizes feelings of safety and privacy.
- **Skin condition (general):** skin exposure is limited to that required for the operative/invasive procedure.
- **Clinical documentation:** personnel are identified and limited to authorized staff only; personal belongings are identified and secured; only authorized personnel have access to patient records.
- **Patient satisfaction:** patient and family verbalize satisfaction with privacy measures.

EXAMPLES OF INTERIM OUTCOME STATEMENTS:

- The patient verbalizes satisfaction with level of privacy provided throughout surgical experience.

POTENTIALLY APPLICABLE NURSING DIAGNOSES:

- Ineffective therapeutic regimen management (X33)
- Low self-esteem (X46)

NURSING INTERVENTIONS AND ACTIVITIES:

Initiates traffic control (I81).
Restricts access to patient care area to authorized individuals only.
- Keeps doors to OR or procedure rooms closed except during movement of patients, personnel, supplies, and equipment.
- Restricts access to surgical suite to authorized personnel only.
- Records names of all individuals who participate in surgical procedure.

Secures patient's records, belongings, and valuables (I115).
Protects patient's clinical records and personal property. Releases belongings and valuables to patient or designated individual.
- Verifies presence of patient records, belongings, and valuables in secured area.
- Encourages family member to keep valuables following facility policy, procedure, or protocol.
- Explains clinical processes to patient/family member.
- Encourages questions regarding processes.
- Completes record of disposition of belongings and valuables following facility policy, procedure, or protocol.

Maintains patient's dignity and privacy (I150).
Protects the patient's privacy (eg, keeps OR doors closed, only exposes body as needed for care). Treats the deceased with respect and provides privacy area for family viewing of the deceased.

- Reviews patient record.
- Obtains interpreter if needed.
- Obtains information regarding current philosophical, cultural, and spiritual beliefs and values towards health and health practices.
- Recognizes patient's philosophical, cultural, and spiritual beliefs and effect on perioperative plan.
- Responds to patient's questions honestly and in terms the patient can readily understand.
- Protects patient's privacy by keeping doors closed and only exposing patient's body as needed to provide care.
- Advocates for respectful conversation during procedure.
- Provides cover, warmth, and comfort:
  - During transfer from unit to surgical suite,
  - Intraoperatively, and
  - During transfer to postoperative unit.
- Provides and maintains respect for deceased.
- Provides a protected area for viewing deceased.
- Evaluates patient's comfort level.

Maintains patient confidentiality (I151).
Limits access of patient information to appropriate members of health care team.
- Maintains patient's record following facility policy, procedure, or protocol.
- Obtains consent before engaging in direct patient care activities.
- Limits discussion of patient information to:
  - Appropriate members of the health care team.
  - Appropriate areas of facility.
- Restricts access to patient care areas to authorized individuals.
- Does not display patient's name with surgical procedure in unrestricted area.
- Protects electronic data.
- Assures human subjects protection for patients enrolled as research subjects.
- Obtains consent before transferring or sharing information to other providers and/or third parties.

COMPETENT CARE

OUTCOME O26 **The patient is the recipient of competent and ethical care within legal standards of practice.**

OUTCOME DEFINITION: Care providers in the perioperative environment provide health services within their legal and ethical scope of practice. Health care professionals are responsible for meeting legal, institutional, professional, and regulatory standards.

INTERPRETIVE STATEMENT: The perioperative patient is entitled to qualified and skilled care providers. Health care professionals are responsible for maintaining requirements and qualifications for competent practice.

OUTCOME INDICATORS:

- **Administrative policy:** clinicians practice in a manner consistent with credentialing policies; records are maintained and document professional nursing staff competence, licensure, and continuing education; perioperative care plans are based on ethical concepts and principles; variances in care are documented and corrective action taken.
- **Patient satisfaction:** patients report that care is competent, ethical, and within legal standards.

EXAMPLES OF INTERIM OUTCOME STATEMENTS:

- The patient voices satisfaction with delivered care.

POTENTIALLY APPLICABLE NURSING DIAGNOSES:

- Risk for injury (X29)
- Risk for infection (X28)

NURSING INTERVENTIONS AND ACTIVITIES:

Provides care without prejudicial behavior (I102).
Applies standards of nursing practice consistently and without bias (eg, disability, economic background, education, culture, religion, race, age, and gender).
- Recognizes personal biases.
- Identifies barriers to communication.
- Determines knowledge level.
- Verifies patient's ability to understand information.
- Appears relaxed and unhurried in interactions with patient.
- Provides culturally sensitive nursing care.
- Obtains interpreter if needed.
- Offers therapeutic communication techniques such as touch, active listening, and empathy.
- Maintains the patient's privacy and dignity.
- Offers comparable care to all patients in all settings.
- Encourages family member participation in discussions and care processes.

Provides care respecting worth and dignity regardless of diagnosis, disease process, procedure, or projected outcome (I100).
Provides for spiritual comfort, arranges for substitute nursing care when personal values conflict with required care, and respects patient's decision for surgery.
- Verifies presence of barriers to communication.
- Listens to patient and encourages communication.

- Identifies cultural and spiritual beliefs and values.
- Provides an environment that facilitates understanding.
- Obtains interpreter as appropriate.
- Demonstrates consistency in delivery of care to all patients.
- Fosters patient/family member participation in development and implementation of care plan.
- Maintains confidentiality of patient information.
- Provides privacy through physical protection.
- Evaluates patient's responses.

Shares patient information only with those directly involved in care (I116).
Protects patient information by completing operative record accurately and shares information in a manner that ensures patient confidentiality.
- Maintains patient confidentiality.
- Discusses patient information only with members of health care team who need the information.
- Refrains from discussing patients in public areas.
- Obtains patient consent before initiating direct care activities.
- Protects patient information.
- Completes records accurately and objectively.
- Honors patient's request to withhold information from family member.
- Releases patient information only to properly identified individuals and in compliance with established policies, mandates, or protocols.

Acts as a patient advocate by protecting the patient from incompetent, unethical, or illegal practices (I1).
Respects the "Patient's Bill of Rights," complies with facility policies of competent performance, complies with federal regulations (eg, OSHA), state nurse practice acts, accrediting agencies (eg, JCAHO), and adheres to professional standards of practice (eg, AORN), and confirms clinician's privileges and credentials. Intervenes to protect the patient's safety.
- Demonstrates competency to function in a professional role as a registered professional nurse in the OR as evidenced by the following:
  - Demonstrates competency to assess patient's physiological health status.
  - Demonstrates competency to assess the psychosocial health status of the patient/family/significant other.
  - Demonstrates competency to formulate nursing diagnosis based on health status data.
  - Demonstrates competency to establish patient goals based on nursing diagnosis.
  - Demonstrates competency to implement nursing actions according to prescribed plan.
  - Demonstrates competency to participate in patient/family members teaching.
  - Demonstrates competency to create and maintain multiple sterile fields.
  - Demonstrates competency to provide equipment and supplies based on patient needs.
  - Demonstrates extensive knowledge of anatomy and physiology. *(RNFA)*
  - Demonstrates competency to perform sponge, sharps, and instrument counts.
  - Demonstrates competency to administer medications and solutions as prescribed.
  - Demonstrates competency to physiologically monitor patient during surgery.
  - Demonstrates competency to act in emergency situations.
  - Demonstrates competency to monitor and control the environment.
  - Demonstrates competency to respect patient rights.
  - Demonstrates competency to perform nursing actions that demonstrate accountability.
  - Demonstrates competency to evaluate patient outcomes.
  - Demonstrates competency to measure effectiveness of nursing care.
  - Demonstrates competency to continuously modify plan of care based on new data.
- Functions within scope of nursing practice in accordance with state nurse practice act.
- Delegates duties only to competent appropriate personnel.
- Maintains credentials as RNFA, practices within state regulations and facility policy. *(RNFA)*
- Integrates expanded nursing role specialty skills with surgical team. *(RNFA)*

CONSISTENT CARE

OUTCOME O27   **The patient receives consistent and comparable care regardless of the setting.**

OUTCOME DEFINITION: The patient receives consistent and comparable care regardless of the setting and from the appropriate care providers. The patient's care is delivered in a nondiscriminatory and nonjudgmental manner according to published legal, facility, professional, and regulatory standards.

INTERPRETIVE STATEMENT: The perioperative patient receives care that fosters a positive self-image and preserves personal dignity. Caregivers respect patients and provide nondiscriminatory and nonprejudicial care.

OUTCOME INDICATORS:

- **Administrative policy:** care is consistent with professional and regulatory standards of care and the facility's human rights policy.
- **Performance improvement:** quality improvement indicators demonstrate consistent quality of care across patient populations.
- **Patient satisfaction:** patients report high levels of satisfaction with the delivery of care.

EXAMPLES OF INTERIM OUTCOME STATEMENTS:

- The patient voices satisfaction with interactions with professional and ancillary staff members throughout perioperative period.

POTENTIALLY APPLICABLE NURSING DIAGNOSES:

- Low self-esteem (X46)
- Spiritual distress (X54)
- Decisional conflict (X12)

NURSING INTERVENTIONS AND ACTIVITIES:

Provides care in a nondiscriminatory, nonprejudicial manner regardless of the setting in which care is given (I99).
Adheres to AORN, Joint Commission on Accreditation of Healthcare Organizations, and other standards of care. Provides comparable levels of care regardless of the setting in which care is given (eg, inpatient, outpatient, public, private, home, emergency department).
- Identifies barriers to communication.
- Determines knowledge level.
- Verifies patient's ability to understand information.
- Appears relaxed and unhurried in interactions with patient.
- Obtains interpreter as appropriate.
- Offers therapeutic communication techniques such as touch, active listening, and empathy.
- Offers explanation of each action.
- Maintains the patient's privacy and dignity.
- Offers comparable care to all patients in all settings.
- Encourages family member participation in discussions and care processes.

Preserves and protects the patient's autonomy, dignity, and human rights (I97).
Confirms consent, implements facility advance directive policy, and supports patient's participation in decision making.

- Establishes rapport
- Identifies barriers to communication
- Determines knowledge level.
- Verifies patient's ability to understand new information.
- Appears unhurried.
- Identifies values and beliefs.
- Provides care in a nonjudgmental manner.
- Offers therapeutic communication techniques such as touch, active listening, and empathy.
- Offers explanation of each action.
- Encourages family member participation in discussions and care processes.
- Evaluates patient's response to care provided.
- Provides culturally sensitive nursing care.
- Obtains interpreter as appropriate.
- Verifies patient's understanding of American Hospital Association's "Bill of Rights" and do not resuscitate (DNR) orders.
- Provides information as needed.
- Includes family members in teaching and decision making according to patient preference.
- Ensures communication of patient's decisions and preferences to members of health care team.
- Provides privacy.
- Maintains confidentiality.

Provides care without prejudicial behavior (I102).
Applies standards of nursing practice consistently and without bias (eg, disability, economic, background, education, culture, religion, race, age, and gender).
- Identifies barriers to communication.
- Determines knowledge level.
- Verifies patient's ability to understand information.
- Appears relaxed and unhurried in interactions with patient.
- Provides culturally sensitive nursing care.
- Obtains interpreter as appropriate.
- Offers therapeutic communication techniques such as touch, active listening, and empathy to allay patient's anxiety.
- Maintains patient's privacy and dignity.
- Offers comparable care to all patients in all settings.
- Encourages family member participation in discussions and care processes.

	RESPECT
OUTCOME O28	**The patient's value system, lifestyle, ethnicity, and culture are considered, respected, and incorporated in the perioperative plan of care.**

OUTCOME DEFINITION: The perioperative plan of care reflects the uniqueness of each patient, and social or economic status, personal attributes or lifestyle, culture, ethnicity, or level of health are considered and respected and reflected in the nursing plan of care.

INTERPRETIVE STATEMENT: The implementation of the perioperative plan of care incorporates, but is not limited to, the patient's:
- cultural and/or ethnic practices,
- spiritual or religious beliefs,
- psychosocial barriers and/or support systems,
- physical and/or cognitive limitations,
- language barriers, and
- age or developmental stage.

OUTCOME INDICATORS:

- **Cognition:** communicates personal needs related to lifestyle, religion, ethnicity, and culture.
- **Affective response:** verbalizes individual needs and indicates whether they are met.
- **Clinical documentation:** plan of care addresses patient's preferences and needs; cultural/religious practices that influence care are recorded; required interpreter services are facilitated; clinical documents reflect age-specific, functional, physical, or cognitive needs.
- **Patient satisfaction:** states that care is individualized and provided in a nondiscriminatory, nonjudgmental manner.

EXAMPLES OF INTERIM OUTCOME STATEMENTS:

- The patient verbalizes satisfaction with delivered care throughout perioperative experience.
- The patient voices satisfaction with interactions with professional and ancillary staff throughout perioperative experience.
- The patient/family member states that care is individualized and provided in a nondiscriminatory, nonjudgmental manner.

POTENTIALLY APPLICABLE NURSING DIAGNOSES:

- Impaired physical mobility (X34)
- Spiritual distress (X54)
- Low self-esteem (X46)

Identifies and reports philosophical, cultural, and spiritual beliefs and values (I57).
Assesses philosophical, cultural, and spiritual factors valued by the patient. Incorporates pertinent information in the plan of care and reports to other members of health care team as appropriate.
- Identifies barriers to communication.
- Determines knowledge level.
- Verifies patient's ability to understand information.
- Provides sufficient time for patient to process the information.
- Appears relaxed and unhurried in interactions with patient.
- Provides culturally sensitive nursing care.
- Validates current beliefs and values.

- Obtains interpreter as appropriate.
- Obtains information regarding philosophical, cultural, and spiritual beliefs and values towards health and health practices.
- Recognizes varying philosophical, cultural, and spiritual practices and beliefs and their effects on health and health practices.
- Encourages family member's participation in discussions as appropriate.
- Encourages family members to remain in perioperative area while patient is receiving care.
- Assesses influence of cultural and spiritual practices that may affect individual behavior and incorporates them in plan of care.
- Integrates value system/cultural beliefs into plan of care.

## Chapter Five

Applying the PNDS in the Practice Setting

The various contributions in this chapter illustrate applications of the PNDS vocabulary in real-world perioperative clinical settings and situations. The articles were written by perioperative nurses who have implemented or developed clinical or educational applications of the PNDS. The topics range from a general introduction to specific step-by-step directions for using the PNDS in clinical practice, education, and management.

Strategies to use the PNDS and examples of clinical records, educational plans, care plans, critical pathways, competency evaluations, and policies and procedures using the PNDS are discussed. All of these authors are enthusiastic about the potential the PNDS brings to the practice of perioperative nursing. They share with you their pioneering work, realism for implementation, and encouragement to begin the process of moving to a PNDS world.

❧

EXEMPLAR I: Implementing an Electronic Perioperative Nursing Care Record

You've been challenged with leading or assisting with the development of an electronic perioperative nursing care record. Researching established perioperative documentation systems in other facilities could provide insight and hints of those pitfalls to avoid. There are many hospitals with fine examples of perioperative electronic health records (EHRs) using a variety of vendor software. Reading the *PNDS @ Work* book called "Building a perioperative patient record" (Denver: AORN, 2004) also will give some valuable clues. It clearly recommends developing an improved written record before beginning screens for a new electronic nursing care record.

Certainly sources such as the PNDS book itself and the other books in the *PNDS @ Work* series will be some of your most valuable assets. Searching the Web sites of professional associations such as the American Society of PeriAnesthesia Nurses and the American Association of Critical-Care Nurses will also provide additional resources for validation of standards of care documentation questions and issues. As you begin to gather information, it may be helpful to create a file for loose papers and articles as well as an electronic file of downloaded materials.

Cynthia E. Yarborough, RN, CNOR
Physician Systems Support
WakeMed Health and Hospitals
Raleigh, North Carolina

ASSESSMENT/PREASSESSMENT

Approach this challenge as you would any patient-identified problem by using your nursing skills set and the nursing process: Assessment, Planning, Implementation, and Evaluation. Begin by gathering subjective data for your assessment. Talk with the nursing staff. What do they like about their current documentation? What do they dislike? How do *they* think the documentation screens should be laid out? Should similar components like the time elements be grouped together, or should the layout follow a chronological order?

It is critical to obtain staff input. These individuals will use the documentation daily. Certainly professionals can adapt and use any form of electronic documentation, but you will be doing your peers a disservice by not involving them in the design. Documentation that is not user-friendly could potentially impact the overall productivity of the OR and ancillary areas. We will return to the role that staff can fill in this process.

Continue in the assessment mode by gathering information from nurse managers, supervisors, and directors for the areas that will be impacted by the incorporation of an electronic record. What are the data elements that they need incorporated for data collection? What information will they want captured for reporting purposes? Will they want to measure staff productivity? Delays? Do they want to capture the amount of time of each delay? What are the challenges they face now with data analysis? These elements will need to be incorporated into the design.

Is it a goal of this electronic documentation implementation to combine multiple facilities with their own methods of documentation into one format? Certainly this will compound the complexity of the project ahead. Will this new documentation span the entire perioperative phase, including preadmission testing, or will this be operative information alone? Are there process improvements that this new documentation will be expected to achieve? Are there components that must be incorporated to meet the requirements of the Joint Commission or other regulatory agencies? Identifying the data component "must haves" before beginning the documentation design will prevent surprises and revisions that can be costly both in labor hours and dollars.

Also obtain the expectations of ancillary departments. Will there be any special requirements from the medical records department for this project? Is your facility moving toward a completely electronic health record (EHR)? Will there be an expectation for an export of the perioperative record into another format? Or will a print product initially be required? Will other units in your facility need access to the electronic documentation? Engage your IT department early in the process. What level of involvement can they provide? Does the IT department have any upcoming plans or projects that could impact the forward momentum of your electronic documentation project? Will there be interfaces to other systems as part of this implementation? What about the lab and radiology billing? How will these departments intersect with your electronic record?

Objective data gathering begins with collecting current copies of electronic or paper documentation. If there are multiple facilities involved, obtain documents from all locations. Identify the similarities and differences among the various documents. If the documentation will span preoperative, intraoperative and postoperative care, is there redundant information? Can the information be captured once and available in other phases without requiring re-entry by staff?

Current Hardware Assessment

Your current computer hardware will need to be assessed. Do you already have servers in place to run a applications? What about computer workstations? Will nursing staff share workstations in the preoperative and postoperative areas, or will these areas need one workstation per nurse? If computer workstations already exist in all areas, remember to verify that the operating system and processor are compatible with the new software recommendations. If other areas of your facilities use computerized documentation, evaluate the type of workstations they are using. Are they mobile? Are the screens easily read? Are they ergonomically correct? Some areas may use laptops while others have a small desktop workstation with an LCD monitor. The combinations are many. The challenge is to identify what will work best in all of the areas moving to the new electronic documentation.

Assessment of Current Process

Analyze current processes by diagramming patient flows and tasks associated with the surgical process. Having a thorough understanding of the processes to be automated by electronic documentation and being able to articulate those processes will be key to achieving success. Document the "who, what, when, where and how." Capture every step in a process. Who is completing the documentation? What components are they responsible for documenting? When are they completing the documentation? Weeks, days, or hours before, or is the documentation immediate? Where is the documentation occurring? Over the phone, across a desk, at the bedside? Begin with the first point of contact from scheduling through to the charge generation and reporting. Is information entered now that flows to downstream systems for billing purposes? Will this process continue, or will it be possible to automate some or all of these processes? Only by understanding the existing culture can a determination be made as to what impact a change may produce.

While you are in this fact-gathering phase, you will hear, "Well, I wish the new system could . . . ." Use these comments to develop a wish list for future review and possible incorporation.

PLANNING GOALS AND OUTCOMES

After the assessment phase, the needs and the desired outcomes are more easily identifiable. This assessment will lay the groundwork to develop the goals desired through implementing an electronic record. Clearly defining the goals will facilitate the decision-making process when comparing various software offerings. By listing the desired requirements the application software will need to accommodate, you lay the foundation for evaluating various software products.

Selecting the Software

This information is often included on a "request for information" or a "request for proposal" and submitted to software vendors for their comments and responses. Side-by-side comparison of features and functionality of each software package being considered will assist in the selection of the application software that best meets the needs of your organization. One caution: what appears adequate on paper to meet your requirements may not equate to an application that performs well when in use. Features of the software can be most accurately evaluated by seeing the software in action. This may require having demos of the software at your facility or actually visiting facilities where the software is in productive use to see it in action. If the software selection has already occurred before the assessment and your involvement, all is not lost. With a thorough assessment completed, you will have a clearer picture of the needs and components that will need to be considered as you move forward.

Perioperative Program Design

With the software selected and installed to the server(s), you will now begin the process of designing your perioperative documentation. During the install of the server software, consider creating both a test and a production environment. Most software vendors will strongly advise having separate environments for testing and productive use. Later, after the system is in productive use (ie, live), the test environment may be very different from the production environment because of upgrade and new release testing. Providing a training environment that mirrors the production

environment may prevent confusion for new individuals being trained on the documentation.

Engaging the Staff

An initial part of the planning phase should include selecting the individuals that will comprise the key design team. Consider having staff nurses from the various service specialties as part of the core team. With their expertise in their respective clinical areas, these individuals will help ensure that the newly created document will more closely fill the documentation requirements of all service lines. The team will also benefit from having nursing staff who are considered the strongest in their clinical documentation skills as design team members.

Often, when moving from handwritten documentation to electronic, the newest nurses to the operative arena are most eager to accept the challenge to assist with the task of migrating the handwritten documentation to an electronic format. Attempt to enlist your more experienced nursing staff. Even though some of these nurses may be some of the most resistant to using computers in the perioperative setting, their attention to documentation details and their understanding of the plan of care for a patient undergoing a surgical procedure will be invaluable assets. Not only can these nurses serve as leaders during the design process but also during the training and implementation phases.

Remember that if multiple facilities will be combining into one documentation record, staff from each site should be involved. Even though adding more team members will add additional challenges, when the time arrives to move the documentation into the implementation phase, the benefit of having a larger pool of "superusers" will be realized.

IMPLEMENTATION

The design team needs to be led by an individual or individuals who can keep the design team focused and on target. Discussions around documentation elements can veer off track easily, and the team leader will need to direct the group back on task. With clearly defined goals and a project plan that lists the tasks to be completed, the problem of "scope creep" can be avoided. Scope creep occurs when during the implementation process the project veers off course, causing delays and additional costs. If the project does not have a deadline for completion, the project can continue to add facets and complexity. Most software implementations, however, especially those where the software vendor is involved, will have a defined, expected completion date. There may even be monetary penalties for extending past the contracted completion date.

Administrative Support

It is critical that the project have the full support of the perioperative management team. Supervisors and managers may need to be involved to ensure that the design, training, and implementation team members are relieved from staffing responsibilities to attend planning sessions and meetings as required. They may need to be consulted when the design team have issues that they are unable to resolve or options that require a decision by management. Management will also need to show that they are united and committed to the task of moving to an electronic nursing care record. If staff members sense that the management team is reluctant to move toward an electronic format, they will attempt to make a case for why they cannot or should not move to electronic documentation with the assumption that management will abandon the project.

With the build team developing the design of the documentation, it is helpful for them to see screen examples or a mock-up of their record as it is being designed. Hopefully the software will allow various means of selecting and entering information into the screens. Drop-down selection boxes, checkboxes, radio buttons, and partial-key look-ups will enable staff to chart more efficiently and with accuracy. Also helpful is a medical spell-check component for information that nursing staff must type into the record.

Incorporating PNDS Into the EHR

While in the implementation design process, determine how PNDS will be included into the nursing documentation. The arrangement of how PNDS is incorporated into your record will depend largely on the design of the application software you are implementing. Some application software arrives with PNDS outcomes and interventions preloaded into the database. Other application software may not have PNDS as a component and may even have restrictions on the amount of data that can be captured due to field limitations. The ideal design would have PNDS outcomes available and visible throughout the continuum of perioperative care in each phase of the electronic record. The interventions and activities specific to the particular phases of the patient's perioperative experience would be dispersed and intermingled throughout the documentation. Others may choose to place all of the PNDS components into one specific area of the documentation rather than scattered throughout the screens. Your design team may have strong opinions one way or another. Much will depend on whether you have decided to follow a chronological flow of documentation or whether you have chosen to group parts of the documentation together in special areas.

Think of the PNDS as a huge care plan. You want to select the patient outcomes that your facility is striving to achieve. If you are a pediatric facility, maintaining body temperature is important, so perhaps you select normothermia as one of your PNDS outcomes to include in your electronic record. If you do mostly orthopedics, then freedom from injury related to surgical position would be important. (See **Table 5-1**.)

It is possible to include all of the freedom from injury outcomes by using the Safety Domain, "Freedom from physical injury" (D1), which includes all the safety outcomes. Don't forget to include presurgery in your outcomes selection, "The patient demonstrates knowledge of the expected responses to the operative or other invasive procedure." The preoperative teaching should be documented in the electronic record.

Once you have a standard set of outcomes that fits your patients, default them into every patient's record along with the PNDS interventions associated with these outcomes. This routine set of outcomes can then be customized based on the preoperative assessment of the patient and the scheduled procedure. Ideally, each procedure would have a set of outcomes and interventions matched to the most commonly scheduled procedures that could default to the electronic record along with the supply pick list. The preoperative nurse would document the activities and interventions completed in the preoperative phase that are directed at moving the patient toward the desired outcomes. For example, cataract patients need many medications; thus, the preoperative nurse would pick "Freedom from medication injury" as an outcome for a cataract patient.

Next, the operative nurse reviews the desired outcomes and adds or modifies the planned outcomes accordingly. He or she also would document the interventions and activities completed in the operative phase that are related to the desired outcomes.

For example, cataract patients never have electrosurgery used during their procedure, so "Freedom from electrosurgery injury" would not be applicable to that patient. If the same documentation continues into the postoperative phase, the interventions and activities completed in the postoperative phase need to be documented. At the close of the patient's perioperative experience, the outcomes would be indicated as completed or achieved. Should the outcomes not be met, the perioperative nurse would document why the outcomes could not be achieved or determined at the close of the nursing documentation.

TABLE 5-1: PNDS Outcome for Positioning the Patient

OUTCOME O5: Patient is free from signs and symptoms of injury related to positioning.

	Source of information	Type of information	Examples
RISK FACTORS Elderly patient population Decreased mobility related to degenerative joint disease (DJD) Poor skin integrity due to aging process Potential for decreased core temperature due to exposed surgical site	Age Nursing notes Skin integrity assessed Temperature	Numeric Free text Dictionary/Table Numeric or varied character	Example: 75 Text Examples: good, fair, poor, see nursing notes Examples: 98 or 98F
ASSESSMENTS Pertinent patient history Chart review of laboratory findings Decreased mobility and range of motion due to DJD Baseline temperature and blood pressure (BP) taken Skin integrity assessed Electrocautery pad site assessed	Patient history Lab review Nursing notes Temperature BP Skin integrity assessed Electrocautery pad site intact preoperatively	Multi-lined Yes/No or checkbox answer Multi-lined Yes/No or checkbox answer Free text Numeric Dictionary/Table Dictionary/Table	Examples: (Checkboxes) Diabetes, CHF, Asthma, MI, CRF Examples: (Check boxes) CBC: Y/N; labs within normal limits Y/N Text Example: 98 Example: 120/80 Examples: good, fair, poor, see nursing notes Yes/No, not applicable
INTERVENTIONS Patient positioned per protocol Safety strap applied Electrocautery pad applied Warming blanket applied Postoperative bed with positioning devices secured	Position Safety strap on Electrocautery pad site Electrocautery pad site intact postoperatively Warming devices Temperature setting Patient discharged via:	Multi-lined checkbox response, possibly linked to positioning device field Dictionary/Table Dictionary/Table Dictionary/Table Dictionary/Table Numeric Dictionary/Table	Examples: supine, prone, lateral; if lateral, then device field activated including following: kidney rest, overhead arm board, axillary roll. Yes/No, not applicable List of potential sites: Yes/No See nursing notes, n/a Linked to hospital inventory of devices Examples: cart, hospital bed, specialty bed.
OUTCOME/EVALUATION Pt is free from signs and symptoms related to positioning (O5)	PNDS and interim outcome statements	Multi-lined checkbox response	

This process can be accomplished quickly if the PNDS is seeded into the software database being used. Then as the nurse documents on the record the electrosurgery cautery unit identification, the outcome "Freedom from electrical injury" automatically populates the outcomes evaluation page.

Conserving Nurse Time

Another feature that may help the busy perioperative nurse is trigger reminders that serve to remind users to complete the documentation fields that are invalid or empty. During the very busy final minutes of an operative case, remembering to complete the documentation for final counts, procedure end times, and immediate post-procedure information can be a challenge. It is easy to miss a data field when completing the documentation. Most programs will have built-in features that allow for field checking for this reason.

Will it be possible to build a nursing electronic record that meets the documentation needs of the 10-minute myringotomy case and the 8-hour trauma case? There may be data fields that the perioperative nurse will not need to document for every type of case, such as implants or laser settings, but these fields nevertheless will need to be present in the record. Will the new documentation accept "inbound" information such as data from bedside physiologic monitors? Especially in the PACU area, this feed of information can be an invaluable time-saver as well as allow staff to focus on patient care rather than entering vital sign data every 5 to 15 minutes.

Testing and Evaluation

Lay out the screen designs for your new documenttation incorporating all the required elements that have been identified. After the new documentation has been placed into the application software, begin testing the screens for flow and performance. Check the documentation to determine whether the individual documentation fields are performing as anticipated? What happens when the character limit on a field element is met? Does the field allow more data to be entered than can be stored in the database? What happens when documentation fields are left blank? If the documentation will need to be printed, test all same scenarios by printing. On the printed document, validate whether data fields overwrite each other. Does data stay within the page margins? Thorough testing cannot be overstressed.

Policies/Procedures

During the record build phase is an ideal time to discuss how current policies and procedures surrounding documentation may change. Again using the design team, revise the policies that will change and have those ready to present to staff when the education begins on the new documentation. Introducing how procedures and policies will change during the new documentation education will assist staff in making the transition to the new documentation. Determine what will be your downtime procedure. Computerized systems need maintenance and do occasionally fail. Develop your downtime plan and communicate this procedure/policy to staff during their hands-on training. Use the hands-on staff training to further test and evaluate the stability of the new documentation.

Training Staff

When beginning staff training on the new documentation, consider using design team members to assist with the classes. Because of their experience during the development of the documentation, the design team members will have in-depth knowledge of why the screens or fields were designed in a particular manner. They will be able to relay this information to their peers during the training sessions. Training on the new documentation should allow ample time for class participants to complete a full patient record and still have time for questions and answers. Small class sizes and a computer workstation for each individual being trained will facilitate productive training sessions and promote the staff's comfort level with the new documentation. Consider evaluations of the class and self-assessments for staff to monitor their understanding and identify future training needs.

To prepare staff members who have never used a computer for documentation, seek basic computer classes for these individuals before their attendance for documentation training. Collaborate with the educator to begin using the PNDS during inservice programs. This will help the staff understand that the PNDS is not something new but only another way to say what they already do. Adding 24/7 online educational offerings on PNDS may also be useful to staff.

Provide written documentation instructions and manuals for class attendees to take with them after training class. Give handouts that can be used as "cheat sheets" for things like shortcuts or when the computer goes down.

If possible, allow staff members to continue to practice documentation in the test environment after their training session. Encourage them to use their documentation from a case they completed using the old manual method and enter this data into the new system. This will help them become more familiar with the placement of data elements on the screens. If the written documentation closely mirrors the screens, it is not as difficult for staff to remember. Continued practice in the new electronic documentation after their training session will help prevent staff from forgetting the information they learned in class. Staff may also identify issues that can be resolved before the go-live.

Preparing to Go Live

Some suggestions to improve the chances for success during the first few days of the go-live include
- increasing staffing levels temporarily,
- identifying superusers who are available to assist other staff,
- having dedicated IT resources available, and
- enlisting the assistance of vendor support representatives.

Nursing staff will naturally be apprehensive about using the new computerized documentation at first. Enlist the staff members who were part of the design team as floaters to assist them when questions arise. Consider allowing one nurse to handle documentation while another nurse performs the normal tasks. Be sure to include communication with physicians; keep them informed about what is happening and when to expect a disruption of their usual routines.

If your go-live plan includes multiple facilities, consider the possibility of moving toward productive use in phases, either one facility at a time or one perioperative phase at a time. Trainers, educators, and superusers from the other sites that will go live at a later time or who have already moved to the new documentation can assist their peers.

Develop a strategy for go-live that will demonstrate to staff the commitment that this project will be successful. Perception is key. Staff will need to feel well prepared and sufficiently supported during the go-live event. This will greatly enhance their perception of the project and will lessen the impact to productivity. Reminder note cards can be attached to computer screens during the go-live to help staff with key functions of the new system. The focus needs to be on supporting the staff and easing their apprehensions.

Reporting/Data Collection

After the new documentation is in productive use, data collection and reporting from the new documentation can begin. Many documentation software applications will be packaged with predesigned reports or with a report development tool embedded or both. The types of information that can be collected are limited only by the data that is documented. The nursing saying "If it's not documented, then it wasn't done" becomes even more evident when electronic documentation is implemented. If a needed data element is not completed or left blank, data cannot be collected accurately for reporting purposes. Because of this, you may want to consider selecting fields in your documentation that will be mandatory for completion if the application software allows.

Be careful using mandatory fields, however. Mandatory fields will force the nurse to enter a value in the data field, even if that value is a "none" or an "n/a" response. All mandatory fields must have an entry before the chart can be closed, and an inappropriate mandatory field may compel the nurse to enter inaccurate data to close that patient record.

EVALUATION

For those involved in the planning and development as well as the go-live, it is beneficial to have a post-live evaluation. Look back to see if the goals identified early in the assessment phase were achieved. Begin to identify improvements that can be made later with enhancements or software upgrades. Being able to look back over the entire implementation process at the obstacles that were overcome and the camaraderie that has developed between facilities and departments will be rewarding.

Keep in mind that software is like the weather: it's ever changing. Improvements, enhancements, and new features will continue to be released. Implementing an electronic nursing documentation record can be challenging, but the rewards and the benefits of moving to an electronic format will prove to be tremendous. Over time, staff members will become so accustomed to it that they will complain bitterly because of system downtime. When you hear them grumbling about having to complete their nursing records the "old-fashioned" way—by handwritten methods—you'll know the project was a resounding success!

EXEMPLAR 2:
Applying PNDS to Perioperative Documents

Every day our patients put their trust in us as professionals to provide their care. Broad societal changes have brought new expectations for contemporary changes. Technological advances bring to light new knowledge and related requirements overtaking earlier ones. We use a variety of tools to demonstrate ongoing processes that validate the incorporation of knowledge into everyday practice.

Policies and procedures, job descriptions, and competency forms are examples of referent materials that individual institutions develop to guide the work of practitioners in the facility. Policies and procedures reflect standards of practice that incorporate community standards, supporting the facility philosophy and evidence-based practices that show relevance. Job descriptions identify the general expectations of a specific job and offer a summary of role responsibilities, reporting structure, and required qualifications and describe working conditions. Competency forms reflect expectations or outcomes of performance and the essential measurable criteria that reflect how the expectations/outcomes have been met. Samples of these types of documents can be found in **Appendix B** in this publication.

The PNDS offers a nationally recognized, standardized nursing vocabulary to use in the various department referent documents. As with any basic vocabulary, broad use of the same terms assists in developing familiarity and ongoing recognition of its key points. Human factor specialists report that consistency of language will improve patient safety and minimize risk of human error. If the policy and procedures, competencies, and job descriptions are all written in the PNDS language, nurses will see the link among department requirements, job specifications, and daily practice and understand how their actions contribute to patient outcomes.

Because PNDS elements are a database of our practice components, they set the stage for this computerized language. Documents can be uploaded

Paula Morton, RN, MS
Director of Perioperative Services
SwedishAmerican Health System
Rockford, Illinois

and immediately available to staff nurses. For example, if a nurse has a question about whether a surgery requires sponges or certain instruments and whether sharps must be counted, the cursor can be placed over the count procedure field and the departmental policy and procedure on counts called up on the screen. A novice nurse can study the competency requirements for a case assigned for the next day. A newly hired but experienced nurse who used PNDS in another hospital could look at a plan of care and know the expectations for that care, thus reducing the length and cost of orientation.

Using the PNDS in all of these documents offers consistency in practice and consistency in communication that allows for transfer of knowledge and assimilation into practice. This same consistency demonstrates reduction in risk of injury and achievement of expected patient outcomes.

APPLYING PNDS TO CLINICAL PRACTICE

The PNDS vocabulary serves all phases of perioperative practice, from preoperative preparation through discharge to the home instructional phase. Nurses who work in the preoperative holding area, in the operating room, and in the postanesthesia care unit all position the patient. The position (eg, semi-Fowler or lithotomy) and the activities selected to accomplish positioning may differ, but the intervention "Position the patient" (I96) is the same. The same is true for checking the surgical consent. No matter in what phase of the surgical experience they work, all perioperative nurses "Verify consent for planned procedure" (I124). When the nurse in preoperative holding says to the interoperative document nurse, "I checked the consent," both know what actions were taken if the PNDS language is incorporated into their department referents.

Practitioners in the clinical practice areas developed the PNDS. It is not new terminology. Rather, it is what nurses caring for surgical patients said they do every day. The PNDS truly reflects what perioperative nurses do, actualization of what they do, and the thought processes that yield results. It includes terms familiar to every perioperative nurse, patient outcomes, nursing diagnosis, and interventions taken to achieve those outcomes. Some describe the PNDS as a "great big care plan " from which nurses can build a plan specific to a particular patient having a particular surgical procedure. Once nurses begin to use the language, it is easy to understand why referent department materials should incorporate the PNDS into documents that direct nurse employees in their daily work. This paper illustrates how one hospital used the PNDS vocabulary to transform its staff nurse/novice nurse competency tool into that standardized language.

DEVELOPING COMPETENCIES WITH PNDS

Professional literature abounds with approaches and methods of competency assessment. All focus on the objective measurement of an individuals' ability to perform desired goals.[1] McConell[2] defines *competence* and *competency* by stating that *competence* refers to an individual's capacity to perform job responsibilities, while *competency* focuses on an individual's actual performance in a particular situation. The former evaluates knowledge and skill. The later verifies one's ability to integrate knowledge and skill, to perform and apply knowledge, and to apply standards. AORN defines competencies as "the knowledge and skills and abilities necessary to fulfill the professional role functions of a registered nurse in the operating room."[3]

Kuehn and Jackson[4] speak to movement from the traditional model of validating competencies with educational components to one that uses quality patient outcomes. Their premise is that standards and competencies are based on patient needs and the quality assessment data is based on institutional implementation of adopted standards. They state, "If the data shows patient outcomes and process indicators are being met, it is reasonable to assume the staff is competent. If not met or adverse outcomes realized, other data must be analyzed."[4] Both the "Competency outcomes and performance assessment

(COPA) model"[5] and the "Synergy model"[6] developed by the American Association of Critical-Care Nurses (AACN) focus on the outcomes or results of activities completed.

Shifting from learning objectives to outcome-focused competencies with patient outcomes as significant indicators is shown in the AACN "Synergy model" and the Kuehn and Jackson work. The PNDS clearly identifies the outcomes we expect our perioperative patients to attain. Transposition of our expectations for patient care outcomes to expected nurse competencies can easily be accomplished. In other words, freedom from signs and symptoms of position injury (O5) can easily be translated to a competency statement that indicates that the nurse will be competent in protecting the patient from injury due to surgical positioning.

Performance measures are discrete, observable behaviors that identify actions the nurse is expected to do. The PNDS has nursing interventions with a list of activities that usually are steps to accomplish the intervention. For example, "performs skin preparation" (I94) requires several activities. The nurse must select the appropriate microbial solution, prevent pooling of the solution, and so forth. These activities are a series of actions that include both cognitive and psychomotor nursing actions or series of actions. The intervention statements readily translate to measurable criteria necessary to achieve the competency statement that was derived from one of the PNDS outcomes.

Early work on the PNDS aligned perioperative interventions with the outcome statements. The Interventions Subcommittee identified the outcome statement each intervention was "most closely linked to" and redefined the definitions as necessary. The reference offers examples for each outcome statement. For example:

O5   The patient is free from signs and symptoms of injury related to positioning.
I64   Identifies physical alterations that may affect procedure specific positioning.
I96   Positions the patient
I38   Evaluates for signs and symptoms of injury as a result of positioning.

O8   The patient is free from signs and symptoms of injury related to transfer/transport.

I118   Transports according to individual need.

I42   Evaluates for signs and symptoms of skin and tissue injury as a result of transfer /transport.[1]

Each intervention then has a sequential listing of activities that indicate what the nurse does for that intervention. For example, under "I118—Transports according to individual need," activities listed are:

- Correctly identifies the patient.
- Performs or directs patient transfer from the admitting area or nursing unit to the operative or invasive suite holding area.
- Admits patient to the operative or invasive procedure suite.
- Performs or directs patient transfer from the holding area to the OR procedure room.
- Assists with transfer of patient from the OR procedure room to the postanesthesia care unit (PACU).
- Performs or directs patient transfer from the OR procedure room to the nursing unit after local anesthesia.
- Performs or directs transfer of the patient with special needs.[1]

SURVEY PROCESS

Our initial goal was to transform our current competency tool into one using the standardized PNDS language. While our behavioral criteria replicated the interventions from PNDS, the outcomes were listed as broad global statements. We wanted to indicate which PNDS outcomes were most important in achieving our departmental standard of care. This would be followed with a check of relevance of these interventions to outcomes. Upon review of the results, the final document was placed on the competency tool template, which requires verification statements for how the measures were evaluated.

In an effort to validate this approach and framework, two different surveys were completed. Two categories of data were assessed using these tools: *nursing process competencies* and *safety/infection control competencies*. The first tool was to assess outcome statements; the second tool was to check the relevance of activities to those outcome statements.

The draft tools were distributed to a convenience sample of 31 perioperative practitioners in two different facilities. Respondents included individuals from the preoperative assessment area, intraoperative practitioners, and postanesthesia care providers. Our plan was to evaluate the commonalities and variances in responses from providers in two locations:

Site	Type facility	Location	Respondents			
			Preop	*Intraop*	*Postop*	*Total*
A	Community	Midwest	2	8	6	16
B	Academic	Northwest	4	4	7	15

The first tool, "Nursing process competencies to outcomes," asked participants to rate their degree of agreement with the importance of the outcome listed to nursing process activities completed daily. (See **Exhibit 5-A** at the end of this exemplar.) Completion of the activities is considered the measurable action that demonstrates achievement of competency. A 1–5 point Likert scale was used, with 1 as very low in importance and 5 as very significant in importance. This format was replicated for the category *safety/infection control.*

The second tool, "Nursing process: Competency/outcome behavior criteria/interventions," asked the participants to rate the degree to which the interventions were relevant to the practice outcomes of competent care. The same 1–5 Likert scale was used. (See **Exhibit 5-B.**) Once again, this format was replicated for the category *safety/infection control.*

RETURN RATE AND OVERALL RESULTS

Nursing Process Competencies to Outcomes

Site A: The return rate was 95%, or 15 tools. Review of the statements revealed that the participants agreed or strongly agreed the outcome was important to their competency of practice in all but one category. That single outlier was an undecided response for O11, "The patient has wound/tissue perfusion consistent with or improved from baseline."

Site B: The return rate was 93%, or 15 tools. Review of data from the second site identified that 13%–26% of respondents (3 individuals) identified for each outcome in "not important" rank to daily use of nursing process. Review of areas of practice shows that all but one individual were practicing in the preadmission assessment or postanesthesia care areas.

Nursing Process: Competency/Outcome Behavior Criteria/Interventions

With review of the statements, participants identified interventions relevant to their competency evaluation. Assessment and implementation components follow.

O23 The patient participates in decision affecting the perioperative plan of care.

Six interventions were listed. Percent identified as relevant/very relevant:

Site A: I135 – 93%, I136 – 88%, I36 – 100%, I113 – 100%, I114 – 100%, I90 – 100%.

Site B: I135 – 70%, I136 – 40%, I36 – 60%, I113 – 60%, I114 – 60%, I90 – 70%.

O24 The plan of care is consistent with the individualized perioperative plan of care.

Four interventions were listed. Percent relevance:

Site A: I30 – 100%, I66 – 100%, I1 – 100%, I24 – 88%.

Site B: I30 – 60%, I66 – 73%, I1 – 86%, I24 – 90%.

O11 The patient has wound/tissue perfusion consistent with or improved from baseline.

Two interventions were listed. Percent relevance:

Site A: I15 – 100%, I60 – 93%.

Site B: I15 – 70%, I60 – 80%.

O29 The patient demonstrates and/or reports adequate pain control.

Three interventions were listed. Percent relevance:

Site A: I16 – 100%, I71 – 100%, I169 – 88%.

Site B: I16 – 80%, I71 – 70%, I169 – 70%.

O10 The patient is free from signs and symptoms of infection.

One intervention was listed. Percent relevance:

Site A: I21 – 100%.

Site B: I21 – 70%.

O14 The patient's cardiac status is consistent with and/or improved from baseline.

Three interventions were listed. Percent relevance:

Site A: I66 – 100%, I59 – 100%, I120 – 100%.

Site B: I66 – 90%, I59 - 93%, I120 – 93%.

O15 The patient's respiratory status is consistent with and/or improved from baseline.

Five interventions were listed. Percent relevance:

Site A: I66 – 100%, I60 – 100%, I87 – 100%, I120 – 93%, I110 – 100%.

Site B: I66 – 80%, I60 – 80%, I87 – 86%, I120 – 86%, I110 – 90%.

O30 The patient's neurological status is consistent with and/or improved from baseline.

One intervention was listed. Percent relevance:

Site A: I144 – 100%.

Site B: I144 – 86%.

O12 The patient is at or returning to normo-thermia at the conclusion of the immediate postoperative period.

Two interventions were listed. Percent relevance:

Site A: I131 – 100%, I78 – 93%.

Site B: I131 – 93%, I78 – 80%.

O13 The patient's fluid/electrolyte and acid base balance is consistent with and/or improved from baseline.

Six interventions were listed. Percent relevance:

Site A: I132 – 100%, I8 – 93%, I23 – 93%, I2 – 93%, I89 – 93%, I111 – 93%.

Site B: I132 – 90%, I8 – 80%, I23 – 70%, I2 – 70%, I89 – 80%, I111 – 90%.

O2–O8 The patient is free from signs and symptoms of physical injury.

Five interventions were listed. Percent relevance:

Site A: I118 – 100%, I123 – 100%, I96 – 100%, I138 – 93%, I122 – 100%.

Site B: I118 – 66%, I123 – 100%, I96 – 66%, I138 – 66%, I122 – 93%.

O25 The patient's right to privacy is maintained

Two interventions were listed. Percent relevance:

Site A: I81 – 100%, I116 – 100%.

Site B: I81 – 63%, I116 – 93%.

O14 The patient's cardiovascular function is consistent with and/or improved from baseline.

One intervention was listed. Percent relevance:

Site A: I144 – 93%.

Site B: I144 – 70%.

O15 The patient's pulmonary function is consistent with and/or improved from baseline.

One intervention was listed. Percent relevance:

Site A: I45 – 93%.

Site B: I45 – 80%.

O30   The patient's neurological function is consistent with and/or improved from baseline.

One intervention was listed. Percent relevance:
Site A: I146 – 93%.
Site B: I146 – 80%.

O12   The patient is at or returning to normothermia at the conclusion of the immediate postoperative period.

One intervention was listed. Percent relevance:
Site A: I55 – 93%.
Site B: I55 – 80%.

O29   The patient demonstrates and/or reports adequate pain control.

One intervention was listed. Percent relevance:
Site A: I54 – 93%.
Site B: I54 – 80%.

O13   The patient's fluid/electrolyte and acid base balance is consistent with and/or improved from preoperative baseline levels.

One intervention was listed. Percent relevance:
Site A: I153 – 93%.
Site B: I153 – 80%.

O24   The patient's care is consistent with the individualized perioperative plan of care.

One intervention was listed. Percent relevance:
Site A: I27 – 100%.
Site B: I27 – 70%.

Safety/Infection Control Competencies to Outcomes

Site A: The return rate was 82%, or 14 tools. Three were discarded for incomplete data. The participants agreed or strongly agreed that the outcomes are important to their competency in practice.

Site B: The return rate was 80%, or 12 responses. Six were discarded for incomplete data. The participants agreed or strongly agreed the outcomes were important to their competency in practice.

Safety/Infection Control: Competency/ Outcome Behavior Criteria/Intervention

In review of the statements, participants identified interventions relevant to their competency evaluation.

O10   The patient is free from signs and symptoms of infection.

Site A: I21 – 92%, I70 – 84%, I22 – 61%, I94 – 76%, I97 – 61%, I98 – 76%, I85 – 69%, I81 – 76%, I3 – 92%, I7 – 100%, I2 – 100%, I83 – 84%, I84 – 61%.

Site B: I21 – 66%, I70 – 83%, I22 – 66%, I94 – 83%, I97 – 83%, I98 – 83%, I85 – 66%, I81 – 66%, I3 – 66%, I7 – 50%, I2 – 50%, I83 – 83%, I84 – 83%.

O20   The patient is free from signs and symptoms of injury due to extraneous objects.

Site A: I118 – 92%,. I143 – 76%, I11 – 84%, I72 – 76%, I73 – 61%, I74 – 69%, I75 – 69%, I76 – 69%, I77 – 76%, I78 – 76%, I138 – 69%, I122 – 84%, I93 – 61%, I9 – 61%.

Site B: I118 – 83%, I143 – 83%, I11 – 83%, I72 – 83%, I73 – 100%, I74 – 83%, I75 – 83%, I76 – 83%, I77 – 83%, I78 – 66%, I138 – 83%, I122 – 83%, I93 – 83%, I9 – 83%.

ANALYSIS OF SURVEY RESULTS

Both facilities are working with automated records. Site A has two different systems, one in the operating room and one for preop/postop; they are not PNDS-based. Site B has an integrated program among all three areas and is PNDS-based. Both basic records contain outcome statements, but activities completed may not be phrased as intervention statements. Both have perioperative plans of care that reflect PNDS language, with outcomes, nursing diagnoses, and interventions. Representatives from both facilities state that the preassessment and postanesthesia staff are not as familiar with the PNDS language as the operating room staff.

Nursing Process Competency Tools

Review of the data collected by the tool "Nursing process competencies to outcomes" revealed two individuals from Site B who questioned the importance of the outcomes to daily practice by answering "neutral" or "uncertain." Drilling down into the data revealed that these were preassessment or postanesthesia care staff. The importance of outcome O10, "The patient is free from signs and symptoms of infection," was questioned by four individuals, all of whom were either preassessment or postanesthesia staff.

Review of the data collected by the tool "Nursing process: Competency/outcome behavior criteria/ interventions" shows higher relevance ratings for Site A. Three respondents from Site B challenged the relevance of the interventions to the outcomes; from one to six individuals responded "neutral" or "uncertain" for each statement. Drilling down into the data revealed that eight of the respondents were either preassessment or postanesthesia care staff, and one respondent was an intraoperative practitioner.

Safety/Infection Control Tools
Review of the data collected by the tool "Safety/ infection control competencies to outcomes" revealed individuals from both facilities who provided incomplete surveys, which resulted in their responses being discarded. Again, since most of the interventions are geared to the intraoperative phase of care, this may reflect the practice areas represented. For example, one participant assigned low importance to the outcome O10, "The patient is free from signs and symptoms of infection."

Review of the data collected by the tool "Safety/ infection control: Competency/outcome behavior criteria/interventions" revealed that the percentage relevance scores are lower for all outcomes in both facilities. In general, participants challenging the relevance of these outcomes work in the preassessment and postanesthesia care areas.

CONCLUSION

This small survey offers a starting point for a much broader review of the documentation process. The tools used in the clinical setting usually reflect competency expectations and the activities required to demonstrate that achievement. The positive results of agreement and relevance suggest this may well be possible with outcome statements and interventions.

The data readily demonstrate differences for practitioners in different areas of perioperative practice. All may not have the same training or exposure to PNDS. Documentation may vary significantly in each area and may or may not reflect PNDS language. Perhaps the activities required to implement an intervention need to be specific to the perioperative phase (eg, preoperative assessment or postoperative recovery). We need to consider

competencies reflective of the practice in those areas for specific categories of care and build tools to include those competencies.

Each practice setting varies in actual processes completed. There will be different degrees of emphasis on specific activities. One example is that nationally all facilities are focusing on correct site surgery. Consequently, it is logical that this would be a competency that is routinely evaluated. Other aspects of care, such as "manages specimen collection," may not be as critical and may not require routine competency evaluation.

To develop your own tool, select components deemed most important in your environment and the behavior criteria/ interventions that reflect those critical examples relevant to the outcome. Consensus on the behavior criteria/interventions may depend on issues most relevant to your facility. **Exhibit 5-C** demonstrates how we transposed our tools onto a competency template for use in the clinical setting.

This small starting point can begin our look at the broader applications in clinical practice. The language conforms to the intent of the competency process. The PNDS can be extrapolated to other relevant documents used for our practice. Consistency in language can link how the nurse's actions contribute to patient outcomes. Broader-scale studies will help expand this validation process and reinforce the relevance of application. We look forward to working with our colleagues to continue this journey of progressive change and advancement of our language.

References
1. S Beyea, ed, *Perioperative Nursing Data Set: The Perioperative Nursing Vocabulary*, second ed (Denver: AORN, 2002).
2. E McConnell, "Competence vs competency," *Nursing Management* 32 no 5 (2001)14.
3. "Competency statements in perioperative nursing," in *Standards, Recommended Practices, and Guidelines* (Denver: AORN, 2007), 21-95.
4. L Kuehn, K Jackson, "Using nursing standards to evaluate competency," *Nursing Management* 28 no 8 (1997) 32K, 32N, 32P.
5. C Lendberg, "The framework, concepts and methods of the Competency Outcomes and Performance Assessment (COPA) Model," *Online Journal of Issues in Nursing* 4 no 3 (Sept 30, 1999); *http://www.nursingworld.org/MainMenuCategories /ANAMarketplace/ANAPeriodicals/OJIN/TableofContents/Volume 41999/No3Sep30/COPAModel.aspx* (accessed 3 Sept 2007).
6. M Curley, "Patient-nurse synergy: Optimizing patients' outcomes," *American Journal of Critical Care* 7 no 1 (1998):64-72.

EXHIBIT 5-A: Nursing Process Competencies to Outcomes		
Competency/Outcome		**1=low, 5 = high**
Demonstrates use of the nursing process in the delivery of patient care.		
O23 The patient participates in decision affecting the perioperative plan of care.		1 2 3 4 5
O28 The patient's value system, lifestyle, ethnicity, and culture are considered respected and incorporated in the perioperative plan of care.		1 2 3 4 5
O24 The plan of care is consistent with the individualized perioperative plan of care.		1 2 3 4 5
O11 The patient has wound/tissue perfusion consistent with or improved from baseline.		1 2 3 4 5
O29 The patient demonstrates and/or reports adequate pain control.		1 2 3 4 5
O10 The patient is free from signs and symptoms of infection.		1 2 3 4 5
O14 The patient's cardiac status is consistent with and/or improved from baseline.		1 2 3 4 5
O15 The patient's respiratory status is consistent with and/or improved from baseline.		1 2 3 4 5
O30 The patient's neurological status is consistent with or improved from baseline.		1 2 3 4 5
O12 The patient is at or returning to normothermia at the conclusion of the immediate postoperative period.		1 2 3 4 5
O13 The patient's fluid/electrolyte and acid base balance is consistent with and/or improved from baseline.		1 2 3 4 5
O2–O8 The patient is free from signs and symptoms of physical injury.		1 2 3 4 5
O25 The patient's right to privacy is maintained.		1 2 3 4 5
O26 The patient is the recipient of competent and ethical care within the standard of practice.		1 2 3 4 5

EXHIBIT 5-B: Nursing Process— Competency/Outcome Behavior Criteria/Interventions		
Competency/Outcome	**Behavior Criteria/Interventions**	**1 = low, 5 = high**
Demonstrates use of the nursing process in delivery of patient care.		
O23 The patient participates in decision affecting the perioperative plan of care	I135 Determines patient's knowledge level. I136 Assesses readiness to learn. I36 Identifies barriers to communication. I113 Screens for physical abuse. I114 Screens for substance abuse. I90 Notes sensor impairments.	1 2 3 4 5 1 2 3 4 5 1 2 3 4 5 1 2 3 4 5 1 2 3 4 5 1 2 3 4 5
O24 The plan of care is consistent with the individualized perioperative plan of care.	I30 Develops individualized plan of care. I66 Identifies physiologic status. I1 Acts as a patient advocate by protecting the patient from incompetent, unethical or illegal practice. I24 Verifies consent for planned procedure.	1 2 3 4 5 1 2 3 4 5 1 2 3 4 5 1 2 3 4 5
O11 The patient has wound/tissue perfusion consistent with or improved from baseline.	I15 Assesses factors related to risks for ineffective tissue perfusion. I60 Identifies baseline tissue perfusion.	1 2 3 4 5 1 2 3 4 5
O29 The patient demonstrates and/or reports adequate pain control.	I16 Assesses pain control. I71 Implements pain guidelines. I169 Implements alternative methods of pain control.	1 2 3 4 5 1 2 3 4 5 1 2 3 4 5
O10 The patient is free from signs and symptoms of infection.	I21 Assesses susceptibility for infection.	1 2 3 4 5
O14 The patient's cardiac status is consistent with and/or improved from baseline.	I66 Identifies physiologic status. I59 Identifies baseline cardiac function. I120 Uses monitoring equipment to assess cardiac status.	1 2 3 4 5 1 2 3 4 5 1 2 3 4 5
O15 The patient's respiratory status is consistent with and/or improved from baseline.	I66 Identifies physiologic status. I60 Identifies baseline tissue perfusion. I87 Monitors changes in respiratory status. I120 Uses monitoring equipment to assess respiratory status. I110 Recognizes and reports deviation in blood gas studies.	1 2 3 4 5 1 2 3 4 5 1 2 3 4 5 1 2 3 4 5 1 2 3 4 5
O30 The patient's neurological status is consistent with or improved from baseline.	I144 Assesses baseline neurological status.	1 2 3 4 5
O12 The patient is at or returning to normothermia at the conclusion of the immediate postoperative period.	I131 Assesses risk for inadvertent hypothermia. I78 Implements thermoregulation measures.	1 2 3 4 5 1 2 3 4 5
O13 The patient's fluid/electrolyte and acid base balance is consistent with and/or improved from baseline.	I132 Identifies factors associated with increased risk for hemorrhage or fluid and electrolyte loss. I8 Administers prescribed medications and solutions.	1 2 3 4 5 1 2 3 4 5

EXHIBIT 5-B: Nursing Process
Competency/Outcome Behavior Criteria/Interventions *(continued)*

Competency/Outcome		Behavior Criteria/Intervention		1 = low, 5 = high
		I23	Collaborates in fluid management.	1 2 3 4 5
		I2	Administers blood product therapy as prescribed.	1 2 3 4 5
		I89	Monitors physical parameters.	1 2 3 4 5
		I111	Recognizes and reports deviation in diagnostic studies.	1 2 3 4 5
O2– O8	The patient is free from signs and symptoms of physical injury.	I118	Transports according to individual need.	1 2 3 4 5
		I123	Verifies allergies.	1 2 3 4 5
		I96	Applies safety devices.	1 2 3 4 5
		I138	Implements protective measures prior to operative or invasive procedure.	1 2 3 4 5
		I122	Uses supplies and equipment within safe parameters.	1 2 3 4 5
O25	The patient's right to privacy is maintained.	I81	Initiates traffic control.	1 2 3 4 5
		I97	Maintains patient's dignity, modesty, and privacy and protects confidentiality of patient information.	1 2 3 4 5
O2– O8	The patient is free from signs and symptoms of physical injury.	I38	Evaluates for signs and symptoms of physical injury after an operative or invasive procedure, transfer, or transport.	1 2 3 4 5
O14	The patient's cardiac status is consistent with and/or improved from baseline.	I44	Evaluates postoperative cardiac function.	1 2 3 4 5
O15	The patient's respiratory status is consistent with and/or improved from baseline.	I45	Evaluates postoperative pulmonary function.	1 2 3 4 5
O30	The patient's neurological status is consistent with or improved from baseline.	I146	Evaluates postoperative neurological status.	1 2 3 4 5
O12	The patient is at or returning to normothermia at the conclusion of the immediate postoperative period.	I55	Evaluates response to thermoregulation measures.	1 2 3 4 5
O29	The patient demonstrates and/or reports adequate pain control.	I54	Evaluate response to pain management interventions.	1 2 3 4 5
O13	The patient's fluid/electrolyte and acid base balance is consistent with and/or improved from baseline.	I153	Evaluates response to administration of fluids and electrolytes.	1 2 3 4 5
O24	The plan of care is consistent with the individualized perioperative plan of care.	I27	Ensures continuity of care by evaluating the patient's response to the plan of care.	1 2 3 4 5

EXHIBIT 5-C:
Sample Competency Template Using PNDS

Performance results were determined by one or more of the following:

1. Medical record documentation
2. Described or demonstrated behavior
3. Performance improvement monitoring
4. Absence of negative patient outcomes

5. Continuing competence assessment
6. Patient satisfaction results
7. Direct observation
8. Documented education with a posttest

Meets Expectations. Signature and date required.						Method
	Does Not Meet Expectations; Improvement Needed *(explain)*. Signature and date required.					
		Not Applicable. Signature and date required.				
			Demonstrates use of the nursing process in delivery of patient care			
			O23	The patient participates in decisions affecting the perioperative plan of care	I135	Determines patient's knowledge level	
					I136	Assesses readiness to learn	
					I36	Identifies barriers to communication	
					I113	Screens for physical abuse	
					I114	Screens for substance abuse	
					I90	Notes sensory impairments	
			O28	The patient's value system, lifestyle, ethnicity and culture are considered, respected, and incorporated in the perioperative plan of care	I63	Assesses the intellectual, emotional, and social components of the patient and ensures all important components will be incorporated into the nursing plan of care.	
			O24	The plan of care is consistent with the individualized perioperative plan of care	I30	Develops individualized plan of care	
					I66	Identifies physiologic status	
					I1	Acts as a patient advocate by protecting the patient from incompetent, unethical, or illegal practice	
					I24	Verifies consent for planned procedure	
			O11	The patient has wound/perfusion consistent with or improved from baseline	I15	Assesses factors related to risks for ineffective tissue perfusion	
					I60	Identifies baseline tissue perfusion	
			O29	The patient demonstrates and/or reports adequate pain control	I16	Assesses pain control	
					I71	Implements pain guidelines	
					I169	Identifies baseline tissue perfusion	
			O10	The patient is free from signs and symptoms of infection	I21	Assesses susceptibility for infection	
			O14	The patient's cardiac status is consistent with and/or improved from baseline	I66	Identifies physiologic status	
					I59	Identifies baseline cardiac function	
					I120	Uses monitoring equipment to assess cardiac status	

EXHIBIT 5-C: Sample Competency Template Using PNDS *(continued)*

							Method
Meets Expectations. Signature and date required.							
	Does Not Meet Expectations; Improvement Needed *(explain)*. **Signature and date required.**						
		Not Applicable. Signature and date required.					
			O15	The patient's respiratory status is consistent with and/or improved from baseline	I66 I60 I87 I120 I110	Identifies physiologic status Identifies baseline tissue perfusion Monitors changes in respiratory status Uses monitoring equipment to assess respiratory status Recognizes and reports deviation in blood gas studies	
			O30	The patient's neurologic status is consistent with or improved from baseline	I144	Assesses baseline neurologic status	
			O12	The patient is at or returning to normothermia at conclusion of immediate postop period	I131 I78	Assesses risk for inadvertent hypothermia Implements thermoregulation measures	
			O13	The patient's fluid/ electrolyte and acid base balance is consistent with and/or improved from baseline	I132 I8 I23 I2 I89 I111	Identifies factors associated with an increased risk of hemorrhage or fluid and electrolyte loss Administers prescribed medications and solutions Collaborates in fluid management Administers blood product therapy as prescribed Monitors physical parameters Recognizes and reports deviation in diagnostic studies	
			O28	The patient is free from S/S of physical injury	I118 I123 I96 I138 I122	Transports according to individual need Verifies allergies Applies safety devices Implements protective measures prior to operative or invasive procedure Uses supplies and equipment within safe parameters	
			O25	The patient's right to privacy is maintained	I81 I97	Initiates traffic control Maintains patient's dignity, modesty, and privacy and protects confidentiality of patient information	
			O26	The patient is recipient of competent and ethical care within the standard of practice	I102 I116	Provides care to each patient without prejudicial behavior Shares information only with those directly involved in case	
			O28	The patient is free from S/S of physical injury	I38	Evaluates for signs and symptoms of physical injury after an operative or invasive procedure, transfer, or transport	

EXHIBIT 5-C: Sample Competency Template Using PNDS *(continued)*

Meets Expectations. Signature and date required.							
	Does Not Meet Expectations; Improvement Needed *(explain)*. Signature and date required.						
		Not Applicable. Signature and date required.					Method
			O14	The patient's cardiovascular function is consistent with and/or improved from baseline	I44	Evaluates postop cardiac function	
			O15	The patient's pulmonary function is consistent with and/or improved from baseline	I45	Evaluates postop pulmonary function	
			O30	The patient's neurologic function is consistent with and/or improved from baseline	I146	Evaluates postop neurologic status	
			O12	The patient is at or returning to normothermia at the conclusion of the immediate postoperative period	I55	Evaluates response to thermoregulation measures	
			O29	The patient demonstrates and/or reports adequate pain control	I54	Evaluates response to main management interventions	
			O13	The patient's fluid/electrolyte and acid base balance is consistent with or improved from baseline levels established preoperatively	I153	Evaluates response to administration of fluids and electrolytes	
			O24	The patient's care is consistent with the individualized perioperative plan of care	I27	Ensures continuity of care by evaluating the patient's response to the plan of care	

EXEMPLAR 3: Teaching Experienced Nursing Staff the Value of the PNDS

Adult learners are most interested in learning a subject that has immediate relevance to their job or personal life. The PNDS provides both new and experienced perioperative nurses a relevant information infrastructure to link and communicate their unique contributions to positive patient outcomes and quality care. It makes evidence-based perioperative nursing practice *visible* by describing a concrete set of interventions from which to draw and serves as a *quality cross check* to identify the critical interventions and activities that have been employed.

TEACHING THE PNDS

The Target Population
The first step in teaching the PNDS is to define and analyze the target population. Who are the students? Are they new to perioperative nursing or do they have years of experience? What is their attitude toward learning? Are they motivated to learn? What knowledge does the target population have? Assessing what learners already know and determining what they need to know will help establish the course content.

The educator also needs to consider the age of the target population. The view we hold of the world, the way it is, and the way it should be is formed during the first 10 to 15 years of life. Therefore, to some extent comfortable generational interaction depends on an individual's birth date (**Table 5-2**).

For the first time in history, five generations are in the work force together. The challenge is to package the education so that every learner benefits. Select a variety of learning materials and activities that appeal to a broad age range. For instance, those born after 1961 will respond to video tapes, CDs, and DVDs best because they can control the content by fast-forwarding anything they don't want to view or listen to. However, this may lead to gaps in their knowledge, so methods to determine how much material they absorbed may be required. Those born between 1943 and 1960 respond to classroom learning that includes group work as a

Kathie G. Shea, RN, MSN, CNOR
Educator, Perioperative Services
Children's Hospital and Research Center
Oakland, California

component because it is more personal and interactive. The imperative is to develop tools/activities to explain a concept so that it appeals to more than one developmental life stage.

Characteristics of the Adult Learner
For instruction to be effective, the following characteristics of adult learners must be taken into consideration:

Adult learners are independent and self-directed. The educator needs to involve them actively in the learning process by allowing the participants to assume responsibility for presentations and group leadership. The educator's job will be to act as a facilitator, guiding participants to increase their own knowledge rather than supplying them with facts. Break the class into planned or random teams, give them all the same case study, provide them with selected handouts on the PNDS, and ask them to work together to identify nursing diagnoses, patient outcomes, or interventions. Have each group leader share the work with all the participants. This format allows for the content to be presented from multiple perspectives and promotes active knowledge construction over passive transmission of information.

Adult learners have life experiences and knowledge that may include work-related activities, family responsibilities, and previous education. Since adults construct knowledge based on experience, the educator needs to connect learning to this knowledge/experience base. Understanding what learners bring to the learning situation is the beginning of helping them build new knowledge. Generally nurses who have been practicing perioperative nursing for some time will have a rich background of knowledge and experience to share with newer nurses. A story based on previous experience can make the concept come alive. For this reason, it would be wise to compose a mix of new and experienced individuals for small group work.

Adult learners are relevancy-oriented. They must see a reason for learning something. To be of value to them, the PNDS must be made applicable to their work or other responsibilities. Develop objectives that are related to concepts the participants are familiar with. Recognize the importance of vocabulary; adults often struggle with new terms. The words *domain, interim outcomes, nursing interventions,* and even *nursing diagnoses* may represent new or fuzzy concepts to adult learners who have been out of school for several years.

Adult learners are practical. They prefer to focus on the aspects that are most useful to them in their work. It may be shocking to the educator, but they actually may not be interested in knowledge for its own sake. How the PNDS will be useful to them in their daily work must be clearly communicated. Will it help them document their care more efficiently? Report or communicate the care the patient has received? Describe what outcomes the patient has achieved? Supply the language or framework for a departmental continuous quality improvement study?

Adult learners need to be shown respect. As mentioned earlier, adults bring a wealth of experience to the classroom. By acknowledging and encouraging the sharing of their experiences, knowledge, and opinions, the educator helps learners feel valued.

DESIGNING THE INSTRUCTION

Begin by deciding what the learners should be able to do at the conclusion of instruction. This will provide a useful starting point for shaping the program. Remember that learners need to know the end result that is expected before they can begin practicing the task. Must they identify nursing interventions? Link interventions to nursing diagnoses or patient outcomes? Use the language in a policy and procedure, competency, or care plan? The possibilities are unlimited, so carefully analyze the task and design the instruction around the task. Notice the repetition of the words "the task" rather than "the PNDS." Those who have been teaching the PNDS for some time have favorite anecdotes, demonstrations, and tools. They like teaching the PNDS and could probably hold forth for hours. However, **do not**

try to teach all there is to know about the PNDS in one class! The extra knowledge is really an obstacle rather than a necessity because adults prefer single-concept classes that focus heavily on the application of the concept to relevant problems. Continuously take into account adult learning theory during instruction design.

- Recognize that adults want their learning to be problem-oriented, personalized, and relevant to self-direction and personal responsibility.
- Build in time to briefly and succinctly explain why specific things are being taught.
- Develop learning activities/formats in the context of the tasks to be performed, not facts to be memorized.
- Find ways to connect the new knowledge with previous knowledge and experience.
- Identify and define new terminology and link it to real-world definitions.
- Use case studies and game show formats or group competitions that allow for practice opportunities instead of long lectures with periods of prolonged sitting.
- Vary the learning materials and activities to stimulate as many senses as possible and allow for a variety of learning styles and previous experience. Remember, some adults learn better by visualizing the material, while others prefer auditory or kinesthetic presentation of new information.
- Design instruction that allows learners to discover things for themselves and practice skills. Practice is a powerful way to learn how to apply concepts. However, it is a deterrent if the educator is not readily available to recognize correct and incorrect performance and provide effective feedback that does not destroy the learner's motivation or self-esteem.
- Build the esteem of the learner, clarify misconceptions, and answer questions.

DELIVERING THE CONTENT

To this point, the audience has been analyzed from a variety of perspectives and the instruction has been painstakingly designed based on adult learning principles (see **Exhibit 5-D**). It is now time to consider what nearly all educators enjoy most—delivering the content. What are the essentials of good teaching?

Teaching is about having a passion for helping people learn. If the educator isn't excited, the students won't be, either.

Teaching is about substance. It is about treating the learners as consumers of knowledge and bridging the gap between theory and practice. Good teaching is also about listening and questioning and remembering that each student is different. It's about eliciting responses from the quiet students and helping them develop confidence in their oral communication. It's about pushing learners to excel and at the same time respecting them and remaining professional.

Teaching is about being flexible. A teacher should have the confidence to adjust to changing circumstances. Teaching is not about following a fixed agenda; it may require deviating from the planned content if something else makes for better learning.

Teaching is about style. Successful teaching is entertaining yet substantial. A good teacher is comfortable working the room and interacting with every learner in it. Don't be afraid to use humor; a harmless joke at the educator's own expense often can break the ice and create a more relaxed learning environment.

Teaching is about caring, nurturing, and developing the skills of the students. It includes devoting time to every student by designing a program that has strong content, well-prepared materials, and activities to enhance the instruction.

Teaching is about having fun. Successful teachers enjoy interacting with students and watching everything come together. Teaching is about the satisfaction of looking into the eyes of a student and seeing the light go on.

Educators must determine whether they are dynamic, motivating facilitators or "talking heads" who drone on and on from behind a podium with eyes fixed on a slide projector. The latter has work to do to become effective with adult learners. Adults respond to teachers who speak at their level, who answer their questions, and who allow them to interact with other students. The key to teaching experienced staff members is to let them discover that the PNDS is not something new; it's just a way to describe what perioperative nurses do for their patients every day.

TABLE 5-2: Generational Interaction		
When the learner is a Boomer (born 1943–1960)	**When the learner is a Generation Xer (born 1961–1981)**	**When the learner is a Millennial (born after 1981)**
OPTIMISTIC	SKEPTIC	REALISTIC
• Know their names and show them that you care about them. • Fairness is important; be nice. • Tell them they are important; they want to be "stars" and shine in your classroom. • Give them a chance to talk; they want to show you what they know. • Dialogue and participation are key. Don't be authoritarian; don't try to boss them around. • Be democratic; treat them as equals. • Acknowledge what they know and ask them lots of questions so they can demonstrate what they know. • Give them opportunities to work in small groups. • Treat them as though they're young, even if they aren't. • Avoid calling them "sir" or "ma'am," which they may take as an insult. • Respect their experience.	• Humor is important; provide a fun and relaxed place to learn. • Give it to them straight. Be direct and truthful; avoid "political correctness." • Talk with them, not at them. • Be on top of your game—know your stuff and demonstrate it clearly. You can't push image without substance. • Gear info to specific and practical outcomes; what you are teaching must have practical value. • Show them how education can help them get ahead, get a better job or more money, or that will improve their situation in some way. • Provide clear statements of what is expected and what they need to do to be successful. • Incorporate state-of-the-art technology and know how to use it. • Materials must be visual and dynamic; use headlines, bullets, and graphics.	• Provide supervision and structure; they expect teachers to know more than they do. • Offer frequent and immediate feedback; they want more attention from authority figures. • Provide multiple focal points; incorporate teamwork to let them move around and interact with each other. • Materials must be lively and dynamic; Millennials are visually similar to Xers, and technology is expected. • Provide backup information for them to read or use as reference. • Focus on skills and information that will help make their working lives less stressful and increase their marketability. • Model good people skills; they often need training in getting along with others.

Sources: P D Hart, *New Leadership for a New Century: Key Findings from a Study on Youth, Leadership, and Community Service* (Washington, DC: Peter D. Hart Research Associates, 1998); N Howe, W Strauss, *Millennials Rising: The Next Great Generation* (New York: Vintage Books, 2000); S A Kallen, *The Baby Boom* (San Diego: Greenhaven Press, 2002); B R Kupperschmidt, "Understanding Generation X employees," *JONA* 28 (1998) 36-43; S R Santos, K Cox, "Workplace adjustment and intergenerational differences between Matures, Boomers, and Xers," *Nursing Economics* 18 (2000) 7-13; B Tulgan, *Managing Generation X: How to Bring Out the Best in Young Talent* (New York: W W Norton and Company, 1995); K Wieck, M Prydun, T Walsh, "What the emerging workforce wants in its leaders," *The Journal of Nursing Scholarship* 34 no 3 (2002) 283-288.

EXHIBIT 5-D: Sample Education Program

Introduction to the Perioperative Nursing Data Set

Objectives
1. Define the PNDS.
2. Discuss the value of the PNDS as a standardized nursing vocabulary.
3. Identify patient outcomes, nursing diagnoses, and nursing interventions based on a hypothetical scenario.

Course Content Outline   *Time Frames*

I. What is the PNDS?   (5 minutes)
   A. Standardized nursing vocabulary
   B. Description of perioperative nursing process
   C. Dictionary
   D. Comprehensive set of descriptive terms

II. Value of the PNDS   (5 minutes)
    (Audience participation with examples)
    A. Increases patient safety because it is a uniform language for describing care and documentation; reduces misunderstanding and miscommunication
    B. Meets clinical information system requirements for standardized terms and definitions
    C. Describes/measures nursing contributions to patient care
    D. Validates patient outcomes
    E. Provides for retrieval of data and a structure to manage and analyze data
    F. Provides the knowledge base for clinical decision-making
    G. Makes nursing visible to legislators, policy makers, and finance officers

III. Structure of Perioperative   (10 minutes)
     Patient-Focused Model
     A. Domains
        1. Safety
        2. Physiological Responses
        3. Behavioral Responses: Family & Individual
        4. Health System
     B. Patient Outcomes
        1. Outcome Indicators
        2. Interim Outcomes
     C. Nursing Diagnoses
     D. Nursing Interventions
        1. Activities to accomplish those interventions

E. What the PNDS is not
   1. PNDS is a large care plan designed to cover all perioperative cases
   2. Select the outcomes/interventions needed for your patient

IV. Case Study Activity/Discussion   (35 minutes)

V. Final Review of Key Concepts   (5 minutes)

Course Materials
- PowerPoint slides
- Handouts: Case study, selected pages from PNDS

Sample Case Study

Patient Profile on Assessment—Mrs. Reed
Mrs. Reed is a pleasant 78-year-old female. She is 5'1" tall and weighs 78 pounds. Her skin appears thin with bruising on both forearms. Her temperature is 99° F. She is allergic to plastic tape, which causes skin blisters. She has generalized osteoarthritis and is an insulin-dependent diabetic. Her current medications are NPH insulin, Indocin, Celebrex, Ambien, and a multivitamin. Previous surgeries include a left mastectomy, a right total hip arthroplasty, and an appendectomy. Her lab work reveals a WBC of 18,000, Hgb 9, and blood glucose of 105. She is widowed and lives alone independently. She has a son who lives in the next state. Her admitting diagnosis is possible bowel obstruction. The planned operative procedure is bowel resection with possible diverting colostomy.

Group #1. Identify potential concerns/nursing diagnoses for this patient. Develop a mock hand-off communication report for the PACU nurse caring for the patient postoperatively.

Group #2. What overall outcome is applicable for this patient with regard to positioning? Are there any applicable interim outcomes? Are there any additional outcomes to be concerned about for this patient? If so, list them.

Group #3. Describe the key nursing interventions/activities when positioning this patient. Are there any additional interventions/activities recommended for certain implementation? What outcome would those interventions target?

Sample answers are provided on the following page.

EXHIBIT 5-D: Sample Education Program *(continued)*

Possible Responses to Case Study

Group #1

Potential Nursing Diagnoses	Rationale
Infection, risk for (Safety Domain)	Possible contamination from bowel intraoperatively. Diabetes. ↑ WBC, ↓ Hgb.
Mobility, impaired physical (Safety Domain)	Osteoarthritis. Previous total joint replacement.
Perioperative positioning injury, risk for (Safety Domain)	Weight. Diabetes, osteoarthritis. Previous total joint replacement.
Peripheral neurovascular dysfunction, risk for (Safety Domain)	Weight. Diabetes.
Skin integrity, risk for impaired; or skin integrity, impaired (Safety Domain)	Diabetes. Previous bruising. Current medications.
Nutrition; less than body requirements, imbalanced (Physiological Responses Domain)	Weight. Widowed, lives alone. Possible ↓ mobility/activity → ↓ appetite.
Tissue perfusion, ineffective (Physiological Responses Domain)	Diabetes. Advanced age; potential for CV disease, microadenopathy.
Anxiety (Behavioral Responses: Family & Individual Domain)	Impending surgery (fear of unknown, postoperative pain). No family close by.
Body image disturbance (Behavioral Responses: Family & Individual Domain)	Possible colostomy.
Home maintenance impaired (Behavioral Responses: Family & Individual Domain)	Loss of mobility due to osteoarthritis. Change in functional ability. No family support.

Information to include in the hand-off report:

Name, age, operative procedure, drains, allergies, diabetes, Accu-Chek result, osteoarthritis, previous operative procedures and any deficits caused by them (eg, decreased range of motion due to total hip arthroplasty, lymphedema related to mastectomy), preoperative forearm bruising, current skin condition including tissue perfusion (capillary refill), movement of extremities, areas of hyperemia, blood products available, preoperative psychological state that is significant. Note: listen to the anesthesia care provider's report and be prepared to add information such as vital signs, estimated blood loss, and total amount and type of fluids given.

Group #2

1. Overall outcome: *The patient is free from signs and symptoms of injury related to positioning.* (O5)
2. Interim outcomes (based on O5):
   - The patient's pressure points demonstrate hyperemia for less than 30 minutes.
   - The patient has full return of movement of extremities at time of discharge from the OR.
   - The patient is unable to move lower extremities secondary to spinal anesthesia at time of transfer to PACU.
   - The patient's peripheral tissue perfusion is consistent with preoperative status at discharge from the OR.
   - The patient is free from pain or numbness associated with surgical positioning.
3. Other outcomes:
   - Free from infection (O10)
   - Understanding of expected responses to operative procedure (O31)
   - At or returning to normothermia (O12)

Group #3

1. Key nursing interventions:
   - Identifies physical alterations that require additional precautions for procedure-specific positioning. (I64)
   - Verifies presence of prosthetics or corrective devices. (I127).
   - Positions the patient. (I96).
     Have learner name several activity statements related to this intervention (eg, selects positioning devices based on patient's identified needs; reviews chart for information on patient's weight, preexisting medical conditions, previous surgeries, and laboratory results; assesses function limitations while patient is awake; maintains body alignment).
   - Evaluates for signs and symptoms of injury as a result of positioning. (I38)
2. Other nursing interventions:
   - Implements thermoregulation measures. (I78, O12)
   - Verifies consent for planned procedure. (I124, O23)
     Many other examples are possible.

As the three groups discuss the case study, help them recognize that the PNDS reflects their clinical reality. Close the discussion by repeating the key points.

─────────────────────────────── ❧❧ ───────────────────────────────

EXEMPLAR 4: The Value of the
PNDS to Student Nurse Learning

At the onset of nursing education and employment, students are eager to learn the language of health care. Use of new language is like joining a club where the insiders are a select group of people who are "in the know." We teach students to record health histories and physical exams using coded shorthand and abbreviations that communicate most effectively with other health care providers. Patients and their families usually do not understand or speak this language shared only among health care professionals. As students become able to perform skills and read the coded word, they gain confidence in their abilities as nursing professionals.

Use of a specific vocabulary associated with perioperative nursing will further imbue the student with an insider's understanding of perioperative nursing. The Perioperative Nursing Data Set is the method of gathering, organizing, and documenting information about the care given during a surgical or other invasive procedure. It is important to include the PNDS along with other new forms of organizing data so learners understand that it is one of many forms helping students and graduate nurses manage information in clinical settings. The way students are taught encourages them to be flexible and adaptable to new learning.

Students differ from licensed nurses in that they usually do not stay for long periods in one clinical setting. Instead, they rotate through a variety of hospitals and clinical sites, all with their particular forms of documentation. Including the PNDS in teaching plans early in a student's perioperative experience will help students view these clinical applications as similar to others as they learn additional forms of organizational language and documentation, such as functional health patterns, nursing diagnoses, nursing interventions, nursing outcomes, and the development of nursing care plans.[1] Students also have the advantage of an early inculcation of health care languages that does not require the more difficult learning of retraining.

Linda M. Sigsby, RN, MS, CNOR
Assistant Professor of Nursing
College of Nursing, University of Florida
Gainsville, Florida

TEACHING THE PNDS

Being aware of student learning styles will facilitate teaching the PNDS. Students with an auditory learning style may prefer to hear lectures and participate in group discussions. Students who have a preference for a visual/verbal learning style may choose to read about the model. Those who use visual/nonverbal learning styles may prefer to view the Perioperative Patient-Focused Model (Chapter 2, exhibit 2-A) or use concept mapping.[2] Tactile/kinesthetic learners appreciate in-class demonstrations and hands-on learning experiences. A wise teacher includes content from all four learning styles in a class to meet the learning needs of all students.

With the patient and his or her significant others brightly centered in this graphic model, it is easy to see how perioperative nursing's primary focus is the patient. Domains, patient outcomes, nursing diagnoses, and nursing interventions radiate out from the patient thus showing the step-by-step use in three-fourths of the model. The remaining one-fourth of the model shows how important the environment is to the surgical patient. The domain is the health system. The desired outcomes in this section are benchmarks often set in clinical pathways. Reports in the health system help identify problems represented by the next radiating section of circle. In the outside ring, structural elements represent ways of modifying the outcomes or benchmarks.

One of the major strengths of the PNDS is that it reinforces how nursing care plans are routinely used in clinical applications. Students often believe nursing care plans with nursing diagnoses and other components are just educational assignments with little relevance to "real" nursing. They are unaware that documentation to nursing care plans meets the Joint Commission and state boards of nursing requirements. Some who are vocal about negative aspects of care plans have failed to identify applications in other clinical settings. The PNDS underscores use of assessment, planning, intervention, and evaluation information in the perioperative clinical area with surgical clients (**Table 5-3**).

To use the care plan, the student fills in each column starting at the left and progressing to the right. To use the PNDS, the student starts with the centrally located patient, moves through domains to establish measurable outcomes, and continues through the rings to nursing diagnoses and to the perimeter ring of the circle that is nursing interventions. The following is an example of how to introduce students to the PNDS during a first or early-in-curriculum experience in the operating room.

Introducing Students to the PNDS

Due to the newness of the unit, the fast-paced environment, and the amount of technology, help the students focus by reminding them that, like any other unit, they are learning about patient care. Thus, the student begins using the model with the patient. Reinforce this by asking for their first impressions with the question, "What can go wrong for the patient in the OR?" Ask the students to group like answers together and think of a category that includes most of the responses. This is a good way of teaching conceptual thinking. If students are unable to do this, refer them to the model and ask if a response is a safety concept or a physiological, behavioral, or health systems concept. When given the title, they can usually identify the PNDS domain that relates to their patients' problems as noted in the parentheses following each bulleted item. Building on their previous surgical experiences with popular media programs, personal experiences, professional experiences, students might respond with the following:

The patient might
- Fall off the narrow table. (Safety)
- Have surgery on the wrong site. (Safety)
- Get an infection. (Safety)
- Get burned. (Safety)
- Have pain. (Safety, Physiological, Behavioral)
- Have high anxiety. (Behavioral)
- Get too cold. (Physiological)
- Bleed too much. (Physiological)
- Have someone fall on him or her. (Safety)

Students often have the most difficulty categorizing pain. If the student believes that the patient will have pain due to an extremely long surgery, the student will use the safety domain. If the student thinks of pain as due to resection of large muscle masses, he or she will often choose the physiological domain. And if the student says that pain is "whatever the patient says it is," then the behavioral domain will be selected.

TABLE 5-3: Comparing the Structure of a Nursing Care Plan and the Perioperative Patient Focused Model

Assess	Analyze	Plan	Implement	Evaluate
Collect objective and subjective data from cognitive, affective, and physical domains.	Cluster information into meaningful patterns. Establish actual or potential nursing diagnoses.	Set realistic goals and measurable outcomes related to nursing diagnoses. Plan interventions related to outcomes.	Apply a variety of psychosocial and physical activities to patient care to impact the patient outcome.	Measure the effectiveness of the care plan and revise.
Patient Assessment	**Domain**	**Nursing Outcomes**	**Nursing Diagnoses**	**Nursing Interventions**
• Acuity of the patient • Psychosocial behavior exhibited • Surgical intervention • Expected duration of the surgery • Position of patient during case.	Select appropriate domain: • Safety *or* • Physiological responses *or* • Behavioral responses *or* • Health System	State measurable goals and objectives for the surgical patient. The outcome will be clearly identified through use of outcome indicators.	Identify actual or potential nursing diagnoses.	Initiate nursing activities specific to the surgical patient to help meet the specified outcome.

The next ring in the perioperative model is patient outcomes. What patient outcome would be desired for any patient with problems in the safety domain? All students would want their patients to be safe with no falls, burns, or infections. As also used in nursing care plans, PNDS patient outcomes must be stated in specific, measurable terms. Skin integrity might be measured preoperatively, at the conclusion of the operative intervention, at discharge from the postanesthesia care unit (PACU), or in a follow-up phone call made to the patient's home. In any case, it needs to be stated so all nurses will know when the plan will be evaluated.

If students have studied nursing diagnoses, ask if the diagnoses for these situations are actual or potential nursing diagnoses. Nursing diagnoses are related to patient outcomes. An actual diagnosis has three parts: a nursing diagnosis followed by a "related to" statement followed by "as evidenced by" information. A potential nursing diagnosis includes the term "risk for" and omits "as evidenced by" because the evidence has not yet occurred and thus there is no evidence yet.

Example 1. Impaired skin integrity related to a motor vehicle accident as evidenced by multiple abrasions and large ecchymotic areas over anterior and posterior trunk and all four extremities.

Example 2. Risk for impaired skin integrity related to patient obesity and lengthy surgical procedure.

The outer ring of the PNDS model represents nursing interventions. These interventions are activities the nurse will perform to impact the

surgical patient's outcome positively. The activities the nurse will perform using the nursing care plan will likely be those used in medical-surgical units, while the perioperative nurse will use interventions specific to the perioperative units. The principle of care remains the same, but the products used in the intervention may be specific to the unit (**Table 5-4**).

Using the nursing diagnosis, risk for impaired skin integrity related to length of surgical procedure, the medical-surgical nurse might float the heels off the bed sheets and cover the heels with a slick transparent dressing to decrease friction with movement and the possibility of tissue breakdown. The perioperative nurse would probably secure gel boots to the feet or apply egg crate foam to protect tissue. In either case, nurses are attempting to use universal principles of care regardless of clinical site to protect soft tissue and bony prominences from pressure and to protect against shearing pressure with movement.

The three outer rings of the Perioperative Nursing Data Set are very similar to the comparable sections on the nursing care plan. As soon as students learn how to do a nursing care plan and have been introduced to the PNDS, they will be able to discern the common relationships between use of the PNDS and nursing care plans.

Relating the PNDS to Curricular Content
Whenever the PNDS is introduced to the student, the subject of the PNDS needs to relate to the content being taught in the curriculum.[3] The more relevant the content is to the student and the curriculum, the better the chance that the student will be able to make meaning out of the information and thus meet the student's learning needs. If the student is in the

TABLE 5-4: Comparison of Care Plan and PNDS Nursing Interventions

Nursing Outcome: Prevent skin breakdown during surgical intervention
Nursing Diagnosis: Risk for Impaired Skin Integrity Related to length of surgical procedure.
Nursing Interventions: *(focusing on feet)*

Using the Nursing Care Plan	Using the Perioperative Patient Focused Model
• Place a protective transparent film over the heels to decrease friction during movement. • Float heels by elevating them off the mattress using a pillow or blanket under the calf of the patient's legs. • Place pillow between or under legs to elevate feet from mattress.	• Secure gel-filled boots to each foot to pad foot surfaces and prevent articulation of bony prominences with each other. • Use egg crate or other padding material to prevent surfaces from producing pressure. • Place padding between lower legs to keep feet separated and in appropriate alignment.

perioperative area in the first semester, a good place to begin is with vital signs. The skills of monitoring temperature, pulse, respirations, and blood pressure are taught immediately after hand washing and universal precautions. The fifth vital sign is pain, an area even very young students understand and are concerned about. Pain is associated with surgery, so students are interested in alleviating pain. It is also a current and major focus of the Joint Commission in the acute care setting, and as a result, it is an important subject both in education and in practice.

The thought process and application of content on pain can be documented using the Perioperative Patient Focused Model.[4] Filling in the rings of the model helps the student work through the process using critical thinking. It also shows how content might be documented (**Table 5-5**).

If the student has progressed in the curriculum and is taking a research course, the PNDS application would be different. One of the difficulties researchers have is consistent meaning among terms used in research studies. The Perioperative Nursing Data Set is a standardized language created in part for the purpose of furthering research and scholarship in the surgical setting. Terms need to be consistent if they are to be compared; otherwise there is no reliable way of drawing a comparison. Does the term *thermal regulation* used in one study really mean hyperthermia, and in another study hypothermia?

A student learning activity that will underscore this problem is to divide the class into small groups to access key words in various databases including Medline and CINAHL. Are they different or the same, and how do the meanings compare? When students have their scientific examples from the literature, ask how temperature was measured? How many studies used scales assessed on the forehead, rectum, bladder, or auditory canal forms? Ask who were the makers of the measurement equipment, because we all know some equipment is more reliable than others. Is it the same equipment used in the student's clinical facility?

Suppose the learning goals were different and focused on evidence-based practice. The goals would be to identify clinical problems and manage them through science, use a systematic application of information, and seek the measurement value of

TABLE 5-5: An Application of the PNDS Model With Pain

Patient-Focused Assessment on Pain

Behavioral Domain	Physiological Domain
• Cries, cries out, grimaces, shows fear	• Increases or decreases B/P
• Identifies pain level on scale	• Increases or decreases respirations
• Uses protective stance	• Increases temperature
• Assess for cultural expressions of pain	• Diaphoretic

PATIENT OUTCOME:
Attain and maintain a comfort level tolerable to the patient = Pain Control

Outcome Indicators: Behavioral Domain	**Outcome Indicators:** Physiological Domain
• Lies quietly	• Stable vital signs
• Moves as instructed	• Stable or declining requests for medication
• Peaceful expression on face	• Decreased diaphoresis
• Follows requested instructions	• Asleep/resting
Nursing Diagnoses: • Impaired comfort • Alterations in comfort • Acute pain • Chronic pain	**Nursing Interventions:** • Assess vital signs and pain scales • Reposition patient • Administer pain medications • Reassess effect after medication administration • Apply heat/cold therapies • Allow verbal expressions of concern • Use of therapeutic touch

consistent use of terms. Students might be channeled toward showing a relationship between the AORN *Standards, Recommended Practices, and Guidelines* and other evidence-based sources.[5] The ultimate academic goal is to use scientific interventions to solve clinical problems.

People often mention the cold temperature of the operating room, and observers often request additional attire to keep warm. Temperature is one academic content area of vital signs, but this example is at a higher level of expectation and student performance than earlier examples. At this point in the curriculum, nursing students know that hypothermia is a serious problem causing hypotension, bradycardia, coagulapathy, acidosis, decreased healing, and increased infections. Asking students to resolve the clinical problem "What is the best way of maintaining the patient's body temperature?" requires the student to seek answers using scholarly best practices (**Table 5-6**).

While developing learning activities for students, it is also useful to select patient care content that is applied broadly and relates to multiple clinical sites. The beauty of this scholarly learning example is that thermoregulation has broad application and relates to a variety of clinical situations and is not specific to perioperative nursing. The patient on a medical-surgical unit lying under the air conditioner vent, one who has fallen through the ice on a winter pond, and the person exposed to cold weather when inadvertently locked out of his or her home all share the same health problem and similar nursing needs.

Perhaps the student is taking an undergraduate leadership course and is interested in learning how orientation for a new graduate might take place in the surgical environment. The student could be directed to find the employer's job description and compare it with PNDS outcomes and interventions lists. Students near graduation also have substantial education that supports an interest in patient advocacy and would identify outcome "Participates in decisions" (O23) or "Privacy rights" (O25) as representative of this interest. Once the outcome is identified, the student can be assured of nursing actions required by reviewing examples of PNDS use listed under that outcome. At the same time, the PNDS could be used to identify guidelines for performance and evaluation. Interventions serve as clear guidelines for expected performance. Today the PNDS is embedded in several computerized documentation programs specific to the operating room. Their ease of use and readability has provided a time-efficient and safer form of legal and ethical documentation.

TABLE 5-6: Student Learning Activity for an Evidence-Based Practice Course

Clinical Problem: What is the best way of maintaining the patient's body temperature?

Directions: Divide the students into pairs and ask each pair to select one of the following items for study:
- Turn up the heat in the operating room before the patient arrives.
- Heat the operating room early; reduce the temperature when draping occurs.
- Use forced-air blanket warmers.
- Use under-body warmers.
- Use heated-bath blankets.
- Use warmed intravenous fluids
- Others?

Further questions: Once selected, the pairs will search databases such as CINAHL, Medline, or PubMed to determine key terms used in their search.
- How were they able to focus their literature search?
- How did using randomized controls and stipulating animal versus human temperature controls narrow searches?
- Was Cochran Systematic Review helpful?

In a total class discussion, ask students for their optimal choice to answer the clinical question and cite their rationale for the choice. How did the consistency of language used in the PNDS facilitate this activity?

Nurses in graduate education courses are gaining knowledge about the business of surgical services through perioperative advanced practice nursing. Whether enrolled in master of science in nursing (MSN) degree programs or doctor of nursing practice (DNP) education, students are preparing for the management of health care personnel and other applications of the PNDS informatics programs. These advanced practice nurses are interested in creating organizational change, providing high quality services at reasonable costs, establishing and measuring quality indicators, and predicting trends in perioperative health care delivery.

Elements of the PNDS are coded for ease of use and retrieval. Outcomes are coded with an O and a number specific to that one outcome. Likewise, "D" and a number signify a specific domain, intervention (I), and nursing diagnoses (X). Use of coding not only makes language consistent and clearly defined, but it also creates a system for easy retrieval.

The structural elements that have been gathered on perioperative documentation forms for the last several years now can have new meaning. Using computer documentation with the PNDS allows the manager to identify which nurses are consistently able to start rooms on time while controlling for anesthesia or surgeon delays and identifying the cause of the delay.[6]

In one quality assurance program, antibiotic timed administration data was gathered to participate in the surgical infection prevention program. In preparation for becoming a Trauma I center, the facility experimented with the availability of scheduling and staffing one surgical suite in any 24-hour time period.[6] In the PNDS heath system domain, this program could serve as an example for students to gather and manipulate data from the structural elements listed on documentation forms to impact benchmarks of customer satisfaction and reduced time delays.

SUMMARY

The PNDS model is an easy-to-use tool for teaching and learning opportunities with students in undergraduate and graduate education. Content learned with the PNDS can be as diversified as the curriculum, moving from simple to complex. To use the PNDS most effectively, the content needs to match the academic content in the curriculum, thus meeting student and academic needs. PNDS applications that focus on universal nursing care principles will broaden use to other than surgical settings.

While it may be tempting to explain how the model can be used in its totality, a little at a time may be more useful. Sections of the PNDS can be used in skills lab, clinical courses, elective courses, and student-selected practicum experiences to apply learning opportunities to and from the surgical environment. In the beginning, the PNDS provides an organizational framework for planning surgical patient care. Lists of interventions provide a new student with ideas on what and how to apply activities to reach the nursing goal or objective set for the patient. The standardized, coded, and computer-programmed language of the PNDS can promote easy retrieval of data for use in research, evidence-based practice, staff evaluation, quality improvement, and managerial change and decision-making. This model helps students understand the variety of uses purposeful legal and ethical documentation can have for the patient, staff, and health care organization.

References
1. L Sigsby, "A knowledge comparison of nursing students in perioperative versus other rotations," *AORN Journal* 80 no 4 (2004) 699-707.
2. S V M Kleinbeck. *PNDS @ Work: Encouraging Perioperative Clinical Experiences* (Denver: AORN, 2005).
3. L Sigsby, "Avoiding problems when establishing a student learning experience in perioperative nursing," *Nurse Educator* 28 no 1 (2003) 1-2.
4. L Sigsby, "Effective learning about the concept of pain from a perioperative clinical rotation," *Pain Managment Nursing* 2 no 1 (2001) 19-24.
5. *Standards, Recommended Practices, and Guidelines* (Denver: AORN, 2007).
6. T Macheski, "Uncorking the delay bottleneck," paper presented October 2004 at the AORN Chapter 1016 meeting, Gainesville, Fla.

EXEMPLAR 5: Teaching the Language of Perioperative Nursing to the Novice

Y ou may have observed and worried about strange behaviors and affects of new employees during their orientation period. You may have noticed that those in orientation seem depressed or irritable; they may experience decreased appetite, difficulty sleeping, or other manifestations of anxiety during their orientation. Chrisman[1] noted that novice perioperative nurses who move to a new operating room experience culture shock. A transcultural analysis of complex new environments reveals belief and behavior patterns (eg, language) disrupt one's basic social cues and lead to culture shock. This response appears to be greater in the OR. The transcultural nursing principle derived from studying those suddenly immersed in a new environment is to learn the language, the perioperative language.

The PNDS provides a structured, uniform language for teaching the practice of perioperative nursing. The PNDS provides wording and definitions for nursing diagnoses, interventions, and outcomes, thereby providing clinicians with the same terms to describe patient care across multiple settings. As the PNDS becomes more widely used across geographic locations, the language gap will close as the PNDS is accepted as the universal nursing language.

The logistics of teaching the language of the PNDS to the novice perioperative nurse is less complicated because they have not yet developed an OR language of their own. It becomes more challenging with the experienced perioperative nurse who begins to learn the language incrementally as it is introduced by integrating the language into in-service programs. These items might include the intraoperative care of a specific patient population, departmental policy and procedures, job descriptions, and nursing plans of care.

The focus of this article is a five-tiered method for teaching the PNDS to the novice perioperative nurse, nursing intern, student, or staff nurse new to the perioperative setting. It consists of an introduction to the PNDS, clinical observation, naming nursing activities, identifying data elements, and a final project.

Cecil A. King, RN, MS, CNOR
Advanced Practice Nurse
Sinai Hospital of Baltimore
Baltimore, Maryland

FIRST TIER: INTRODUCTION TO THE PNDS

The first tier is to introduce the learner to the Perioperative Patient Focused Model and the PNDS. Before the first clinical observation day, interns and students are assigned the computer-based training offered by AORN online at *http://www.aorn.org /Education/ContinuingEducation/FREEOnline Education/PerioperativeNursingDataSet*. The free continuing education program provides the learner with an overview of the perioperative model and the PNDS. In addition, novices are given a handout example of how the PNDS is applied to an adult plan of care.[2] The handout is an article that uses the PNDS to describe the patient care provided during a simple cystoscopy procedure.

SECOND TIER: CLINICAL OBSERVATION

The novice's completion of the computer-based training lays the foundation for the second tier of learning, clinical observation, during the second week of training (**Table 5-7**). The objectives for the clinical observation are as follows:

- Describe the four domains of the Perioperative Nursing Data Set.
- Identify the construct of the PNDS.
- Demonstrate application of the PNDS in describing a patient.

The learners are assigned to observe an entire surgical case from beginning to end. They are not to deliver care but only to shadow the circulating nurse, making notes on an Observation Activity Form about what they see the circulating nurse doing in the domains of Safety, Physiological, and Behavioral Responses in the care of the patient. These activities and interventions are noted on the Observation Activity Form as they correspond to the respective

TABLE 5-7: Perioperative Lesson Plan				
OBJECTIVES	**CONTENT**	**TIME FRAME**	**FACULTY**	**METHOD**
1. Describe the four domains of the Perioperative Nursing Data Set.	1.1 Perioperative Patient Focused Model 1.2 Development/Importance of PNDS 1.3 Taxonomy 1.4 Describe Data Elements 1.5 Application to Practice	10 min	Cecil A. King	Lecture Handouts Overhead Discussion
2. Identify the construct of the PNDS.	2.1 Outcomes 2.2 Outcomes Indicators 2.3 Interim Outcomes 2.4 Nursing Diagnoses 2.5 Nursing Interventions and Activities	30 min	Cecil A. King	Lecture Handouts Overhead Discussion
3. Demonstrate application of the PNDS in describing patient.	3.1 Clinical Assignment of PNDS, Weeks 1 & 2 3.2 Review Clinical Assignment 3.3 Discuss Nursing Interventions and Activities provided to the patient in the clinical area	30 min	Cecil A. King	Overheads Discussion Clinical Assignment

domain and outcome(s) listed. For example, *Implements protective measures prior to operative and invasive procedure* (I138) is the intervention (ie, data element) specific to reviewing the preoperative checklist. Novices may log this on the Observation Activity Form in their own words during the observation. **Table 5-8** details the PNDS Clinical Observation Assignment given to the novices.

THIRD TIER: NAMING NURSING ACTIVITIES

The Observation Activity Form (**Table 5-9**) is provided to the novices for recording those nursing activities they observe performed in caring for the patient. This is the third tier of the lesson plan, where the novice uses the PNDS to name those activities and interventions that comprise the care of the patient.

FOURTH TIER: IDENTIFYING DATA ELEMENTS

The first class day following the clinical observation is the fourth tier of learning. This is a classroom discussion of what the novice observed during clinical. During this class the instructor and novice review the observed activities using a projected blank overhead. As the novice report what they saw the circulator do for the patient, the instructor will write it in on the projected overhead (see example). In this

way the activity is reviewed in class, with the instructor and novice identifying those data elements (ie, specific language) that describe the nursing interventions performed for the patient. This method of identifying specific interventions related to the corresponding patient outcome is reinforced in each class and clinical exercise.

This exercise is the foundation leading to the fifth and final tier of the lesson plan—the student's final paper (**Table 5-10**). In this project, a case is presented and a plan of care developed for a specific patient using the plan of care format illustrated in **Table 5-11**.

Instructor overhead: Identified data elements		
DOMAIN	**OUTCOMES** • Outcome Indicators	**NURSING INTERVENTIONS AND ACTIVITIES**
Safety	**O2.** The patient is free from signs and symptoms of injury caused by extraneous objects.	Applies safety devices **(I11)** • Safety belt above knees

EXAMPLE: The instructor writes in the identified data elements describing the nursing activity noted during the clinical observation.

TABLE 5-8: PNDS Clinical Observation Assignment

Clinical Week 2: This assignment will be completed during the second week of the program and is the focus of the clinical observation during week 2. You are not to deliver care to any patient. You will be assigned to observe at least one case from the very beginning to the end, including transfer to PACU. Finish your observation by 2 PM to allow yourself time to complete the Observation Activity Form. Describing the role of the scrub person is not part of this exercise.

OBJECTIVES:
1. Observe and shadow a circulating nurse in the OR. *Describe how the circulating nurse uses the nursing process to prioritize and sequence care of the patient.*
2. Demonstrate basic application of the PNDS in describing patient care.
3. Identify nursing interventions and activities performed by the circulating nurse during the care of the patient.

Assignment: There are four parts.
1. Computer-based training program (CBT) that you must complete; show your certificate of completion the following Friday in class.
2. Clinical Observation
3. Written Observation Activity Form (OAF)
4. Classroom discussion of your observational experience; what you learned from this assignment.
5. Application of the PNDS in the Perioperative Case Study paper.

Computer-Based Training:
You are responsible for completing the AORN computer-based training module on the Perioperative Nursing Data Set (PNDS). When you complete the module, print the certificate as evidence that you completed this portion of the assignment. Access the site by logging on at *http://www.aorn.org/PracticeResources/PNDS*. Follow the instructions for a nonmember.

Clinical Observation Activity:
You are scheduled for a clinical observation day during week 2 of the program. Refer to your class schedule for specific dates and times. You are to observe the work of the circulating nurse in the OR. You are not to deliver patient care during this assignment. The procedure that you are assigned to observe must be completed during your observation. In other words, you are to observe at least one procedure from the circulator's first encounter with the patient through and including, transfer of the patient to the care of the PACU nurse. During the observation, **you are responsible for identifying nursing interventions and**

activities performed by the circulating nurse as articulated in the PNDS. The purpose of this assignment is to develop your understanding of the basic responsibilities of the circulating nurse.

Written Observation Activity Form (OAF):
You will complete a written OAF (**Table 5-9**) for the clinical observation day. You are required to complete this form on the day of observation The educator/CNS at your clinical site may require that it be turned in to them for review; check with the educator/CNS at your clinical site for specific expectations.

Plan on finishing your observation by 2 PM to allow time to complete the OAF. Suggestions for preparing to complete this assignment include reviewing the PNDS book, completing and exploring other resources about the PNDS online, and other recommended readings.

A few outcomes have been listed for you on the OAF. List the corresponding nursing interventions and activities performed by the circulating nurse for those outcomes. You may identify additional outcomes; list these as described in the PNDS. Focus on identifying and listing nursing interventions and activities for each outcome. Those activities of the circulating nurse that you list should describe the role of the circulating nursing in the care of the patient. When you identify what the nurse did, write this down as you observe it. Do not quote something out of the PNDS or a textbook; focus on what the circulating nurse actually did for the patient.

In the same column as OUTCOMES are **outcome indicators**. Outcome indicators are assessment factors that denote evaluation of the patient. Jot down in this column what outcome indicators the circulating nurse uses to determine if the interventions achieved the intended outcomes. You may refer to the PNDS for examples of outcome indicators as they correspond to various interventions and activities of care.

Recommended Reading:
Petersen, C, ed. *Perioperative Nursing Data Set: The Perioperative Nursing Vocabulary,* revised second ed. Denver: AORN, 2007.
King, C A; Veit, K. "Perioperative Nursing Data Set for the adult having a cystoscopy." *Seminars in Perioperative Nursing* 10 no 1 (2001) 4753.
Rothrock, J, ed. *Alexander's Care of the Patient in Surgery,* 12th ed. Philadelphia: Mosby, 2003.

Grading: This is a pass/fail activity and a required part of your observations during week 2.

TABLE 5-9: Observation Activity Form		
Procedure observed: _____	*Intern:* _____	*Date:* _____
DOMAIN	**OUTCOMES** • Outcome indicators	**NURSING INTERVENTIONS AND ACTIVITIES**
Safety	**O2.** The patient is free from signs and symptoms of injury caused by extraneous objects.	
	O3. The patient is free from signs and symptoms of chemical injury.	
	O4. The patient is free from signs and symptoms of electrical injury.	
	O5. The patient is free from signs and symptoms of injury related to positioning	
Physiologic Reponses	**O12.** The patient is at or returning to normothermia at the conclusion of the immediate postoperative period.	
Behavioral Responses	**O25.** The patient's right to privacy is maintained.	
	O31. The patient demonstrates knowledge of the procedure.	
Health System	**O10.** The patient is free from signs and symptoms of infection.	

© Inova Health System 2003. Adapted with permission.

FIFTH TIER: SYNTHESIS OF LEARNING

Having the novice perform a case study and present the patient care as a formal paper and oral presentation facilitates synthesis of learning. This is the culmination of the course, whereby the novices are able to demonstrate application of the PNDS in the care of a patient across the continuum of care.

Novices are assigned to pick a patient (ie, procedure) for whom they have a particular interest and follow this patient across the continuum of care from the point of preanesthesia evaluation through postoperative day 1 or 2. Given this requirement, novices are encouraged to care for a patient who will remain in the medical center two to three days postoperatively. The novice is to perform the role of the circulator during the procedure for the case study patient to implement the plan of care and evaluate those outcomes listed on the plan of care.

The student and faculty use the guidelines presented in **Table 5-10** in planning and evaluating the project. The novice then presents the case study and plan of care to the class and faculty during the last week of class.

CONCLUSION

Using this tiered method to introduce the student to the PNDS and integrating the language throughout their training teaches novices a standardized language while challenging the students to critically think about what perioperative nurses do for their patients. Working with the experienced nurse to use the data set in developing a plan of care will not only further validate the value of the RN, but it will also demonstrate to staff the value of a standardized language.

As the language of the PNDS (eg, data elements) are further integrated into the syllabus, lesson plans, policies and procedures, competencies, and job descriptions, educators will further advance our profession through the application of a national uniform-structured language linking patient outcomes to the care provided by the perioperative nurse.

References

1.   N J Chrisman, "Cultural shock in the operating room: Cultural analysis in transcultural nursing," *Journal of Transcultural Nursing* 1 no 2 (1990) 33-39.

2.   C A King, K Veit, "Perioperative Nursing Data Set for the adult having a cystoscopy, *Seminars in Perioperative Nursing* 10 no 1 (2001) 47-53.

TABLE 5-10: Synthesis of Learning Project

1. **Preoperative Assessment**   10 points
   1.1. Participates in the preanesthesia assessment in the outpatient clinic.
   1.2. Documents assessment and preoperative teaching.
   1.3. Develops a plan of care identifying nursing diagnoses and appropriate nursing interventions and activities within the PNDS specific to those outcomes unique to the patient of study. *Note:* Caution the learner and faculty not to rework the entire PNDS, but to focus on those outcomes and interventions unique to the specific patient and procedure (eg, positioning for spine patients more so than patient in the supine position).
2. **Case presentation and pathophysiology** 10 points
   2.1. Presenting those assessment findings pertinent to the care of the patient during the perioperative period.
3. **Discussion** of the surgical procedure and indications relevant to the patient's diagnosis.   10 points

4. **Perioperative nursing process**   15 points
   4.1. Discussion of nursing activities that may not be captured in the plan of care.
   4.2. Inclusive of surgeon's preference lists, special equipment, other disciplines (eg, radiology), specimens, etc.
   4.3. Documentation and completion of operative record. Attach a copy of operative record, pathology requisition, implant record, etc.; White out and remove any patient identifiers from the attachments.
5. **PLAN OF CARE**   25 points
   5.1. This is the principle focus of the paper and should provide a clear picture of the perioperative care planned for the patient.
   5.2. The care plan must use PNDS data elements indicating the criteria used to evaluate if outcomes were met, including an explanation of variances. The care plan template (**Table 5-11**) is given to the student on disk to provide structure for the care plan.

6. **References** 15 points
   6.1. The paper must reference the AORN recommended practices and PNDS data elements.
   6.2. References must include at least one perioperative nursing or peer-reviewed journal article published within the past 5 years.
7. **Paper formatting requirements** 5 points
   7.1. 5–7 pages in length, excluding cover page.
   7.2. Cover page with student name, facility, date.
7.3. Word-processed, doubled-spaced, using 12-point font and one-inch margins.
7.4. The paper must use the plan of care template provided.
7.5. Minimum of 2 references required (see item 6)
8. **Overall evaluation** Maximum of 10 points
   8.1. Meeting due date *(specify)*.
   8.2. Late papers will automatically be deducted 10 points.

TABLE 5-11: Perioperative Plan of Care Template			
Domain	**Nursing Diagnosis**	**Perioperative Nursing Interventions**	**Patient Outcome**

❦

EXEMPLAR 6: Encouraging Use of PNDS in Specialty Procedure Units

Invasive procedures are routinely performed in operating rooms and a variety of specialty procedure suites (eg, endoscopy suites, cardiovascular labs, and interventional radiology suites) across the nation. The registered nurses working in these departments have many things in common with perioperative RNs. Each is concerned about assessing the patient and implementing a plan specific to his or her physiologic and behavioral needs. The ultimate goal of all professionals is to keep the patient safe during invasive procedures (eg, colonoscopies, cardiac catheterizations, arteriograms, and computed axial tomography–guided needle biopsies).

Many invasive-procedure RNs are represented by a specialty professional nursing organization. These organizations, such as the Society of Gastroenterology Nurses and Associates (SGNA), American College of Cardiovascular Nurses (ACCN), American Society of PeriAnesthesia Nurses (ASPAN), and American Radiological Nurses Association (ARNA), have mission statements and practice standards unique to the patient populations they serve. These organizations interact and collaborate with AORN, each other, and other professional nursing organizations for the common purpose of improving health care services provided to their unique patient populations.

The objective of this text is to present some of the commonalities among the nursing professionals delivering care to the invasive-procedure patient and to suggest the PNDS as the universal vocabulary for documentation on all of these types of patient cases. Increased creative ideas and innovation could result if nursing professionals from all specialties had the ability to compare outcomes and share their talents and expertise to improve the quality of health care across the country.

THE COMMON THREAD: THE PATIENT

The common thread that unites all nurses is the patient. RNs who provide nursing care in specialty procedure units and the OR have a common characteristic, a specific patient type: the patient

Mary A. Salreno, RN, MSN
OR Business Manager
Sharon Regional Health System
Sharon, Pennsylvania

undergoing a high-risk invasive procedure. While the RNs' practice areas may be different, the nursing care standards, guidelines, and standards of patient care are remarkably similar. The universal themes running through the standards are the same:

- patient safety,
- protecting patient rights,
- monitoring physiological responses, and
- providing patient education.

These common themes are represented in the patient care domains of the PNDS. Consider the magnitude of the impact on the health care industry if all RNs could share and compare patient outcomes related to safety and the invasive procedure patient. This can be accomplished only through a common vocabulary set, and the PNDS is the answer. Recognized by the American Nurses Association (ANA), the PNDS is a standardized nursing vocabulary that addresses the perioperative patient experience from preadmission to discharge.[2] As information technology continues to grow, a codified language is going to be required for a nurse to document on a patient record.

In this decade, electronic documentation—the paperless patient record—has burst onto the scene with the promise of organized and concise data. However, the "organized data" is useful only if "an apple" is truly "an apple," and only if those "apples" can be extracted and compared in an organized fashion. In electronic documentation and reporting, it's all about the language. "Language" is a systematic means of communicating. Electronic documentation is accomplished through menus, drop boxes, and check boxes that are linked to tables containing data elements that have specific meaning and intent. If the facility wants to electronically retrieve the data staff members put into an electronic document, the language has to be organized and coded. Organized data also facilitates the nursing research process in which the data must be defined, reliable, and valid.

The PNDS is codified and provides a comprehensive structure and design for that common language. The PNDS provides the language that addresses the delivery of nursing care across the entire continuum of the perioperative experience and can be used by all areas or departments performing high-risk invasive procedures.

THE NEED FOR A COMMON LANGUAGE

The future of health care documentation is in electronic/computerized documentation. According to the Medical Records Institute, the factors driving the need for electronic health record (EHR) systems include the need to

- improve clinical processes;
- share information;
- improve patient safety;
- improve clinical data capture and documentation;
- facilitate clinical decision support; and
- meet requirements of legal, regulatory, and/or accreditation standards.[1]

Ideally, practitioners should be able to retrieve data elements easily from an electronic record and share data for purposes of reporting and quality improvement activities. To accomplish these goals, the data elements must be captured in the same fashion, and each element must have a specific, unambiguous meaning. The data between two different patient records must be comparable. PNDS can be the universal language to quantify the outcomes that result from adherence to the standard of care. Using the PNDS, practitioners from all perioperative and specialty areas would have the ability to aggregate, compare, and report data.

Most certainly, the paramount force behind development of a common language between common activities in health care is the consumer and external stakeholder. As the depth of public reporting broadens, many patients take the time to educate themselves about clinical outcomes before seeking services from a particular health care facility. Consumers are demanding information about the quality of services rendered at hospitals. Groups such as the National Quality Forum (NQF), the Joint Commission, and the Leapfrog Group offer the consumer comprehensive assessments and databases on the safety and quality of participating hospitals. The goal of these groups is to improve the quality of health care through measuring performance and encouraging public reporting on safety practices, high-risk procedure outcomes, and compliance to recommended treatment protocols. A hospital's willingness to participate in voluntary public reporting is influenced by reimbursement requirements of third-party payors for public reporting and/or participation in national registries.

In 2004, the Joint Commission published the most detailed hospital performance measurement tool of its kind. *Quality Check* provides the online consumer information about patient safety and quality for its 16,000 accredited organizations.[3] Participation in *Quality Check* is mandatory for hospitals seeking accreditation by the Joint Commission. The Web site compares hospital-to-hospital performance with adherence to the Joint Commission's standards for patients with heart attack, heart failure, pneumonia, and pregnancy-related conditions.

Ultimately, the consumer reaps the benefits of public reporting, which provides information to make informed health care decisions about where to seek high-quality health services. Conceivably, public reporting of specific outcomes related to invasive procedures could be a requirement in the future for many hospitals across the country. PNDS provides a framework and codified language to collect relevant data that can potentially be used for national reporting on specific aspects of invasive procedures in the future.

THE JOINT COMMISSION AND THE INVASIVE PROCEDURE

As stated previously, the common thread of this discussion is the patient undergoing a high-risk invasive procedure. When the Joint Commission published the *Universal Protocol for Preventing Wrong Site, Wrong Procedure, Wrong Person Surgery,* the organization defined the scope of the protocol by defining the invasive procedure as follows:

This Protocol and its Implementation Guidelines apply to all operative and other invasive procedures that expose patients to more than minimal risk, including procedures done in settings other than the OR, such as a special procedures unit, endoscopy unit or interventional radiology suite. Certain routine "minor" procedures such as venipuncture, peripheral IV line placement, insertion of NG tube, or Foley catheter insertion are not within the scope of the Protocol. However, most other procedures that involve puncture or incision of the skin, or insertion of an instrument or foreign material into the body, including, but not limited to, percutaneous aspirations, biopsies, cardiac and vascular catheterizations, and endoscopies are within the scope of this Protocol.[4]

Additionally, LD.3.20 from the *Comprehensive Accreditation Manual for Hospitals* requires that patients with comparable needs receive the same level of care, treatment, and services throughout the organization.[5] The patient undergoing an gastroscopy in the endoscopy suite is required by the Joint Commission to receive the same level of care as the patient in the OR. The nurse in the cardiovascular lab should have similar competencies to the perioperative nurse in the OR. An invasive procedure in the interventional radiology suite is no less an invasive procedure than one in the OR. PNDS is the clinically relevant vocabulary set designed to provide uniformity to nursing documentation across all areas performing high-risk invasive procedures. In addition to uniform documentation, PNDS can provide the infrastructure for nurse competencies, nursing care plans, clinical pathways, education and training, and benchmarking for any of the invasive procedure suites.

PNDS IS NOT THE STANDARD

To understand the purpose of the PNDS, one must first separate the concepts of the "standard" versus the "language." The standard is the established norm—the level of excellence. The language is the vehicle for communication. PNDS is the language that describes the outcome when one adheres to the standard. PNDS is not the standard of care.

It is hoped that RNs reading this exemplar will consider adopting PNDS as the universal vocabulary for nursing documentation of invasive procedure care in specialty procedure units. The recommended practices and guidelines, standards of care, and position statements of the specialty specific professional nursing organizations (eg, SGNA, ACCN) will not change by doing so. Each specialty organization can maintain its mission and unique identity and still agree upon a common language for documentation. It is through the use of a common language that all RNs working in the perioperative setting and specialty procedure units can share and compare relevant, meaningful data for the purpose of improving quality patient care to the invasive procedure patient.

For example, AORN's Standard V: Ethics reads, "The perioperative nurse's decision and actions on behalf of the patients are determined in an ethical manner."[6] Just as AORN, ASPAN, SGNA, and ACCN each have their own unique published standards of nursing practice, all of them have published at least one standard addressing patient rights and ethical behaviors.[7-9] Each organization addresses their unique patient population, but the "words" are all similar.

All PNDS outcomes in the domain of *Behavioral Responses – Patient and Family: Rights/Ethics* could easily be used by all of the professional groups listed to document a positive outcome for adherence to the organizations' practice standard(s). PNDS is the language used to document nursing care, but it is not the standard.

NURSING COMPETENCIES

AORN defines *competency* as "the knowledge, skills, and abilities necessary to fulfill the professional role of a registered nurse in the operating room."[10] RNs working in specialty procedure units must also possess competencies relative to the delivery of patient care in their area of practice. The PNDS can be used in all arenas to not only capture the nursing process, but also to define the performance expectations of the RN.

The Joint Commission requires organizations to provide competent staff and to assess and maintain those competencies. Competencies are directly related to patient safety including, but not limited to, medication administration, proper use of equipment, skills such as phlebotomy and dysrhythmia interpretation, and age-specific activities based on the patient population served. PNDS interventions are measurable and therefore appropriate for defining competency of a nurse. The RN in the endoscopy suite assisting the gastroenterologist with a colonoscopy keeps the patient in a safe environment. Examples of nurse interventions followed by the unique identifier code include

- confirming the patient's identity before the invasive procedure (I26),
- using supplies and equipment within safe parameters (I122),
- verifying allergies (I123),
- positioning the patient (I96), and
- administering prescribed medications as ordered (I8).

The registered nurse in the cardiovascular lab assisting the cardiologist with the insertion of a pacemaker keeps the patient free from infection by

- implementing aseptic technique (I70),
- performing skin preparations (I94),
- initiating traffic control in the suite (I81), and
- administering care to the wound sites (I4).

The interventions are measurable through documentation, direct observation, and/or critical thinking test scenarios and can provide the foundation for defining the competency of all RNs working in specialty procedure units as well as the perioperative setting. Using these and the other codified interventions in the PNDS as statements to evaluate nurse competencies, RNs can define their competency with a common language that quantifies the value of the nurse in the care of the invasive procedure patient. Because this information has a code, it can be extracted, marketed, and compared across health care institutions as well as presented to the external stakeholders and accrediting bodies.

ACHIEVING THE DESIRED OUTCOMES

The competent RN follows policies and procedures and achieves desired outcomes. PNDS is the language that describes these desired outcomes. If two or more invasive procedure suites across a facility want to compare their infection control outcomes, all the areas must have the data documented in a uniform manner. The documentation elements must have the same

definitions across all areas being compared. The outcome criteria and nursing interventions must have the same specific, defined definitions. In addition, and certainly the most important point, the nurse documenting must know and understand the elements and definitions.

The nurse achieves the goal by individualizing the activities associated with the interventions, based on the patient's needs. By design, the PNDS provides for individualization of the specific activities for each intervention performed by the nurse to meet the desired outcome. The nurse can define the activities performed based on the needs of the patient and the population being served while maintaining uniformity of the desired outcome and nursing interventions. Even in the absence of electronic documentation, the nurses in all areas could develop a plan of care using the uniform vocabulary set, thereby making it comparable.

For example, using outcome O2, "The patient is free from signs and symptoms of injury caused by extraneous objects," nurses in the OR, endoscopy suite, cardiovascular lab, and interventional radiology suite could use some if not all of the interventions associated with this outcome to define the plan of care:

- Implements protective measure prior to operative or invasive procedures (I138)
- Confirms identity before the operative or invasive procedure (I26)
- Implements universal patient identity protocol (I156)
- Applies safety devices (I11)
- Implements protective measures to prevent skin or tissue injury due to thermal sources (I76)
- Implements protective measures to prevent skin/tissue injury due to mechanical sources (I77)
- Manages specimen collection and disposition (I84)
- Uses supplies and equipment within safe parameters (I122)
- Records devices implanted during the operative or invasive procedure (I112)
- Performs venipuncture (I95)
- Maintains continuous surveillance (I128)
- Evaluates for signs and symptoms of physical injury to skin and tissue (I152)

The safety devices applied to an adult patient in the cardiovascular lab will differ from the safety devices used on a pediatric patient in the OR, but the intervention is the same: "Applies safety devices" (I11). The activities (or devices applied) are different. For another example, the nurse in the OR setting positions a surgical patient in lithotomy using stirrups, and the nurse in the endoscopy suites may position an endoscopic retrograde cholangiopancreatography patient first prone and then reposition several times during the procedure. Once again, the intervention "Positions the patient" (I96) is the same for both, yet the activities are different.

PERIANESTHESIA NURSES: THE CONTINUUM OF CARE

The continuum of care for the invasive procedure patient is incomplete without the perianesthesia nurse. Immediately following the invasive procedure, these are the nurses who carry on with the responsibility of keeping the patient safe. The range of skills, expertise, and knowledge of these nurses is very extensive. In the hospital setting, perioperative nurses working in the postanesthesia care unit (PACU) deliver care to all age groups. The intensity of the care provided ranges from the minimally invasive outpatient procedure to the in-hospital patient with multi-system trauma who will be going to the intensive care unit.

Using the PNDS to document nursing care only during the invasive period but not in the PACU limits the usefulness of the documentation from the stand-point of the continuum of care. The PNDS also allows for flexibility because the interventions are not phase-specific. Like the nurse in the OR, the perioperative nurse in the PACU also develops an individualized plan of care (I30), monitors physiological status (I89), and transports according to individual needs (I118).

The following are just a few additional PNDS interventions that PACU nurses implement:
- Positions the patient (I96)
- Assesses pain control (I16)
- Monitors body temperature (I86)
- Monitors change in cardiac status (I158)
- Evaluates neurological status (I146)
- Evaluates response to administration of fluids and electrolytes (I153)

Not using the PNDS across the entire continuum of care would result in fragmentation and inconsistency not only of the documentation, but also of the data. In the electronic documentation world, vendors offer the ability to document in all phases of the perioperative event. Using more than one vocabulary within one specific documentation system, although it may be possible, would be like a bad dream for the software developer. With more than one vocabulary, information can become fragmented, unorganized, and therefore not useful. It makes sense to use one vocabulary set across the entire patient care continuum for the invasive procedure patient.

LET THE REVOLUTION BEGIN!

Although the rapid growth of electronic documentation has emphasized the importance of a common language among areas performing like activities, there is no ready-made, generic, all-purpose documentation format the serves the needs of all departments and patient populations. Electronic documentation is relatively new, and software vendors are still working to capture the essence of the PNDS.

The PNDS itself is also relatively new. All registered nurses working in the perioperative environment and specialty procedure units need to take an active role in its growth and development through their professional nursing organizations. But first, everyone must agree on its use, and everyone needs to understand what PNDS is. This text has made the point that the PNDS can be used as a common language for nursing documentation for the invasive procedure patient. Even though the PNDS is complete and comprehensive language, by design it is dynamic. It continues to change as the health care industry changes.

Imagine the revolution on the health care industry if AORN, ASPAN, ARNA, ACCN, and SGNA, to name a few, adopted the same vocabulary set for the invasive procedure patient. Imagine the impact on public reporting, nursing research, nursing competencies, nursing education, and defining the value of the registered nurse. So, why reinvent the wheel? Instead of each professional group writing its own vocabulary set, RNs working in specialty procedure units could adopt the PNDS as their vocabulary set. And then, let the revolution begin!

References

1. C P Waegemann, *Status Report 2002: Electronic Health Records* (Boston, Medical Records Institute) 2005.

2. *Perioperative Nursing Data Set: The Perioperative Nursing Vocabulary*, second ed (Denver: AORN) 2002.

3. "Care quality: JCAHO launches 'new generation' of quality reporting," *Clinical Strategy Watch* (July 2004). The Advisory Board Company.

4. "Frequently asked questions about the *Universal Protocol for Preventing Wrong Site, Wrong Procedure, Wrong Person Surgery,"* The Joint Commission, *http://www.jointcommission .org/PatientSafety/UniversalProtocol/up_faqs.htm* (accessed 10 Aug 2007.

5. Joint Commission on Accreditation of Healthcare Organizations. *Comprehensive Accreditation Manual for Hospitals.* Oakbrook Terrace, Ill: Joint Commission Resources; 2002.

6. "Standards of perioperative professional practice," in *Standards, Recommended Practices, and Guidelines* (Denver: AORN, 2007) 433-436.

7. *Standards of Perianesthesia Nursing Practice* (Cherry Hill, NJ: American Society of PeriAnesthesia Nurses) 2000.

8. Standards of clinical nursing practice and role delineation statements, in *Standards and Guidelines 2001*, Society of Gastroenterology Nurses and Associates (SGNA), *http://www.sgna.org /Resources/guidelines/guideline8.cfm* (accessed 10 Aug 2007).

9. "The 1998/2004 scope and standards of practice for cardiovascular nurses, educators, and nurse practitioners," in *Scope and Standards of Practice* (Riverview, Fla: The American College of Cardiovascular Nurses) 2004.

10. "Competency statements in perioperative nursing," in *Standards, Recommended Practices, and Guidelines* (Denver: AORN, 2007) 21-96.

EXEMPLAR 7: Generating Knowledge Through Research

Over the past 10 years, nursing research has become increasingly important as the demand for evidence-based decisions in clinical, administrative, and educational nursing practice has increased. Studies continue to emerge that support the impact of nurses on the quality of patient outcomes. It is critical for nurses to define their practice and establish the value that they contribute to the patient's clinical outcomes and experience.

The PNDS provides the taxonomy for naming structures required for basic quality, describing the processes of care that perioperative nurses conduct, and relating the subsequent patient outcomes expected when perioperative nursing processes are completed. The purpose of this exemplar is to describe opportunities to use the PNDS to measure perioperative factors and subsequent outcomes through research.

RESEARCH PROCESS VS QUALITY IMPROVEMENT

The purpose of research is to generate new knowledge (**Table 5-12**). As a profession, nursing has a unique body of knowledge developed through research findings. This unique body of knowledge

Robin Newhouse, RN, PhD, CNOR, CNA
Assistant Dean, Doctor of Nursing Practice Program; Associate Professor, Organizational Systems and Adult Health; University of Maryland School of Nursing, Baltimore

explores, describes, and explains the impact of nursing processes on patient and nurse outcomes. Research designs include quantitative (numbers) and qualitative (words) approaches to understand the concepts of interest. Although this chapter focuses on PNDS as taxonomy for research, it is worthwhile to include a brief discussion on quality improvement.

Quality improvement is a coordinated effort by health care systems to enhance health care processes to produce improved services and health outcomes for the patients served.[3] The purpose is to improve processes of care for a specific patient population within an organization. All perioperative settings are engaged in quality improvement projects and have an organizational model or process to guide them. Research designs, on the other hand, focus on strong control of all variables, inclusion of a sample that will allow generalizability or application of findings to a population, and a sample size that will allow statistical significance. Quality improvement benefits patients through organizational processes and seeks a change for the better, instead of striving for statistical significance, per se.

Numerous organizational factors within the perioperative setting have a significant influence on nurse and patient outcomes. Perioperative nurse leaders are responsible to allocate resources that promote quality care. For example, nursing-specific variables such as nurse certification, 24-hour staffing, the performance of multidisciplinary code drills, nurse staffing, and agency use are important variables. Each variable has an impact in terms of quality and cost. Identifying the best structures, processes, and outcomes to measure interventions and improvements is necessary to advance the quality of health care. The PNDS provides guidance in these relationships. The next step is to use these relationships to measure and improve care through quality improvement initiatives, outcomes measurement, and research.

RESEARCH EXEMPLAR

As the need for evidence-based practice continues, perioperative nurses and administrators need to understand the effect of their decisions. The PNDS provides a framework or taxonomy to understand the impact that staffing decisions have on patient outcomes. It provides a practice-level theory. A practice-level theory is prescriptive and provides guidance for nurses to use in their everyday clinical experience.

In the following sections, a 2005 study by Newhouse and colleagues[1] will be used to demonstrate the use of PNDS in a research process. An abstract of the study appears in **Table 5-13** on the following page. The basic components of the research process are introduction (problem, conceptual framework, purpose, and research questions); method (design, sample, procedure, instruments or measures, and the analysis strategy); results (the descriptive and inferential statistics with tables); and discussion (implications of the study to clinicians, management, or policy makers and theoretical implications for future research). These headings will frame the subsequent discussion.

Introduction
The first step in the research process is to consider the problem and the state of evidence. This requires a critical review of the scientific evidence to determine

> ### TABLE 5-12: Definitions
>
> **Research:** A systematic investigation, including research development, testing, and evaluation, designed to develop or contribute to generalizable knowledge.
>
> *Source:* Code of Federal Regulations §46.102 Definitions *http://www.hhs.gov/ohrp/humansubjects/guidance /45cfr46.htm#46.102.* Accessed 10 August 2007.
>
> **Quality:** The degree to which health services for individuals and populations increase the likelihood of desired health outcomes and are consistent with current professional knowledge.
>
> *Source:* Institute of Medicine, *http://www.iom.edu/focus on.asp?id=8089.* Accessed August 10, 2007.

where research is needed. Part of this critical review is to define the concepts of interest and their relationships in a conceptual framework or theoretical model. When the concepts and relationships are framed, a research question or hypothesis can be generated.

For example, consider the state of evidence related to nurse staffing and patient outcomes. Research has continued to emerge to demonstrate the relationship between nurse staffing and patient outcomes.[2] The perioperative areas were not the focus of these studies, however, so the unique contribution of the registered nurse in the operating room has not been studied. Therefore, the purpose of this research was to identify the relationship between RN staffing factors in the OR and surgical patient outcomes.

The study was guided by the Quality Health Outcomes Model,[4] which frames the relationship among the patient, system characteristics, and patient outcomes. In this model system and patient variables influence the outcome. The research questions were as follows, controlling for patient characteristics (age, gender, comorbidity, severity) and hospital volume:

1. Is the level of RN staffing in the OR related to postoperative complications, mortality, and length of stay?

2. Are certification, RN agency use, 24-hour staffing, or the performance of multidisciplinary code drills related to complications, mortality, or length of stay?

TABLE 5-13: Abstract

Title: Perioperative Nurses and Patient Outcomes: An Exploration of Mortality, Complications, and Length of Stay

Objective: This study examined the relationship between operating room organization (nurse certification, 24-hour staffing, the performance of multidisciplinary code drills, nurse staffing, and staffing agency use) and patient outcomes (surgical complications, mortality, and length of stay) for patients discharged post-abdominal aneurysm repair and aortic-iliac-femoral bypass.

Design: Survey and cross-sectional descriptive correlational.

Population: Discharge abstracts from 1894 patients undergoing abdominal aneurysm repair and aortic-iliac-femoral bypass in 2000–2002 in 32 Maryland hospitals were studied. Perioperative directors provided organizational data via mail survey.

Findings: For hospitals with no night coverage, a lower likelihood of complications was found as compared to hospitals with scheduled assigned staff (OR: 0.54, 95% CI: 0.37 to 0.79). The estimated odds of death decreased 33% per 10% increase in RN agency use (OR: 0.67, 95% CI: 0.56 to 0.80). The proportion of RNs with certification (CNOR) decreased the odds of complications or death by approximately 8% per 10% increase in the proportion of CNOR RNs, although these results were not statistically significant (OR:0.92, 95% CI: 0.84, 1.00 and OR: 0.92, CI:0.82, 1.04, respectively).

Conclusion: Organizational factors within ORs had significant influence on patient outcomes. ORs without staffed night shifts are commonly in smaller nonteaching hospitals with lower volume. These hospitals also serve a lower patient complexity that may not have been captured in this study's risk adjustment methodology. Operating room agency nurses are usually seasoned perioperative nurses with specific expertise in a specialty service (eg, vascular). The use of a higher proportion of CNOR RNs was related to a lower risk of complications, although this finding was not statistically significant.

Implication: Organizational structures and processes are increasingly targeted as opportunities to improve staff morale and patient safety. Agency staffing in the OR has had an impact on outcomes, supporting administrative decisions to fill vacancies with agency nurses. Additional research is needed to study these and other nurse structural factors and their effect on patient care.

Source: Newhouse et al, 2005.

Method

In the method section, the researcher chooses the design of the study appropriate to answer the research question, the sample, the procedure, and the instruments and plans the analysis strategy to answer the questions. In this example, the study is a nonexperimental study using secondary data analysis. The sample was perioperative nurse directors or managers linked to corresponding hospital patient discharge data for 2000–2002 abstracted from a public use database for patients discharged post–abdominal aneurysm repair and aortic-iliac-femoral bypass.

Review of the PNDS guided the description of perioperative practice and subsequent outcomes. Survey items were constructed from nursing interventions of interest. Corresponding outcomes (surgical complications, length of stay, and mortality) were identified, along with linking ICD-9 codes that are available in secondary data. The outcomes included O2 – O8, "The patient is free from signs and symptoms of [physical] injury," and O11, "The patient has wound/tissue perfusion consistent with or improved from baseline levels established preoperatively." **Table 5-14** describes the ICD-9 codes that can be associated with the selected PNDS nursing outcomes.

Surveys were sent to hospital perioperative managers or directors (N=44) who were responsible for ORs from which patients had been discharged post–abdominal aneurysm repair and aortic-iliac-femoral bypass.

Results

The results section presents the analysis through descriptive and inferential statistics, with tables. Thirty-two hospitals responded (73%) representing 1894 patient discharges. The results are adjusted for age, gender, race, comorbidities, rupture, admitting code, extubation, and aortic surgery hospital volume. Complications and length of stay were not statistically significantly related to the percentage of RN agency use; however, the estimated odds of death decreased significantly per 10% increase in RN agency use (OR: 0.77, 95% CI: 0.63 to 0.94). Complications were significantly lower in hospitals where no RN night shift coverage is provided versus a night shift with scheduled assigned staff (OR: 0.54, 95% CI: 0.37 to 0.79). In addition, the estimated odds of complications or death are lower by approximately 8% per each 10% increase in the proportion of RNs with CNOR certification, although these results were not statistically significant.

Discussion

The discussion section includes implications of the study to clinicians, management, or policy makers and theoretical implications for future research. In this study, the background supported the premise that organizational structures and processes are the focus of performance improvement and research as opportunities to improve staff morale and patient safety. Through a nonexperimental design, survey data on nurse staffing variables were linked to corresponding outcomes based on the PNDS framework.

The results indicate that agency staffing in the OR has had an impact on outcomes, supporting administrative decisions to fill vacancies with agency nurses, and that a trend of higher nurse certification (CNOR) is associated with 8% to 10% improvement in complications, though not statistically significant. The implication is that additional research is needed to study these and other nurse structural factors and their effect on patient care. These include the relationship between certification in the OR and patient outcomes and empirical testing of PNDS nursing interventions and their relationship to outcomes.

FUTURE OPPORTUNITIES FOR PNDS USE

The PNDS has virtually unlimited utility for perioperative nurse researchers. Using a standard perioperative nomenclature guided by the concepts presented in the PNDS will build knowledge, allowing comparisons of outcomes between similar concepts. Each concept or variable can be used in a variety of designs. Examples of perioperative management, clinical, and education studies follow using the domain of Safety, Positioning injury.[5] **Table 5-15** specifies the PNDS domain, outcome, and selected nursing interventions.

Safety: Positioning Injury

Lower rates of hospital-acquired pressure ulcers are related to a higher proportion of RNs.[6] These research results have contributed to the support for hospital acquired pressure ulcers as a nurse-sensitive outcome.[7] Perioperative nurses assist with positioning, select positioning aids, assess the potential for risk, plan care, and complete an evaluation postoperatively within their delivery of care. There is virtually unlimited potential for research related to clinical, administrative, or education practice.

PNDS Nursing Diagnosis	Outcome Diagnostic Code and Description
The patient is free from:	**ICD-9-Diagnosis**
O2 – O8 Physical injury related to intended procedure O3 Physical injury related to chemical injury O4 Physical injury related to electrical injury O5 Physical injury related to positioning O6 Physical injury related to laser injury O7 Physical injury related to radiation injury O8 Physical injury related to transfer/transport	41511 Pulmonary Embolus And Infarction 4582 Iatrogenic Hypotension 5121 Iatrogenic Pneumothorax 9991 Air Embolism During The Procedure *E Codes* E8700–8709 Accidental Cut Or Puncture E8710–8719 Foreign Body Left In E8720–8729 Failure In Sterile Precautions E8740–8749 Instrument Failure E8750–8759 Contaminated Blood Fluid Drug Or Biological Substance
O10 Signs of infection	99851 Post Operative Infection 99859 Other Post Operative Infection 9993 Infection Related to Complication of Medical Care
O2 Physical injury related to extraneous objects	E871, E8710, E8711, E8712, E8713, E8714, E8715, E8716, E8717, E8718, E8719 Foreign Body Left In Wound

TABLE 5-14. PNDS Nursing Diagnoses Linked to ICD–9 Codes

TABLE 5-15: Risk for Impaired Skin Integrity		
PNDS Domain	PNDS Outcome	Selected Nursing Interventions
Safety: Positioning	The patient is free from signs and symptoms of injury related to positioning	• Identifies individuals at risk for positioning injury • Examines patient skin condition • Implements measures to prevent positioning injury

Clinical Research Opportunity

Consider that you are interested in determining whether a foam mattress or an alternative gel mattress reduces skin pressure in surgical patients who are positioned supine for more that 2 hours. Under the domain of Safety, Positioning Injury, the outcome is "The patient is free from signs and symptoms of injury related to positioning." The skin assessment should demonstrate hyperemia for less than 30 minutes. A variety of research designs could be used.

Experimental: Subjects will be randomized to one of two mattresses that will be used for their surgical procedure. A skin assessment will be conducted preoperatively, postoperatively and 30 minutes after admission to the PACU.

Quasiexperimental: Each of the two mattresses will be placed in a specific OR, and all subjects who have surgeries in those two rooms will be placed on the mattress assigned to that room. A skin assessment will be conducted preoperatively, postoperatively, and 30 minutes after admission to the PACU.

Nonexperimental: The two mattresses are used in the ORs. All records for patients who have had surgery for more than two hours in a supine position for a period of two months are reviewed. The type of mattress and skin assessment preoperatively, postoperatively, and in PACU are abstracted from the patient record and the mattresses compared.

Education Research Opportunity

Knowing that prevention of pressure ulcers is a nurse-sensitive outcome and that pressure ulcer rates are higher than expected in their facility, the leadership team decides to implement a training program for perioperative staff. Because perioperative staff members work multiple shifts seven days a week, it is often difficult to have all staff members complete training in a timely period. The leadership team is interested in conducting a research study because there is no evidence to support the benefit of a standard class or Web education strategies. The team decides to conduct research to test whether a Web education module is as effective as a class at improving the process of perioperative positioning.

Experimental: Nurses are recruited to join the study and then randomized to the standard education class on perioperative positioning or the Web class. Both groups complete a knowledge test related to positioning content preeducation and posteducation and demonstrate positioning in a simulation lab before and after education. Change in test scores and compliance with total positioning process steps is compared.

Quasiexperimental: Nurses from two different perioperative setting are compared. One setting receives standard education class and the second receives the Web class. Both groups complete a knowledge test related to positioning content preeducation and posteducation and demonstrate positioning in a simulation lab before and after education. Change in test scores and compliance with total positioning process steps are compared.

Nonexperimental: A local hospital that currently offers a Web class on perioperative positioning and one that offers standard education use the same test to evaluate the class. You compare the posttest scores, conduct an observation of the process steps, and compare total test and process scores.

Administrative Research Opportunity

A new pressure-relieving positioning device is now being marketed for high-risk patients. The problem is that it is expensive, not budgeted, and the cost effectiveness of the device is unknown. A study is conducted to determine whether the new device decreases skin pressure and whether it is cost effective.

Experimental: Subjects will be randomized to the standard positioning aids or the new device to be used for their surgical procedure. A skin assessment will be conducted of bony prominences preoperatively, postoperatively, 30 minutes after admission to the PACU, and day 5 postoperatively. Direct surgical time to position the subject will be measured. Outcomes are the occurrence of pressure ulcers by stage and the cost per case. Cost effectiveness will be assessed by the comparison of the number of pressure ulcers per dollar spent in each group.

Quasiexperimental: Two hospitals have the same protocol for positioning patients. One hospital will use the standard positioning aids and the second hospital will use the new device for the surgical procedure. A skin assessment will be conducted of bony prominences preoperatively, postoperatively, 30 minutes after admission to the PACU, and day 5 postoperatively. Direct surgical time to position the subject will be measured. Outcomes will be the occurrence of pressure ulcers by stage, the cost per case, and the rate of pressure ulcer development. Cost effectiveness will be assessed by the comparison of the number of pressure ulcers per dollar spent.

Nonexperimental: One hospital has used the new positioning device and is interested in comparing outcomes with a hospital that uses a standard positioning protocol. The research teams from both hospitals collaborate to compare outcomes by selecting specific surgical cases and reviewing medical records to determine whether there is a difference in the incidence of hyperemia on skin assessment during the immediate postoperative skin assessment.

Summary

These brief examples of potential research represent only one domain, Safety, and one outcome, "Freedom from positioning injury." They are presented with the understanding that all research requires Institutional Review Board review and approval. In addition, for the sake of brevity, only the design and variables were included. Multiple procedural steps in the research process were not included in the content, such as recruitment of subjects, subject consent, control variables, analysis, or specific measures. Multiple physiologic (pressure ulcer formation, hyperemia) and behavioral (demonstration and test scores) responses were presented that can be used as research dependent variables or outcomes.

Guided by the PNDS, the potential studies focused on nursing interventions to decrease the risk of impaired skin integrity (Nursing diagnosis X51). They were presented as a research example for perioperative nurses to demonstrate potential uses of the PNDS in research. Each domain of the PNDS (safety, physiol-

ogic responses, and behavioral responses) presents the same opportunity, including multiple nursing interventions and related patient outcomes. These relationships can be used to test nursing interventions that explain and predict specific patient outcomes.

CONCLUSION

This chapter described research opportunities to measure perioperative factors and subsequent outcomes using the PNDS as a conceptual framework. A research study was used as a research exemplar,[1] and one domain of the PNDS, "Safety: Positioning injury," was used to demonstrate potential research designs to test a variety of variables.

The opportunities for perioperative researchers are unlimited since the PNDS includes unique coding for perioperative nursing diagnosis and a conceptual framework that links perioperative outcomes with nursing interventions. This framework provides a rich source of practice-level theory.

Perioperative nurses provide value to patients through interventions that improve patient surgical outcomes. These quality outcomes represent patient clinical, experiential, and resource-based (eg, cost, length of stay) outcomes. Future work of perioperative researchers is critical to understand best practices, cost-effective care, and the value-added contribution of perioperative registered nurses. Using the PNDS as a conceptual framework for research will provide practice-level variables, advancing the science of perioperative nursing.

References

1. R P Newhouse, M Johantgen, P J Pronovost, E Johnson, "Perioperative nurses and patient outcomes—mortality, complications, and length of stay," *AORN Journal* 81 no 3 (2005) 508-525.

2. M W Stanton, M K Rutherford, *Hospital Nurse Staffing and Quality of Care* (Rockville, MD: Agency for Healthcare Research and Quality, 2004).

3. R P Newhouse et al, "The slippery slope: Differentiating between quality improvement and research," *JONA* 38 no 4 (2006) 211-219.

4. P H Mitchell, S Ferketich, B M Jennings, "Quality Health Outcomes Model," *Journal of Nursing Scholarship* 30 (1998) 43-46.

5. S Beyea ed, *Perioperative Nursing Data Set: The Perioperative Nursing Vocabulary,* second ed (Denver: AORN, 2002).

6. L Unruh, "Licensed nurse staffing and adverse events in hospitals," *Medical Care* 41 (2003)142-152.

7. The National Database of Nursing Quality Indicators (NDNQI), American Nurses Association, *http://www.nursing world.org/MainMenuCategories/ThePracticeofProfessional Nursing/PatientSafetyQuality/NDNQI/NDNQI_1.aspx* (accessed 10 Aug 2007).

EXEMPLAR 8: Helping
Perioperative Nurses Implement the PNDS

Health care today relies on communication among providers to maintain and improve patient safety and provide care. The emphasis on communication has created a growing need for nurses who are skilled in information management. Using technology for information management can save time and money, increase productivity, and improve communication. Computer technology may be incorporated into many areas, and experienced perioperative nurses are often recruited to industry to help hospitals and agencies implement purchased software that will facilitate patient data management, resource management, and interdisciplinary communication.

The standards for nursing informatics have been published by the American Nurses Association.[1] Roles are expanding in hospitals and in the corporate environment. In the hospital, informatics nurses serve as system administrators, project managers, superusers, and trainers. The corporate world offers informatics nurses opportunities as chief nursing officer, product specialist, implementation specialist, project manager, or consultant (see the sidebar "Nursing in the Corporate World").

Nurses interested in the field of informatics should begin with the basics. Computer classes using Windows Office products such as Word, Excel, Access, PowerPoint, and Outlook will benefit all nurses communicating in today's technical environment, and knowledge of them is essential to work in industry. Involvement in an interdisciplinary or departmental system selection committee will provide education and experience not only for information system selection, but also for the process improvement that can be accomplished in conjunction with implementation.

The purpose of this article is twofold. First, it will offer an introduction to the challenges for the nursing informatics professional assisting with the implementation of an OR information system (ORIS). Second, it will provide suggestions for the nurse who is interested in pursuing a career in this dynamic and expanding field.

Jessica L. White, RN, MSN, BC, CNOR
Senior Clinical Product Specialist
SIS – Surgical Information Systems
Alpharetta, Georgia

NEED FOR STANDARDIZED LANGUAGE

Over the years nursing professionals have highlighted the ubiquity of variation in practice and have urged clinicians to move toward evidence-based practice; however, a number of barriers have been identified. These include the rapid rate of medical knowledge development, inadequate access to clinically relevant information at the point of need, increased workload and patient complexity, and difficulty translating the evidence for use with a particular patient.

Perioperative nurses increasingly find themselves in the position of having to demonstrate that the RN has a positive impact on patient outcomes. The language used in nursing care documentation plays a crucial role in validating the effect nursing interventions have on patient outcomes. A standardized nursing language has become essential to ensure that the RN remains the patient advocate and care provider in the perioperative environment.

The PNDS, developed by AORN, can be used to measure and compare outcomes sensitive to nursing care. The usefulness, accuracy, and reliability of this standardized language will be used to plan interventions, measure outcomes, and report indicators that may be variable at any point on a continuum from most negative to most positive over time. Three points of data should be collected and reported to make evidence-based nursing practice usable. Those data points are patient problems (nursing diagnoses), nursing interventions, and outcome achievement.

The database of an information system provides the ability to query all of the data points to analyze intervention leading to positive and negative outcomes. Comparisons can be made over time for individual patients or groups of patients. Standardized language facilitates the ability for benchmarking, thereby establishing best practices.

AUTOMATING THE CARE PLAN

Writing care plans was probably the most dreaded activity faced by nursing students. It appears to be tedious paperwork that only increases sleepless nights. The PNDS takes the basic information taught in nursing programs and expands it into today's modern environment of perioperative services to standardize care, measure outcomes, and develop best practices using the nursing process experienced nurses learned so many years ago.

Nursing is a science performed with protocols and continual critical thinking. Planning care for surgical patients requires a unique body of knowledge that is difficult and time consuming to document. Critical thinking skills are essential for planning and delivery of care. Documentation of this care is crucial in today's environment for nurses to maintain autonomy, to receive recognition of responsibilities, and to develop best practices for patient care.

Perioperative patients experience both actual problems and potential problems. Actual problems with documented signs and symptoms can include inability to cope, hypothermia, and pain. Potential problems with no documented signs and symptoms have risk factors involved that are controlled by the nursing staff. Potential problems include anxiety, risk for injury, and infection and breakdown of skin integrity. Both actual and potential problems should be documented, monitored, and evaluated by the RN because he or she automatically manages these tasks every day. The PNDS provides the means to document, evaluate, and report on them.

One of the past problems with care plans was that they were usually documented separately in the areas of perioperative services (preoperative, intraoperative, and postoperative). An ORIS allows a plan of care initiated preoperatively to be updated and evaluated throughout the perioperative visit. Automation through an information system allows nurses to work more efficiently and managers to allocate resources more effectively while improving patient care. Automated clinical documentation can provide work lists to standardize planned nursing interventions, generate legible documentation, and

automate the selection of nursing care plans for designated groups of patients.

During the implementation of an ORIS, it is crucial to meet with clinical specialists and team leaders to develop a list of potential problems and automate the process of their documentation into the clinical record. The automation of documenting potential problems will decrease documentation time, increase face time with patients, and enhance nursing staff satisfaction with the documentation process. Actual problems are added individually.

NURSING IN THE CORPORATE WORLD

"So you're not a nurse anymore?" This is the question most frequently asked of the industry nurse by friends, family, and coworkers who have heard of the transition from working in the surgical environment daily to working for a perioperative software company.

The adamant answer should be that you are and always will be a registered nurse! Your professional focus, however, has now changed. The personal reward in the daily life of a perioperative nurse was the knowledge that one made a difference in someone's life with every nursing duty performed. Now, however, the work you do will have a positive long-term effect on patient care and improve the tools that perioperative nurses have to do their jobs more efficiently and effectively.

Say goodbye to the 7-to-3 shift with call! Your day can start as early as 6 AM and last until the airlines cooperate and you arrive home. Most corporate jobs require at least 50% travel, but 80% is hardly unusual. You may find yourself leaving on Sunday evening or early Monday morning and returning home on Thursday evening. Fridays are usually spent working remotely from home.

Your reward is the opportunity for travel and the people you meet along the way. Living in or near a city with a large airport and a number of flight options is essential. Becoming a frequent flyer on the airline of choice definitely has its perks. In addition to free tickets for family trips and vacations, there are potentially shorter security lines, upgrades to first class, and the ability to change flights at no cost to get home early. Selecting one hotel chain may add benefits such as upgrades and free nights.

If you love to travel, enjoy meeting new people, and look forward to a new challenge every day, working in industry may be the career you've always wanted. ◘

PROJECT MANAGEMENT AND IMPLEMENTATION

Process improvement or redesign knowledge is essential for optimal project management and implementation of an ORIS. Many hospitals and organizations offer courses in quality improvement. These classes will provide insight into outcomes-based accountability that is focused on the core goal of health care, which is patient care. Using the PNDS allows reporting of outcome data to be used in the planning and improvement of patient outcomes.

A well-implemented and fully used information system will provide hospital administrators the information they need to achieve excellence in patient care. The accuracy and distribution of collected information are components of knowledge management used to monitor and improve processes that support an organization's strategic objectives. Organizations should integrate an ORIS into their care processes.

Working With Vendors

Vendors need to gather essential knowledge of an organization's technological environment and strategic objectives to assist with project management. Current clinical information systems (CISs) in place will allow for discussions of possible interfaces needed to improve interdepartmental communication. What information is currently automated, such as scheduling of cases, preference card documentation, and charging, will provide the vendor with opportunities to identify processes that work and those that need improvement.

In addition, business and clinical objectives must be outlined in the beginning so they can be evaluated after implementation and afterward on an ongoing basis. Hospitals must spend time defining and outlining clinicians' and the organization's needs to select and design an ORIS that is compatible with desired clinical processes.

Role of the Project Manager

The project manager for perioperative services provides leadership and management of the perioperative component of the hospital-wide CIS project. The role involves assessment of current processes, planning and creating a vision for redesign, managing implementation and adoption of redesigned processes, and training and education. Communication with perioperative services and CIS team members is essential in this role.

Implementation of perioperative software is often a catalyst for process redesign. The project manager may act as the leader of the implementation team of clinical and technological experts in developing an implementation plan. An implementation plan will include goals and objectives to be accomplished within a developed time line. Technologically speaking, hardware installation must be organized, and information security and data integrity must be assured.

System preparation will focus on standardization with data definitions, integration of nursing languages, and file and table building. A successful ORIS implementation depends of the alignment of people, processes, and technology. Typical information collected includes procedures, personnel, material usage, case times, counts, diagnosis, drugs, event times, and the outcome of nursing interventions. Computerized documentation forms can be customized to offer continuity in current documentation processes in addition to developing uniform content and compliance with standardized documentation and clinical practice protocols.

Guiding the implementation of an ORIS will include setting expectations with the project manager who will be responsible for the development of new policies and procedures related to security, downtime, work processes, training, and test procedures. Training will involve program development for managers, end users, and new employees as well as refresher courses. Collaboration with managers and staff will provide input into the continual development of up-to-date instruction and user support. Self-directed learning manuals and computer-based training modules offer convenience to busy staff members who are willing to use them to study at home.

Managing Change

New policies, new equipment, and decreasing length of stays are common changes in today's health care environment. Nurses continue to be flexible and innovative in the face of change. Computers may push the limits of the surgical nurse's flexibility related to varying aptitudes of computer technology. The project manager of an ORIS must be prepared for panic and rebellion while implementing the organization's vision of automation. Recognition of that resistance to change will enable the leadership to move beyond the rebellion and consciously and constructively deal with the emotions associated with change.

HOW DO I GET STARTED?

The American Nurses Credentialing Center offers a certification in informatics for baccalaureate-prepared nurses. Three-day courses are available to assist in preparation for the certification exam. These courses also provide the basic information, terminology, and networking the nurse needs to begin the journey into the world of informatics. Exam topics may include:

I.   System Life Cycle
    A.   System planning
    B.   System analysis
    C.   System design
    D.   System implementation and testing
    E.   System evaluation, maintenance, and support

II. Human Factors
    A.   Ergonomics
    B.   Software and user interface

III. Information Technology
    A.   Hardware
    B.   Software
    C.   Communications
    D.   Data representation
    E.   Security

IV. Information Management and Knowledge Generation
    A.   Data
    B.   Information
    C.   Knowledge

V.   Professional Practice Trends and Issues
    A.   Roles
    B.   Trends and issues
    C.   Ethics

VI. Models and Theories
    A.   Foundations of nursing informatics
    B.   Nursing and health care data sets, classification systems, and nomenclatures
    C.   Related theories and sciences

Resources

American Nurses Association (ANA)
http://nursingworld.org

American Nurses Credentialing Center (ANCC)
http://www.nursecredentialing.org

American Nursing Informatics Association (ANIA)
http://www.ania.org

AORN Perioperative Nursing Informatics Specialty Assembly
http://www.aorn.org/Community/SpecialtyAssemblies

Nursing Informatics Online
http://www.informaticsnurse.com

Online Journal of Nursing Informatics
http://cac.psu.edu/~dxm12/OJNI.html   ◻

Evaluation

Evaluation of system implementation is crucial for improvement and strategic planning. Benefits related to return on investment, increased room utilization, enhanced communication, and patient safety should be documented. The benefits of implementing an ORIS are complex and extend beyond the individual patient, nurse, and perioperative unit. The CIS is part of a larger system of standardized documentation and provides a continuous flow of information. The goals of the CIS include being a repository for clinical data, providing clinical decision support, enhancing nursing practice, and validating clinical problem solving, all of which lead to improved patient care.

MAXIMIZING THE BENEFITS OF AN ORIS

The goals in using an ORIS are enhancing nursing practice, identifying clinical problem solving, and improving the quality of care. Additionally, a CIS is implemented to improve communication, standardize documentation, improve accuracy and accessibility of records, and increase compliance with agencies such as the Joint Commission, the US Department of Health and Human Services, and the US Food and Drug Administration.

Scheduling software allows facilities to manage their resources effectively to provide optimum patient care. The process scheduling can be standardized to improve information collection and increase room utilization. Clinical documentation minimizes documentation time while increasing face time with patients. Standardizing documentation will reduce operating costs and improve inefficiencies and inadequate communication.

Surgery software integrated with the CIS provides seamless access to complete patient information. All components of the plan of care may be standardized through the enterprise patient record. This complete record provides the nursing staff with the knowledge necessary to deliver appropriate, efficient, and cost-effective care. Incorporating PNDS into the ORIS provides the standardized data fields necessary to measure ongoing care and plan improvements and develop best practices.

References

1.   American Nurses Association. *Scope and Standards of Nursing Informatics Practice.* Silver Spring, MD: American Nurses Association, 2001.

Selected Resources for Chapter 5:
"Applying the PNDS in the Practice Setting"

Online

Agency for Healthcare Research and Quality (AHRQ)
http://www.ahrq.gov

American Association of Critical-Care Nurses
http://www.aacn.org

> *Synergy model:* http://www.certcorp.org/certcorp/cert corp.nsf/vwdoc/SynModel?opendocument#Basic%20 Informat

American College of Cardiovascular Nurses (ACCN)
Scope and Standards of Practice (2006):
http://www.accn.net/CVN%20Standards.htm

American Nurses Association (ANA)
http://nursingworld.org

> *COPA model:* http://www.nursingworld.org/Main MenuCategories/ANAMarketplace/ANAPeriodicals /OJIN/TableofContents/Volume41999/No3Sep30 /COPAModel.aspx

> *National Database of Nursing Quality Indicators (NDNQI):* http://www.nursingworld.org/Main MenuCategories/ThePracticeofProfessionalNursing /PatientSafetyQuality/NDNQI/NDNQI_1.aspx

American Nurses Credentialing Center (ANCC)
http://www.nursecredentialing.org

American Nursing Informatics Association (ANIA)
http://www.ania.org

American Society of PeriAnesthesia Nurses (ASPAN)
http://www.aspan.org

Association of PeriOperative Registered Nurses (AORN)
http://www.AORN.org

> *Perioperative Nursing Data Set (PNDS):* http://www.aorn.org/PracticeResources/PNDS

> *Perioperative Nursing Informatics Specialty Assembly:* http://www.aorn.org/Community/SpecialtyAssemblies /SpecialtyAssemblyGroups/PONISA

The Joint Commission on Accreditation of Health Care Organizations: http://www.jointcommission.org

> *Universal Protocol:* http://www.jointcommission.org /PatientSafety/UniversalProtocol/up_faqs.htm

> *Quality Check:* http://www.jointcommission.org /AccreditationPrograms/PublicityKit/about_qc_qr.htm

Institute of Medicine: *Health Care Quality Initiative*
http://www.iom.edu/focus on.asp?id=8089

The Leapfrog Group for Patient Safety
http://www.leapfroggroup.org

Medical Records Institute
http://www.medrecinst.com

National Quality Forum (NQF)
http://www.qualityforum.org

Nursing Informatics Online
http://www.informaticsnurse.com

Online Journal of Nursing Informatics
http://cac.psu.edu/~dxm12/OJNI.html

Society of Gastroenterology Nurses and Associates (SGNA)
http://www.sgna.org m

Print

Care quality: JCAHO launches 'new generation' of quality reporting. *Clinical Strategy Watch*. July 2004. The Advisory Board Company.

Competency statements in perioperative nursing. In *Standards, Recommended Practices, and Guidelines*. Denver, Colo: AORN, 2007, 21-95.

Kleinbeck SVM. *PNDS @ Work: Encouraging Periopera-tive Clinical Experiences*. Denver, CO: AORN, Inc. 2005.

McConnell E. Competence vs competency. *Nurs Manage*. 2001;32(5):14.

Newhouse RP, Johantgen M, Pronovost PJ, Johnson E. Peri-operative nurses and patient outcomes—mortality, compli-cations, and length of stay. *AORN J.* 2005;81(3):508-525.

Scope and Standards of Nursing Informatics Practice. Silver Spring, MD: American Nurses Association, 2001.

Sigsby L. A knowledge comparison of nursing students in perioperative vs other rotations. *AORN J.* 2004;80(4):699-707.

Sigsby L. Avoiding problems when establishing a student learning experience in perioperative nursing. *Nurse Educ*. 2003;28(1):1-2.

Sigsby L. Effective learning about the concept of pain from a perioperative clinical rotation. *Pain Manag Nurs*. 2001;2(1):19-24.

Standards of clinical nursing practice and role delineation statements. *Standards and Guidelines*. 2001. Society of Gastroenterology Nurses and Associates, Inc (SGNA).

Standards of perioperative professional practice. In *Standards, Recommended Practices, and Guidelines*. Denver, CO: AORN, Inc; 2007:433-436.

Stanton MW, Rutherford MK. Hospital nurse staffing and quality of care. Rockville, MD: Agency for Healthcare Research and Quality; 2004.

Unruh L. Licensed nurse staffing and adverse events in hospitals. *Med Care*. 2003;41:142-152.

## Chapter Six

The PNDS Dashboard:
Application in Surgical Department Management

Use of the Perioperative Nursing Data Set (PNDS) initially began with a focus on direct patient care clinical activities, such as developing documentation and patient care plans. The evolution of these led to development of competency statements, orientation plans, teaching plans, policy statements, and quality improvement reporting, all using the PNDS. It was a natural step for these activities to lead to more focused work on the application of PNDS in managing surgical departments and the development of structural data elements. This resulted in the development of the Perioperative Dashboard, a management tool, by these two authors.

THE MANAGER'S CHALLENGE

What perioperative nurses do in caring for patients is captured within the PNDS. The Perioperative Patient Focused Model (**Figure 6-1**) is a visual representation of the perioperative world, our circle of influence,

Renae N. Battié, RN, MN, CNOR
Director, Intraoperative Services
Swedish Medical Center
Seattle, Washington

Annette M. Dopp, RN, MBA, CNOR
Director of Perioperative Services
St. John's Hospital
Springfield, Illinois

that illustrates the activities involved in delivering care to perioperative patients. The PNDS is a language, enabling connections among a variety of activities in perioperative care using the outcome statements, whether the outcomes are used in competency statements, policies, or patient care plans (**Figure 6-2**). Imbedding these outcome statements as defined data points across various aspects of perioperative activities allows the profession to begin measuring effectiveness of these activities (**Figure 6-3**). For example, activities supporting O8, "Preventing injury," are articulated in the nurse's job description, competency statements, evaluations, patient care plans, and documentation, and ultimately are integrated into the outcomes measured in quality assurance reports and reflected in unit and institutional policies.

Perioperative nursing leaders face the numerous challenges associated with maintaining their unit's health by balancing the needs of staff members and physicians with the safety, health, and well-being of all their patients. The ability to track a particular set of activities across the patient care environment facilitates the ability for managers to measure effectiveness of resource utilization, both financial and human, in supporting various initiatives. In the past, managers have been able to measure an infection rate and report an overall staff cost without interconnecting these activities. Ultimately, use of the PNDS outcomes offers the ability to balance measures of financial activities with clinical activities and provide a picture of departmental "health," which is the job of the perioperative manager.

FIGURE 6-1: The Perioperative Patient Focused Model

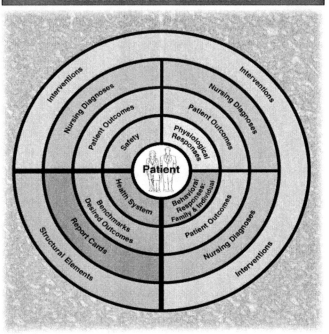

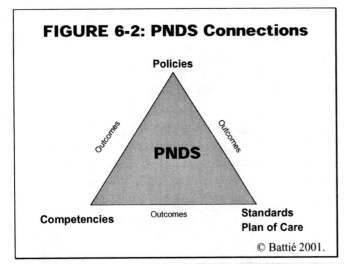

FIGURE 6-2: PNDS Connections

Policies

PNDS

Outcomes

Outcomes

Competencies   Outcomes   Standards
Plan of Care

© Battié 2001.

DEVELOPING THE PNDS DASHBOARD:

BACKGROUND

With the PNDS Health Systems Domain[1] and the Balanced Scorecard Model,[2] pertinent quality indicators can be displayed in a dashboard format and trended over time. The key is to balance clinical, operational, institutional, and financial indicators and learn how each of the indicators correlate. By linking clinical outcomes to health system outcomes, the overall quality of care can be monitored. Data analysis of quality measures can then serve as benchmarks and report cards.[3]

The PNDS Benchmark Database Task Force was charged by the AORN Board of Directors to develop a tool for OR managers and directors to study these indicators in a balanced scorecard approach and to make that tool available in a Web-based format. The objectives of the PNDS Dashboard included

- describing the PNDS Dashboard as a balanced outcomes tool,
- describing the indicators to be measured in quadrants,
- describing trends identified through the data that has been collected, and
- discussing the next steps in repository development to document the impact of the perioperative nurse on patient outcomes.

The original data elements were identified by a review of literature and the PNDS reference book,[1] conducting exploratory task force research, and soliciting expert opinion. The authors developed a dashboard model, the Battié-Dopp Model, as a way to illustrate how key quality, operational, institutional

and financial elements must be in balance for a healthy perioperative unit (**Figure 6-4**).

The dashboard was developed with the intent of being a visual tool to "see" the balance between the clinical and financial "health" of a surgical department. After developers surveyed a panel of experts, data elements that were commonly used in tracking departmental activities were identified and prioritized by importance, occurrence, and value. Definitions were developed for each of these elements (**Figure 6-5**) and were validated by task force members of the original project, as well by means of the results of 1000+ surveys sent to AORN managers and 151 surveys that were completed. The majority of the respondents (46%) were from metropolitan hospital settings. In addition, 29% were from rural hospitals, 17% from freestanding ambulatory surgery centers, and the remainder from hospital-based ambulatory surgery settings, industry, and "other" categories. Hospitals from all across the United States were represented.

Each data definition was validated by asking the following questions:

1. Is this definition easily understood?
2. Will collection of this data field be useful for data analysis?
3. Do you collect this data point?
4. How are you currently collecting this data?

The acceptable responses for the first three questions were *Yes, No,* or *Not Sure.* The acceptable responses for the fourth question included department spreadsheet, written administrative report, computerized database report, hand calculation, and *other—please specify.*

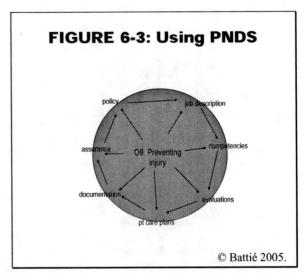

FIGURE 6-3: Using PNDS

policy   job description

assurance

O8 Preventing injury

competencies

documentation

evaluations

pt care plans

© Battié 2005.

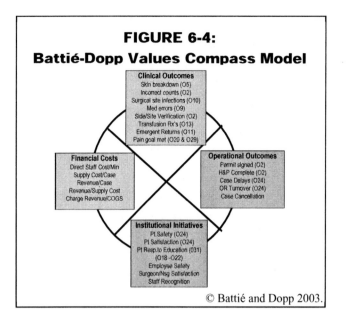

FIGURE 6-4:
Battié-Dopp Values Compass Model

© Battié and Dopp 2003.

The participating respondents overwhelmingly accepted the data definitions (**Figure 6-5**) for clarity at a rate of 98%. The majority (87%) of the respondents believed the data element was useful for data analysis but surprisingly, only 62% of the respondents were currently collecting the information on a regular basis. Most of the financial and case statistics information was collected in a formalized report of some kind and the clinical outcomes were usually collected by hand calculation.

The survey demonstrated that the members polled generally accepted the PNDS Dashboard elements. The definitions developed by the task force are clear and accepted as valid. The membership polled accepts the elements as pertinent information but are not necessarily tracking the indicator at their institution for some reason. This would indicate that further work of the task force should include practical application of the information being collected to demonstrate the usefulness of the data and motivate participants to collect the information in the clinical setting.

The AORN Board of Directors supported the development of this balanced outcomes tool towards the original PNDS goal of creating a repository of data, with the goal of validating the role of the perioperative nurse in quality patient care. With this in mind, a Web-based tool was developed that would allow remote entry of the data points by qualified participants. This was the first step towards actively growing the data repository. Revisions were made based on reviewers comments in 2004 and applied to

the Dashboard tool for use in the Perioperative Dashboard project. (The complete table of definitions is shown in **Exhibit 6-A** at the end of this chapter.)

The Task Force successfully launched a Web-based tool[4] that serves as a national database allowing members to benchmark their facility's health system data against averages for similar health care facilities. It allows internal as well as external analyses of an institution's performance that can be trended over time. Monitoring quality measures permits managers to make data-driven decisions that will lead to improved patient care. The use of the PNDS language encourages consistent and accurate documentation of outcomes data that can be shared between institutions.

DASHBOARD PROJECT DATA ENTRY

To participate in this project, AORN members complete online application on the AORN website. While it is helpful to be a manager or a director, it is not essential. Participants must have support from their facility, both in signing the confidentiality agreement as well as for the resource time involved in participating.

After signing a confidentiality agreement, each participant is given a unique login and a URL that will allow secure connection to the PNDS Dashboard system. AORN uses 128-bit encryption technology via an SSL certificate provided by Thawte, a leader in the Internet encryption industry. The PNDS database that stores the PNDS Dashboard data is protected by a state-of-the-art hardware firewall that prevents any access from the Internet directly to the database.

FIGURE 6-5:
Clinical Data Definitions

Quality Indicator	Data Source	Calculation	Benchmark (Goal)
Incorrect count	#Case records #Reported inj	#Injuries/#CR's	0%
Surgical Site Infection	#Case records #Reported infections	#Infections/#CR's	0%
Medication Error	#Case records #Med-errors	#Errors/#CR's	0%
Transfusion Reaction	#Case Records #Reported incidents	#Incidents/#CR's	0%
Side Site Verification	#Case Records audited #Incorrect documentation	#Incorrect doc/ #CR's audited	0%
Pain Documentation	#Case Records audited #Incomplete documentation	#Inc Doc/#CR's	0%
Pain Goal Met	#Case Records audited #Unsatisfactory Pain Goal scores	#Poor Scores/ #CR's audited	0%

Every new participant must provide demographic information specific to the hospital (**Figure 6-6**). A tutorial is available to participating hospitals that describes the project and the process of data entry. Data elements are described and defined for each data field, and minimum required fields are identified. (**Figure 6-7**) These required fields are necessary for supporting the standard reports available through the Web site. Participants must be able to provide the minimum required data fields to participate. Questions about data fields during data entry can also be answered merely by clicking on the description, which brings up the window with the actual field definition. Each data field has specified ranges that minimize erroneous entry and equations that set up the reporting abilities.

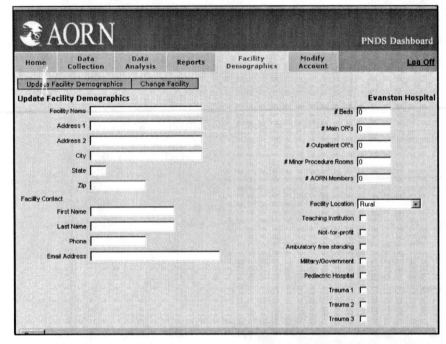

FIGURE 6-6: Demographic Information Required

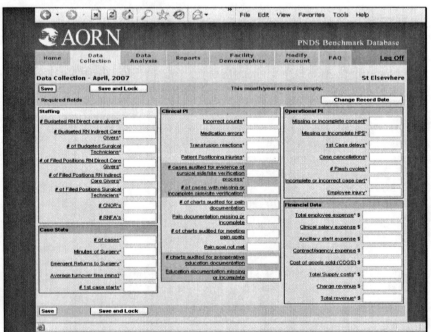

FIGURE 6-7: Minimum Required Data Fields

Trend data for the participant is available in a tracking tool that shows all data entered by month (**Figure 6-8**, below left). Once data has been entered, the reports tab (**Figure 6-9**, below right) can be selected to view information by specific field by looking at a matrix of incident rates in percentage as well as report charts The reports are for both internal (ie, trends within one's own hospital) and external (ie, comparative trends across the group participants) information. Report filters can be used to further refine data comparisons, such as hospital size, type, location, ambulatory, etc.

Care has been taken to protect individual hospital identity, particularly with quality improvement data. External data is available only in aggregate so the hospital's individual data is protected.

Tools available for participants include the tutorial, the data definition table (as well as the online link from each individual field), a frequently asked questions site (one is available on the public website, and additional items are available for actual participants), as well as an email link for additional questions. Monthly conference calls allow participants to ask questions and share challenges of gathering data. In August 2007, there were 88 participating facilities of a variety of sizes and types. Applications to participate continue to increase (**Figure 6-10**).

Once data for the month is completed and reviewed, the participant must "lock" the data, signifying it is complete and available for external reports. Participants may choose to enter data over

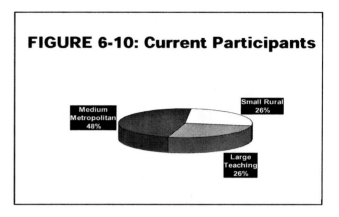

FIGURE 6-10: Current Participants

time or edit previous data by "saving" but not "locking" their data. Prior to locking the data, the data is only usable for internal reports and graphs. Participants are able to put in data over a five-month period of time. If data has not been locked within five months, the data will be lost. This has been done so that participants can reliably know when external data is available to them and those types of reports will have the most complete data included.

IMPLEMENTATION: UNDERSTANDING CORRELATION OF DATA ELEMENTS

So, how does a manager decide what he or she needs to be concentrating on? What are the quality indicators that should be measured on a consistent basis and trended over time? What indicators need to be monitored when a change is initiated?

Active development of both internal and external reports is ongoing, as the data repository grows. Examples of reports are shown in the following scenarios.

FIGURE 6-8: Data Entered by Month

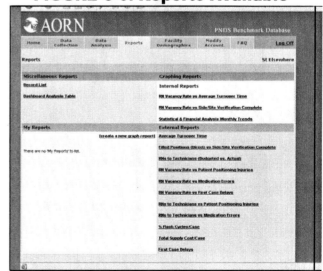

FIGURE 6-9: Reports Available

Scenario #1

The OR director is asked to review employee expense and eliminate unfilled RN positions to reduce costs. Each decision has an effect on the business as a whole and more importantly on the care that is given to the patient.

Topics to consider:

- Financial indicator—What are the overall cost savings?

- Operation indicator—What is the impact on efficiencies of this change?
  - How would a change in traffic flow affect surgical site infection rates?

- Quality indicator—What is the impact on quality of care on patient outcomes due to this change?
  - What would the effect of concentrating on decreasing turnover time do to the incidence of patient errors?

Dashboard reports available:

- Average turnover time could be used as an operational indicator here because reducing staff could impact this activity (**Figure 6-11**).

- RN Vacancy rate could be used as either another operational indicator or a quality indicator to plot against the average turnover time and see the trend—ie, how this rate tends to affect turnover time already, and therefore the anticipated trend of this proposal (**Figure 6-12**).

- RN Filled positions trended against accurate documentation of the Universal Protocol for site identification, a very important quality monitor, could be used to see the impact on quality of care with this change (**Figure 6-13**).

All of these are standard charts that are available on the PNDS Dashboard Web site and that can be used by the participants with this scenario.

Scenario #2

The OR director has now justified keeping these RN positions open, but is asked to consider skill mix change for potential cost savings.

Topics to consider:

- Financial indicator—What are the overall cost savings?

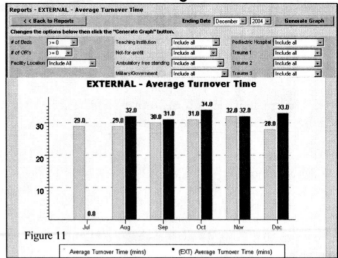

FIGURE 6-11: Average Turnover Time

Figure 11

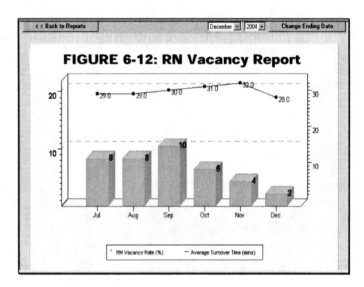

FIGURE 6-12: RN Vacancy Report

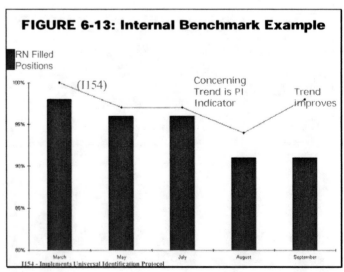

FIGURE 6-13: Internal Benchmark Example

- Operational indicator—What is the impact on efficiencies?

- Quality indicator—What is the impact on quality of care due to changing the RN to Tech ratio?

Dashboard reports available:

- Budgeted to Actual RN-to-technician ratios would be helpful in evaluating one's site against institutions of similar size and activity for potential changes (**Figure 6-14**).

- Surgical Site verification would be useful in tracking the potential impact of decreasing RN ratios on quality of care.

Scenario #3

An institution invests in new improved technology like state-of-the-art minimally invasive surgery equipment.

Topics to consider:

- Financial indicator
  - o Will patient length of stay decrease?
  - o Will it result in increased case volume?

- Operational indicator
  - o What impact will the technology have on length of case and block schedules?
  - o How will staff be trained to handle the technology?
  - o What surgeon training is necessary?

- Quality indicator
  - o Will patient outcomes improve?
  - o How will patients and their families respond?

One of the simplest examples correlating the data elements collected in the benchmark database was a trend noted by a participating site studying the institutional indicator of RN vacancy rate (trended over time) and the quality indicator of side/site verification documentation (**Figure 6-13**). As the vacancy rate went up, the documentation of side/site verification trended down. By monitoring this trend and instituting staff education as a performance improvement project—the documentation of the universal protocol for side/site verification improved. Even though the staffing indicator did not quite recover, the site was able to improve their performance with side/site verification and perhaps decrease the risk of wrong site surgery.

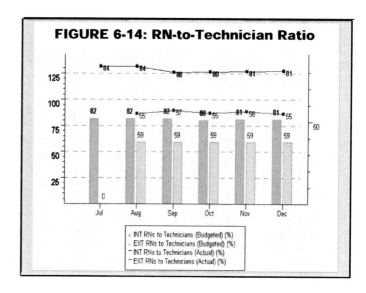

FIGURE 6-14: RN-to-Technician Ratio

Another correlation that can be observed when looking at the RN-to-Tech ratio and turnover time (**Figure 6-12**). Though this is difficult to study as an internal trend because an institution's RN-to-Tech ratio does not usually fluctuate dramatically, one can benchmark performance with like facilities and see the effect of the percentage of RNs on turnover time statistics.

Trending financial indicators has been widely accepted and published in the literature.[5] This allows managers to monitor their fiscal performance, budget for future growth, and monitor increases in supply costs and can help identify errors in financial reports. Commonly studied financial ratios include supply revenue vs cost of goods sold, patient revenue or cost per statistical activity, and total revenue vs total expense.

FUTURE DEVELOPMENT OF THE PERIOPERATIVE DASHBOARD

Future enhancements of the PNDS Dashboard include the ability to enter by uploading a local spreadsheet and separating reports by divisions of a single institution, such as the main OR and the ambulatory OR's within one facility. Another enhancement to come is the ability to leave an internal note attached to a month or a data field, for instance when an OR was down due to construction for a period of time and data is affected.

Additional data fields to include may be refinement of employee safety indicators (splitting out body fluid exposures from on-the-job injuries, for instance), surgical site infection indicators (antibiotic timing, normothermia, glucose control). Additional report development would then be able to track the RN's impact on some of these measures as well.

Future Web-based tools to be explored are a case costing model that would align standard definitions across the various software programs at institutions, profitability studies, and report cards. All of these tools are available within some software programs or institutions, but what the PNDS and this project does for them is allow standardized definitions and models that support accurate comparison and modeling across institutions. It also helps further build the data repository about the importance of perioperative nursing care that underscores all of this work.

As this data repository grows and matures, the research arm of AORN becomes increasingly important as a partner in working alongside this project. Many of the questions and interests of the profession have been hampered by lack of access to data, and this repository truly helps make that dream available. Discussions have begun with the AORN Research Committee to explore directions in this project that would enhance research interests from other areas as well.

SUMMARY

The PNDS is not only a valuable tool for our clinical practice but also an important part of the language set for perioperative nursing leaders. The PNDS is the language of the activities that perioperative nurses do every day. While it certainly covers clinical activities, the understanding of the health systems quadrant is just beginning to grow with the Perioperative Dashboard project, and this will enhance our understanding as a profession of the interaction of clinical and financial indicators.

Using the PNDS supports standardized data gathering that can help individual institutions in viewing balanced outcomes for various initiatives and departmental health. Utilizing a standardized language set when developing quality indicators is an important element to allow for sharing of data between institutions The Perioperative Dashboard project supports the profession in developing a data repository that will enhance our understanding of the value of the perioperative nurse in influencing outcomes. It is an important journey for the perioperative profession, but most of all for perioperative patients who will benefit from these efforts.

Thanks to Susan Kleinbeck, RN, PhD, CNOR, for encouragement and support in finishing this article, and to our many PNDS colleagues who sharpen our work.

References

1. S Beyea, ed,. *Perioperative Nursing Data Set: The Perioperative Nursing Vocabulary,* second ed (Denver: AORN, 2002).

2. R N Battié, A Dopp, "Using the Perioperative Dashboard/ PNDS to demonstrate the RN's impact on outcomes," presentation at the 51st AORN Congress, March 22, 2004, San Diego, Calif.

3. S V M Kleinbeck, A Dopp, "The Perioperative Nursing Data Set—A new language for documenting care," *AORN Journal* 82 no 1 (July 2005) 51-57.

4. "Perioperative Nursing Data Set," *AORN Online, http:// www.aorn.org/PracticeResources/PNDS* (accessed 5 Sept 2007).

5. R S Kaplan, R.S. & D P Norton, D. P. "The balanced scorecard: Measures that drive performance," *Harvard Business Review* 70 no 1 (January-February 1992) 71-79. Reprint #92105.

EXHIBIT 6-A: Data Field Definitions

DATA FIELD	DATA INPUT DEFINITIONS
Staffing	
# Budgeted RN Direct caregivers	Total # of budgeted RN FTEs that touch patient and give direct patient care. This includes but is not limited to in-room RNs and float RNs.
# Budgeted RN Indirect Caregivers	Total # of budgeted indirect RN FTEs (eg, RN manager, educator). If the RN manager is required to provide patient care greater than 50% of the time the full FTE should be included with direct care givers FTE. If less than 50% of time is spent on direct patient care, the full FTE should be counted as indirect. (The # of budgeted direct RNs + the # of budgeted indirect RNs = total # of budgeted RN FTEs.)
# Budgeted Surgical Technicians	Total # of budgeted Surgical Technician FTEs at the patient bedside and/or scrub in for procedures. (The total # of budgeted RN FTEs + # of budgeted surgical technicians = total # of budgeted clinical FTEs.)
# of Filled Positions RN Direct Care Givers	Total # of actual filled RN FTEs that touch patient and give direct patient care. This includes but is not limited to in-room RNs and float RNs. This includes hospital employees and contract RNs such as travel nurses.
# of Filled Positions RN Indirect Care Givers	Total # of actual filled indirect RN FTEs (eg, RN manager, educator). If the RN manager is required to provide patient care greater than 50% of the time the full FTE should be included with direct care givers FTE. If less than 50% of time is spent on direct patient care, the full FTE should be counted as indirect. (The # of filled direct RNs + the # of filled indirect RNs = total # of filled RN FTEs) This includes hospital employees and contract RNs such as travel nurses.
# of Filled Positions Surgical Technicians	Total # of actual filled Surgical Technician FTEs that scrub in for procedures. (The total # of filled RN FTEs + # of filled surgical technicians = total # of filled clinical FTEs.)
# CNOR	# of CNORs on staff.
# RNFA	# of RNFAs within department employed by the facility. If .25% of RN FTE time is spent as an RNFA then include .25 FTE for RNFA calculation.
Case Stats	
# of cases	# of cases performed per month. This is the actual number of individual patients having surgery performed. Multiple procedures performed on one patient are counted as one case.
Minutes of Surgery	Total minutes of surgery time for month is calculated by using patient in room (PIR) to patient out of room (POR).
Emergent returns to surgery	Total number of emergency unplanned return visits to the operating room within 48 hours after POR for initial surgery.
Average turnover time (minutes)	Time PIR for patient #2 minus time POR for patient #1 (average for your facility). *Calculated only between cases scheduled to follow each other.*
# 1st case starts	First cases of the day are defined as the cases scheduled to start at the beginning of the institution's business day. The time the OR or procedure room is available to schedule the first case is outlined by the facility's operational plan (eg, 7:30 or 8 AM) and the number of business days in the month. Example: If the first cases are staggered between 7:30 and 8 AM, all cases scheduled to start during this time are "first cases"—a 9 AM or later start in this scenario would not be counted as a first case. If the department is open for scheduled cases on Saturday, the first cases from the number of rooms utilized that month will need to be added to the total number of first case starts that month. (If Saturdays are only for emergent or urgent unscheduled cases, do not include in the calculation.)
Financial Data	
Total employee salary expense	Total salaries per month as reported on financial report. This includes benefits and should equal the sum of the clinical, ancillary, and contract agency expenses.
Clinical salary expense	Total salary expense for clinical staff = direct patient care and indirect (eg, management, educators) RNs and technicians.

EXHIBIT 6-A: Data Field Definitions (continued)

DATA FIELD	DATA INPUT DEFINITIONS
Ancillary staff expense	Salaries and benefits for non clinical staff.
Contract/agency expense	Expense for contract agency use. (eg, RNs and technicians).
Cost of goods sold (COGS)	Total cost of patient charge items. This is what was paid to the vendor to get the item charged to the patient. (eg, implants or any charge item).
Total supply costs	Total supply costs (includes COGS and all supplies).
Charge revenue (supply)	Revenue from supply charges.
Total revenue	Actual total gross revenue.
Clinical Performance Improvement	
Incorrect counts	# of incorrect counts for month as reported through internal QA.
Medication errors	# of medication errors occurring in the OR and reported through internal QA per month.
Transfusion reactions	# of reported transfusion reactions for month reported through QA per month.
Patient Positioning injuries	# of patient positioning injuries reported through QA per month.
# Cases audited for evidence of surgical side/ site verification process	# of patient charts audited for evidence of surgical side and site verification process as described in facility policy.
# of cases with missing or incomplete side/site verification	The number of case with missing or incomplete side/site verification (eg, documentation, observation).
# of charts audited for pain documentation	# of patient charts audited for pain documentation.
Pain documentation missing or incomplete	# of patient charts missing or incomplete documentation of pain assessment.
# of charts audited for meeting pain goals	# of patient charts audited for meeting pain goals.
Pain goal not met	# of unsatisfactory pain goal scores; pain score is less than adequate (assumes pain scale used).
# charts audited for preoperative education documentation	# charts audited for preoperative education documentation.
Education documentation missing or incomplete	# of charts missing or incomplete documentation of preop education for the month.
Operational Performance Improvement	
Missing or incomplete consent	# of missing or incomplete consents for the month.
Missing or Incomplete H&Ps	# of missing, incomplete and/or out of date H&Ps for the month.
1st case delays	# of first case delays greater than 10 minutes per month (patient in the room greater than 10 minutes after scheduled start time).
Case cancellations (Same Day)	# of cases canceled on the day of surgery for the month.
# Flash cycles	# of flash sterilization cycles for the month.
Incomplete or incorrect case cart	# of incomplete or incorrect case carts for the month.
Employee injury	# of staff injuries reported for the month.

A Brief History of the Perioperative Nursing Data Set

AORN, the Association of periOperative Registered Nurses, is a professional organization of 40,000 nurses committed to providing cost-effective, quality perioperative nursing care. Since 1993, members of AORN have been involved in activities to describe, define, and establish a data set that represents perioperative nursing practice. The organization's initial goal was to develop a unified language so that nursing care could be systematically quantified, coded, and easily captured in a computerized format in the perioperative setting. The ultimate goal was to help perioperative nurses achieve recognition and reimbursement for their unique knowledge, skills, and contributions to perioperative patient outcomes.

This project was originally organized and directed by the AORN Task Force on Perioperative Data Elements (1993–1995). The initial charge of the Task Force was to describe, define, and develop the data elements of perioperative nursing practice that describe nursing practice. From 1995 to 1998, that work was continued by the Data Elements Coordinating Committee (DECC). The cumulative result of these efforts was the Perioperative Nursing Data Set (PNDS).

In February 1999, the PNDS received recognition from the American Nurses Association (ANA) Committee on Nursing Practice Information Infrastructure as a data set useful in the practice of nursing. The PNDS is a clinically relevant and empirically validated standardized nursing language. It consists of data elements that are clearly defined, common to all cases, and consistent across time. The data set relates to the delivery of care in the perioperative setting at any point in time and is appropriate for use in any surgical setting.

BACKGROUND

An awareness of the need for a database describing perioperative nursing began in 1988 with the AORN Critical Issues Committee. The organization's Project 2000 evaluation initiative and the Project Team on the Effectiveness Initiatives both supported this same premise. A four-year organizational evaluation clearly demonstrated the need to identify the relationship of nursing interventions to patient outcomes and the need for a database capable of providing evidence of the value of the perioperative nurse during a patient's surgical experience. To achieve these goals, the AORN Board of Directors established the Task Force on Perioperative Data Elements in November 1993. Fourteen expert perioperative nurses, including staff nurses, nurse managers, computer/informatics specialists, and nurse scientists, began the process of defining the elements of the database.

After a review of existing standardized languages, the Task Force members determined that perioperative nursing practice was not adequately or fully addressed in any available nursing languages or data sets. Task Force members concluded that the North American Nursing Diagnosis Association (NANDA) Taxonomy was the only standardized language that reflected many of the phenomena of concern to perioperative nurses. The NANDA Taxonomy, however, addressed only the diagnostic step of the nursing process and did not address or identify many nursing diagnoses or etiologies pertinent to perioperative practice. Since that time, a number of languages have evolved and have been more inclusive of the roles and responsibilities of the perioperative nurse. The PNDS, however, is the only nursing data set that has the single focus of perioperative nursing and addresses the contributions of professional registered nurses to the care of patients undergoing surgical or invasive procedures.

AORN's development of a standardized language was an important first step toward formally defining the professional roles and contributions of perioperative registered nurses. These roles and responsibilities were often embedded in the clinical practice of perioperative nurses and had not been consistently articulated, formalized, or described in practice settings. Although the nursing process served as the foundation for the provision of nursing care, perioperative nurses had not consistently made those contributions explicit in a formal nursing care plan. In fact, many perioperative nurses struggled with describing how a nursing presence in perioperative settings contributed to positive patient outcomes.

Task Force members believed that a standardized nursing language would provide a structured vocabulary and, thus, a common means of communication. An essential part of the process was identifying terms that were clear, precise, and consistent and that described nursing care in the perioperative setting. Another critical step was explicating the dimensions of professional nursing practice in the perioperative setting. The work of Task Force members was guided by the premise that language development would help perioperative nurses document the care they gave while providing a foundation for examining and evaluating the quality and effectiveness of that care.

Despite high levels of commitment, task force members initially struggled with the conceptualization and meaning of a data element in perioperative practice. Confusion arose from an absence of clear definitions for terms commonly associated with standardized nursing languages. In addition, no other nursing clinical specialty had traversed a similar pathway related to language development. Task Force members carefully and systematically evaluated each step of the process in the context of extant knowledge related to language development. The group proceeded with a full awareness that, although the goals were clear, their course had not been fully mapped.

Initially, the Task Force conducted a systematic review of existing background materials on perioperative nursing practice. The group also agreed on four specific goals, strategies to achieve those goals, and an action plan. Using the consensus process, expert opinion, and extant knowledge, the group established definitions to guide their work activities (**Exhibit A-1**). Next, the group decided to develop a unified data set, rather than a uniform data set, which allowed various terms to be used for the same or similar activities (eg, bovie versus cautery).

The task force accepted the recommendations of Harriet Werley, RN, PhD, FAAN, and colleagues to extend the Medicare Uniform Hospital Discharge Data Set, so the framework chosen for data collection and language development was the Nursing Minimum Data Set (NMDS).[1] Task Force members chose four key components of the NMDS on which to focus future work, which included nursing diagnoses, nursing interventions, nursing outcomes, and intensity of nursing care.

The DECC recognized the need for standardized languages for computerized records and validation of outcome effectiveness. Committee members were dedicated to the premise that uniform systematic

computerized records of perioperative nurse/patient activities must be available and accessible for perioperative nursing to be visible to administrators, financial officers, health care policy makers, and others. The group adopted the motto of Norma Lang, RN, PhD, FAAN, FRCN, "If we cannot name it, we cannot control it, finance it, teach it, research it, or put it into public policy."[2]

A standardized language consists of a collection of data elements. In the PNDS, the data elements include perioperative nursing diagnoses, interventions, and patient outcomes. Subcommittee efforts also addressed related data elements such as structural definitions. A data element is a "unit of data for which the definition, identification, representation, and permissible values are specified by means of a set of attributes."[3] Data elements are characterized by being the smallest unit of information that retains meaning (eg, a raw fact, material, observation). Each data element is a discrete component that describes the concept without requiring further interpretation or information.

Data elements allow for standardization of a language and also permit the language to be managed in an electronic format. Patient-specific information in the medical record is a database that consists of data elements. Defining data elements allows information to be managed in computer software and automated databases. The DECC focused on identifying data elements that defined and described nursing activities that contribute to patient outcomes in the perioperative setting. When these individual data elements were combined, they provided the framework for the PNDS.

DATA ELEMENTS COORDINATING COMMITTEE

In 1995, the AORN Board of Directors accepted the work of the Task Force on Perioperative Data Elements. Committed to continuing the project, the Board of Directors then created the DECC, which then created four subcommittees, each charged with examining, defining, and validating a component of the PNDS:
- diagnoses,
- interventions,
- outcomes, and
- structural elements (previously intensity of care).

A fifth subcommittee was formed to address clinical practice guidelines. The work of this additional subcommittee was reported to the DECC and AORN Board of Directors, but was not integral to the language development efforts.

Before initiating work on the data set, Task Force members and DECC members defined terms and agreed to a general framework to explore and develop each nursing element. The content validity and reliability process for these initiatives included

- a review of the published and nonpublished nursing and non-nursing literature, as well as AORN documents related to each component;
- an examination of perioperative nursing practice—current and predicted future;
- a process for determining inter-rater reliability for accepted terms and definitions;
- a validation study with experienced perioperative nurses as respondents; and
- an integrated product that reflected the specific component that would interface with the other final documents prepared by the subcommittees.

Each subcommittee accepted their various assignments and began the process that led to the eventual development of the PNDS, its subsequent refinements, and submission to the ANA for recognition. The consistent presence of AORN staff members and volunteers ensured that there was continual feedback to all involved on the project and to the AORN Board of Directors.

NURSING DIAGNOSES DATA ELEMENTS

In 1995, the Nursing Diagnoses Subcommittee of the DECC was convened to identify the nursing diagnoses of concern for perioperative nurses. The primary objective of this subcommittee was to identify the clinical judgments that are integral to perioperative nursing practice. To accomplish this, the subcommittee members first developed an operational definition of nursing diagnosis for perioperative nurses using the consensus process. The resulting definition follows:

A nursing diagnosis is a concise clinical judgment label of a perioperative patient problem formulated for the purpose of directing nursing actions intended to achieve the expected outcomes.[4]

After thoughtful consideration and deliberation, the group excluded a phrase from NANDA's definition, "for which the nurse is solely responsible," because of the high degree of teamwork and collaboration in the perioperative arena.

Following that effort, subcommittee members conducted a systematic review of the literature, including the *AORN Journal;* other nursing journals; all current perioperative textbooks; and related psychology, sociology, education, and physical therapy references. That review included pertinent perioperative literature published within the last 10 years and yielded more than 100 perioperative nursing diagnoses that were mentioned at least once in the literature. Based on the context and frequency of each diagnosis in the literature, the Nursing Diagnoses Subcommittee members agreed that only 60 of the identified diagnoses were pertinent to perioperative nursing practice.

The subcommittee members designed and mailed a survey to AORN members in an effort to validate this list of 60 diagnoses. The instrument included the subcommittee's definition for the term *nursing diagnosis* and a definition for each of the diagnostic categories to minimize the risk of personal interpretation by participants. Survey respondents were asked to rank the frequency that each nursing diagnosis occurred on a daily basis in their practice using a scale of one to five, rating items from "never" to "almost all of the time." They also were asked to rank the priority they assigned to that specific patient problem on a scale of one to five from "never needs attention" to "demands immediate attention of the nurse" (eg, a life-threatening situation).[5]

Based on the responses to the frequency and priority, a weighted mean score was calculated for each diagnosis. Using the weighted mean scores, diagnoses were classified as to whether they were

- critical to patient outcomes (ie, occurring in more than half the patients on a daily basis with a high priority for immediate nursing attention);
- primary perioperative nursing diagnoses (ie, occurring in less than half the patients with a moderate to high priority for nursing attention); or
- secondary perioperative nursing diagnoses (ie, occurring in less than half the patients with a low to moderate priority for nursing attention).

The weighted mean scores were used to develop weighted diagnostic labels (**Table A-1**). From this analysis, the nursing diagnoses "risk of perioperative position injury" and "risk of infection" emerged as the only two diagnoses in the high frequency, high priority critical category. The second tier of this ranking procedure categorized low frequency, high priority diagnoses as "primary." A total of 24 diagnoses were identified in this subset. Examples include pain, neurovascular dysfunction, risk of aspiration, risk of injury, hypothermia, and impaired gas exchange. When these diagnoses occur in the perioperative arena, they pose a physical threat to the surgical patient and can result in untoward patient outcomes. These diagnoses represent the foundation of perioperative nursing practice and require nursing intervention when observed.[4]

The final tier of this classification process reflected "secondary diagnoses." These 34 diagnoses do not occur very often, do not require immediate attention, and have a moderate priority. Examples included impaired verbal communication, acute confusion, sensory perception alterations, and decisional conflict. Most of these human responses are not observed during the intraoperative phase, but are phenomena of concern to nurses caring for patients during other phases of the surgical experience.[4]

TABLE A-1: Weighted Diagnostic Labels

Type of diagnosis	Diagnostic label	
Critical nursing diagnoses	Risk for perioperative positioning injury Risk for infection	
Primary nursing diagnoses	Altered protection	Risk for fluid volume deficit
	Pain	Knowledge deficit
	Risk for peripheral neurovascular dysfunction	Ineffective airway clearance
	Risk for aspiration	Impaired skin integrity
	Risk for impaired skin integrity	Impaired gas exchange
	Risk for altered body temperature	Altered tissue perfusion
	Risk for injury	Decreased cardiac output
	Anxiety	Ineffective breathing pattern
	Fear	Fluid volume deficit
	Hypothermia	Fluid volume excess
	Impaired tissue integrity	Altered urinary elimination
	Inability to sustain spontaneous respirations	Impaired physical mobility
Secondary nursing diagnoses	Impaired verbal communication	Urinary retention
	Sensory perceptual alterations	Social isolation
	Ineffective individual coping	Activity intolerance
	Acute confusion	Sexual dysfunction
	Powerlessness	Risk for caregiver role strain
	Altered thought process	Hopelessness
	Hyperthermia	Ineffective thermal regulation
	Post-trauma response	Altered nutrition; less than
	Risk for altered parent/child attachment	Altered nutrition; more than
	Spiritual distress	Caregiver role strain
	Body image disturbance	Ineffective therapeutic regimen
	Altered role performance	Self-esteem disturbance
	Decisional conflict	Altered growth and development
	Anticipatory grieving	Altered sexuality patterns
	Noncompliance	Sleep pattern disturbance
	Ineffective family coping	Ineffective denial
	Impaired home maintenance management	Altered family processes

No diagnoses were classified by respondents as "never occurring," "never requiring nursing attention," or "occurring almost all of the time." There were significant differences in respondents' responses according to the percent of time they spent giving direct care, their primary clinical role, and their education level. The subcommittee members hypothesized that this finding indicated different conceptualization of problems by indirect and direct care providers. Overall, the study confirmed that the primary focus of perioperative nurses is maintaining safety and preventing harm. The findings also demonstrated that the role of the nurse during the intraoperative phase is chiefly one of surveillance. Perioperative nurses must maintain high levels of vigilance to prevent problems and detect early complications.[4] **Table A-2** summarizes the research methods used to establish reliability and validity of the perioperative nursing diagnostic language.

Based on respondents' feedback, the extensive literature review, and the combined expertise of the DECC committee members, a number of additional proposed perioperative nursing diagnoses were identified. The group also noted that a number of nursing diagnoses in the *NANDA Taxonomy* did not include perioperative-related factors or defining characteristics.[6] The recommended new labels included

- infection,
- latex allergy response,
- malignant hyperthermia,
- morbid obesity,
- risk of fall,
- risk of fluid imbalance,
- risk of foreign body injury,
- risk of laser injury,
- risk of thermal injury, and
- delayed surgical recovery.

TABLE A-2: Validation Methods—Nursing Diagnoses

Objective	Approach	Strategy	Reliability
Identify initial list of nursing diagnosis labels.	Systematic review of pertinent literature by expert panel. Identified 60 diagnoses that were relevant to perioperative nursing practice.	Inductive Consensus process	Interrater reliability with > 90% agreement among the panel.
Validate initial list of 60 nursing diagnostic labels.	A survey was conducted to rank frequency and priority of diagnoses label in clinical practice (n = 239).	Survey research Construct validity Content validity	Survey instrument pilot tested prior to implementation.
Identify additional perioperative nursing diagnostic labels that reflect phenomena of concern in the setting.	Survey feedback. Agreement of the expert panel. Systematic review of pertinent literature related to proposed labels.	Construct validity Qualitative analysis of written comments	Interrater reliability with > 90% agreement among the panel.
Validate proposed labels.	Review by diagnostic review committee and NANDA. Validated by expert panel.	Construct validity Inductive	Interrater reliability. Theoretical model explained 42.1% of the variance.
Identify major domains of nursing practice based on nursing diagnostic language.	Exploratory factor analysis. Theoretical discussion by the expert panel.	Quantitative Deductive Construct validity	

The group identified a number of revisions and additions to risk for infection, acute confusion, urinary retention, risk for altered body temperature, hypothermia, sensory/perceptual alterations, anxiety, and knowledge deficit. The intent of this effort was to make existing nursing diagnostic language more reflective of the perioperative clinical experience and the needs of the patient undergoing surgery. All of these suggestions were submitted to the Diagnoses Review Committee of the NANDA in December 1997.

The NANDA accepted four of the new diagnostic categories—latex allergy response, risk for latex allergy response, delayed surgical recovery, and risk of fluid volume imbalance—and have published them in the latest edition of the *NANDA Taxonomy.*[7] These diagnostic labels have been published with the identified etiologies and signs and symptoms, and AORN has been acknowledged for these contributions. Additional diagnoses submitted by AORN were accepted for further review and developmental staging. Recommendations for revisions to existing NANDA labels, related factors, and defining characteristics remain under review by NANDA's Diagnostic Review Committee.

NURSING INTERVENTIONS SUBCOMMITTEE

The work of the Nursing Interventions Subcommittee began with an extensive review of the literature and consultation with practice experts. Task Force members initially identified 145 data elements reflective of perioperative nursing treatments and interventions. Using committee-developed criteria for nursing interventions, the consensus process, and a review of preexisting AORN documents related to patient outcomes, standards of care, and competency statements, task force members refined the list to 115 intervention statements to minimize duplication and redundancy. Most of the intervention statements were derived from the competency statements from the Learner Competency Assessment Tool and the perioperative literature.[8]

Next, committee members decided to survey the membership to validate these data elements by linking outcome standards and nursing interventions. A survey was mailed to a volunteer panel of perioperative nursing experts. The Task Force asked:

In today's health care environment/practice setting, do the treatments/interventions listed demonstrate what a perioperative nurse does to contribute to the outcomes(s) of patients undergoing invasive procedures?

Participants linked the interventions to six outcomes and answered two open-ended questions:

- What nursing actions are not listed? and
- What patient outcomes are not listed?

Respondents to the initial survey reported that traditional nursing performed tasks were more easily represented by the data elements than the professional dimensions of perioperative practice and that nursing actions could be linked to outcomes. From the survey results, it was apparent that there was confusion about the level of abstraction for nursing interventions. Respondents included activities or tasks as interventions rather than identifying interventions at a more conceptual level. For example, "monitors aseptic technique" requires several activities, including checking the integrity of a package and sterilant indicator before completing the intervention. In light of this confusion, Task Force members adopted a carefully determined set of assumptions to guide intervention statement development.

In developing future intervention statements, the Task Force, and later the Nursing Interventions Subcommittee, worked from the following assumptions and criteria.

- Each nursing intervention listed in the PNDS would be operationally defined.
- An operational definition would reflect a concept or variable in terms of the operation or procedure for which it is measured.
- Each definition would include essential cognitive and psychomotor nursing actions or series of actions that compose a nursing intervention.
- The terminology used in the nursing intervention definitions would reflect the accepted terminology of AORN's *Standards, Recommended Practices, and Guidelines.*
- Cognitive and psychomotor nursing actions might not necessarily be documented on the perioperative record.
- Overlapping within and across nursing interventions is acceptable and may be necessary in the development of operational definitions.
- The nursing activity of assessment is considered a nursing intervention.

Based on responses of the survey participants and in the context of these recently established criteria, the members further modified the nursing action statements. The two major objectives of this second survey were to validate that identified interventions are linked to outcomes and identify interventions that would later become an initial minimum data set. This second survey also asked respondents to indicate whether nursing actions contributed to patient outcomes and whether statements required additional revision. Response choices included

- the nursing action is not relevant;
- the statement needs major revision;
- the nursing action is relevant, but needs minor revision; and
- the nursing action is very relevant and is clearly stated.

Analysis of the survey results led to the development of a document titled *Perioperative Nursing Data Elements: Interventions 1.0*, which included 73 nursing interventions, each linked to one of six outcome statements. The identified interventions were deemed applicable across all perioperative settings, to be focused on patient care, and to have future computerized record applications.

The results of these surveys provided the foundation for the initial version of perioperative interventions. The AORN Board of Directors reviewed and approved the document and committed resources for the continued development of a perioperative nursing data set. At this time, the AORN Board of Directors approved the formation of the DECC and charged the group with developing a data set that would include nursing diagnoses, nursing interventions, patient outcomes, and a patient intensity index.

Subsequently, the work on interventions was assumed by the Nursing Interventions Subcommittee of DECC. This group was charged with realigning the perioperative nursing interventions and refining definitions. The group accepted the following intervention guidelines.

- It is critical that all essential cognitive nursing actions be included in the definitions.
- The patient and desired outcome provide the underlying focus of the intervention definition.
- The interventions may be placed into the preoperative, intraoperative, and postoperative phases within the definition.
- Nursing actions may be listed in sequential order.

Work on the intervention statements occurred parallel to the Outcomes Subcommittee members' work related to the revision of the outcome statements. By late 1996, the AORN Board of Directors approved the concepts and intended meaning of the 29 recently validated outcome statements, which were expanded from the original six. At that time, Interventions Subcommittee members decided to realign each nursing intervention with the patient outcome that each intervention was "most closely linked to" and to refine the definitions as necessary.

The panel of expert clinicians on this subcommittee achieved a 90% or better level of agreement with all nursing intervention definitions. This group further refined the document and prepared the *Perioperative Nursing Data Elements: Interventions: Version 2*. The group members began by adding interventions that contributed to outcome achievement that were not listed in the *Perioperative Nursing Data Elements: Interventions 1.0*. These interventions were derived from the responses to the surveys and were validated with an extensive review of the literature and consultation with practice experts. **Table A-3** summarizes validation efforts pertinent to perioperative nursing interventions.

Starting with the original work on the intervention and outcomes statements, members of the Interventions Subcommittee began the process of identifying activity statements. These activity statements further described the interventions and the various nursing actions that composed a particular nursing intervention. The activity statements were derived from a literature and research review of the pertinent perioperative nursing literature and were validated through the consensus process.

Activity statements describe nursing actions that contribute to providing a specific nursing intervention. The activity statements were derived from a systematic evidence-based literature review of the pertinent perioperative nursing literature and validated through the consensus process. For example, the intervention "implementing aseptic technique" comprises multiple activities, such as preventing cross-infection, performing skin preparation, and applying a sterile dressing. Within the PNDS, activities are identified for each intervention statement and, thus, support the achievement of desired outcomes.

NURSING OUTCOMES SUBCOMMITTEE

In 1975, a joint committee of the Association of Operating Room Nurses and the ANA Executive Committee on the Division of Medical-Surgical Nursing Practice collaborated to develop standards of practice for the OR. These guidelines reflected the nature of this specialized area of practice and described assessment factors and patient outcomes. The purpose of this effort was to develop patient outcomes that would establish an approach to evaluate the quality of nursing care in the perioperative setting. These same standards were republished by AORN in 1978 in a document titled *AORN Standards of Practice.*[9]

In 1981, the ANA Executive Committee on the Division of Medical-Surgical Nursing Practice and AORN jointly reviewed and revised the previously published documents. The intent of this effort was to ensure effective nursing care in the OR by establishing quality standards. This revision reflected almost six years of effort by AORN to educate nurses about clinical practice standards and to help nurses evaluate their professional practice. This revision reflected feedback from AORN members regarding the applicability and usefulness of the language and the format of the standards.

These efforts led to later revisions and publication of patient outcome standards for perioperative nursing by AORN[10] and established six outcome standards related to high incidence problem areas for surgical patients. The focus was the OR nurse's scope of responsibility and primarily addressed the intraoperative area. The standard statements also addressed the preoperative and postoperative phases of nursing care. Each statement reflected desired, observable patient outcomes, and interpretative statements for each standard provided guidance for nursing action.

In 1991, these standards were renamed *Patient Outcomes: Standards of Perioperative Care.* AORN defined patient outcomes as observable, measurable,

TABLE A-3: Validation Methods—Nursing Interventions

Objective	Approach	Strategy	Reliability
Identify initial list of 145 perioperative nursing interventions.	Systematic review of pertinent literature by expert panel. Identified 145 interventions that were relevant to perioperative nursing practice.	Consensus process Inductive	Interrater reliability with > 90% agreement among the panel.
Validate perioperative nursing interventions and the linkages between interventions and list of outcome statements.	A survey was conducted to rank the frequency of the interventions and to link the interventions to six outcomes (n = 145).	Survey research Construct validity Content validity	Survey instrument tested prior to implementation.
Identify perioperative nursing interventions not included in initial list.	Survey and list of interventions was revised based on results of first survey. Agreement of the expert panel. Systematic review of the literature.	Construct validity Qualitative analysis of written comments Survey research	Interrater reliability with > 90% agreement among the panel.
Validate revised list of interventions and linkages to outcomes.	Revised survey to determine relationship of nursing actions to patient outcomes and need for further revision of interventions (n = 158).	Content validity Construct validity	Analysis of consistency among respondents.

physiological, and psychological responses to perioprative nursing interventions. This supported the work on data elements. Furthermore, outcomes, interpretive statements, and accompanying criteria served as a framework for measuring and documenting patient outcomes. Perioperative patient outcomes reflected collaborative, interdisciplinary efforts and independent nursing activities. Achieving patient outcomes is of primary concern for the perioperative nurse in assessing, planning, implementing, and evaluating care. The outcomes reflected the nurse's scope of responsibility in all phases of the perioperative period and were guided by ethical, legal, and moral principles.

The Task Force, and later the Nursing Outcomes Subcommittee, specified certain assumptions as they revised and further developed the outcome statements. They assumed that patients, as recipients of care, are entitled to the assurance of privacy, confidentiality, personal dignity, and quality health services. Both groups approached their task using the following additional assumptions.

- Successful achievement of outcomes may depend on the patient's preoperative status.
- The perioperative registered nurse is to be actively involved in identifying potential hazards in the practice setting and implementing appropriate interventions.
- The perioperative registered nurse uses all phases of the nursing process.
- Outcomes are not mutually exclusive and may overlap.
- In the outcome statements, signs refer to objective, observable phenomena and symptoms refer to subjective, patient-reported phenomena.
- The patient has a right to know the risks of surgical or other invasive procedures and the right to be treated by qualified, competent personnel.
- The patient expects to have a surgical or other invasive procedure for an intended therapeutic effect without injury.
- The patient is the primary partner in care. A responsible caregiver, significant other, or family member may perform this role if the patient is unable to do so.

After an extensive literature and research review, the outcome statements were reviewed and revised through the consensus process as part of the original task force survey. Task Force members revised, rephrased, or deleted outcome statements based on the results of the original survey. To measure the appropriateness of patient outcomes, Task Force members included the following subsequent survey questions.

- Is the outcome observable, measurable, singular in nature, and realistic?
- Does the outcome reflect collaboration with interdisciplinary professionals?
- Is the outcome related to the nursing process within the perioperative setting?
- Will the outcome communicate the patient's experience and response to perioperative intervention?

From the results of the this subsequent survey, the Task Force identified 73 nursing interventions, each of which was linked to one of six specific patient outcomes. The Task Force agreed that interventions could be identified and linked to patient outcomes while maintaining a patient focus. The results of this survey round were identified as the Perioperative Nursing Data Elements.[11]

Respondents to this survey round had suggested a number of additions to the outcome statements, including outcomes related to pain control, temperature regulation, cost-effective care, home care preparation, privacy, confidentiality, and quality of care. These suggestions and the results of the earlier survey efforts were instrumental in the Task Force's recommending additional revisions and refinement of the outcome statements.

In 1995, a number of expert clinical nurses were invited to join the Nursing Outcomes Subcommittee with an initial charge to review and revise the existing outcomes document. The subcommittee members agreed that the results of the survey and the "measurble criteria" listed for AORN's 18 perioperative competency statements would provide the starting point.[7] The group wanted to develop outcomes that reflected collaborative, interdisciplinary efforts, as well as independent nursing activities. The ultimate goal was to link the patient outcomes to the nursing interventions.

Using an internal iteration process, and after an extensive literature review, the group expanded the six outcome standards to 29 statements. To validate these statements, they developed a survey in which participants were asked to determine whether each outcome statement and its criteria were useful in practice, teaching, research, and policy development. Participants also were asked to answer yes or no to three statements/questions:

1. The intent of this statement is clear to me;
2. The interpretative statement and criteria support the outcome statement; and
3 Do you currently document information about this outcome?

For the purposes of analysis, the subcommittee members decided to systematically review respondents' level of agreement on the survey. The group decided beforehand to establish the following decision rules as an evaluation framework.

- If there was agreement at the 80% level or greater, an outcome was judged valid and accepted as a data element (ie, outcome statement).
- For all outcome statements for which there was 69% to 79% level of agreement, the specific outcome statement was either accepted as written or reviewed and/or revised by the expert committee before its inclusion as a data element.
- If there was less than a 69% level of agreement, the item was subject to deletion or revision before acceptance as a data element.

Survey data for each of the proposed outcome statements were reviewed by the subcommittee. Areas related to research, teaching, and policy consistently fell below 80% agreement level. Respondents had high levels of agreement for the outcome statements related to being useful in practice. Though there were a number of statements to which the respondents reported high levels of agreement, they also made suggestions to make the outcome statement more measurable or realistic. The expert panel decided to revise and retain each of these outcome statements as they were deemed useful to practice.

The area related to whether information was documented about a specific outcome also had consistently low levels of agreement. In fact, there were only four outcomes for which there were high levels of agreement with regard to documentation (ie, "The patient is free from signs and symptoms of physical injury"; "The patient is free of signs and symptoms of injury due to extraneous objects"; "The patient is free from signs and symptoms of electrical injury"; "The patient is free from signs and symptoms of injury related to positioning"). All statements with low levels of agreement about the clarity of the intent of the statement were examined and revised based on feedback from participants.

All outcome statements for which there was 69% to 79% level of agreement on one or more of the questions were either accepted as written or reviewed and/or revised by expert committee members. This process was conducted using the comments of survey participants, a consensus process, and consultation with clinical practice experts. If there was less than a 69% level of agreement for any one or more of the questions related to each outcome, group members discussed the specific outcome. Outcomes that demonstrated low levels of agreement in more than one area were considered for deletion and revised only if there were strong theoretical arguments for revising and retaining the specific outcome statement. This process resulted in a list of 29 perioperative outcomes. **Table A-4** summarizes perioperative outcome validation efforts.

TABLE A-4: Validation Methods—Nursing Outcomes

Objective	Approach	Strategy	Reliability
Identify initial list of perioperative nursing outcomes.	Systematic review of pertinent literature.	Consensus process Inductive	Interrater reliability with > 90% agreement among the panel.
Review and revise outcome statements.	Review of data obtained from diagnoses and interventions validation surveys by expert panel.	Consensus process	Interrater reliability with > 90% agreement among the panel.
Validate outcome statements.	Survey to stratified randomized sample to evaluate the clarity of the outcome statements and their usefulness in clinical practice (n = 175).	Survey research Construct validity Content validity	Survey instrument pilot tested prior to implementation.

STRUCTURAL DATA ELEMENTS SUBCOMMITTEE

The work of the Task Force on Perioperative Data Elements and the DECC focused its early energies on nursing diagnoses, interventions, and outcomes. Later efforts addressed the structural elements. The Structural Elements Subcommittee conducted a review of the pertinent literature and related research. The breadth and depth of the structural elements in the perioperative arena contributed to the complexity of this group's work.

Two separate surveys were mailed to AORN members to help in the validation of structural data elements. All respondents were members of the Management Specialty Assembly with experience in surgical services management. Respondents were asked to help identify and validate those aspects of perioperative nursing practice that fall into the structural or administrative category. Participants were instructed that the purpose of the survey was to determine a minimum data set that pertained to documenting patient care during the perioperative period.

The survey for this round was a modification of a survey developed by Huber, Delaney, Crossley, Mehmert, and Ellerbe.[12] The survey focused on 11 major categories:

- infection control,
- safety,
- assessment/reassessment,
- resource allocation,
- physiological,
- legal/regulatory,
- surgical procedure,
- units of time,
- implants/explants,
- fluids and electrolytes, and
- anesthesia.

For each of these content areas, a number of data elements were identified. For example, within the category of infection control, the structural elements included were drain(s), wound classification, cultures, skin preparation, preoperative shave, and dressings. Participants were asked to review the categories, definitions, and data elements and respond to three questions.

- Does it need to be documented?
- Is it clearly stated? and
- Is it retrievable?

Overall, the respondents reported high levels of agreement about each data element and whether it needed to be documented, was clearly stated, and was retrievable. Data elements in which there were lower levels of agreement related to patient transportation (ie, mode, accompanied by, report given), room temperature and humidity, procedure classification, and acuity level.

At the time of this effort, a number of other national initiatives on structural data elements were ongoing. One important project development was the Nursing Management Minimum Data Set developed by Huber, Delaney, Crossley, Mehmert, and Ellerbe.[12] Another ongoing effort was standardization of perioperative language for scheduling and monitoring by the American Association of Clinical Directors (AACD). The Structural Elements Subcommittee members monitored progress on these efforts and, by the fall of 1997, it became apparent that the lexicon of AACD should become an integral component of the AORN structural data elements.

As a result, in December 1997, the DECC developed and pilot tested a second survey based on the AACD lexicon "Glossary of Times Used for Scheduling and Monitoring of Diagnostic and Therapeutic Procedures."[13] The subcommittee obtained permission from the AACD to use and print the lexicon as part of their work. The AORN Board of Directors also approved the AACD lexicon for use by DECC. This glossary provides for standardization of terms related to scheduling, utilization, and efficiency and includes procedural times, procedural and scheduling definitions and time periods, utilization and efficiency indices, and patient categories.

Additional structural data elements were developed by the Structural Elements Subcommittee based on results from the earlier surveys and insights derived from management and benchmarking experts. The purpose of the pilot test was to identify weaknesses and any missing structural data elements. For any missing structural data elements, participants were asked to identify the element and include a title, a brief definition, and category. Members of the AORN Board of Directors and Management Specialty Assembly Governing Council pilot tested the survey. The survey was revised and edited based on respondents' comments.

Most respondents reported that all but eight of the 121 structural elements were either very useful or

FIGURE A-1: The Perioperative Patient Focused Model

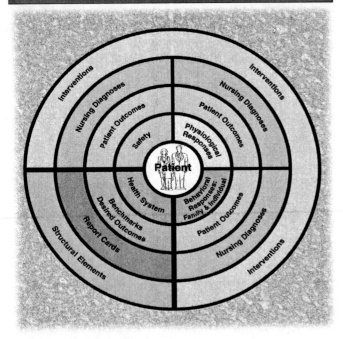

useful. In fact, 65 of the 121 structural elements were reported to be very useful or useful by 75% or more of respondents. The only items that the majority of respondents reported to be only slightly useful or not useful were structkural elements from the AACD glossary. The panel of experts reviewing the results believed that a possible explanation for this finding was that, although the term might exist in the perioperative setting, it was not useful from a nursing management perspective.

Overwhelmingly, respondents reported that the definitions were extremely useful and would be extremely helpful in the development of computerized records. Respondents also reported that having access to such data would be helpful from a management perspective. Based on the findings of this survey, the DECC accepted the terms as defined in the survey instrument. (The AACD lexicon is published in the AORN *Standards, Recommended Practices, and Guidelines.*[14] See **Exhibit A-2** for the additional AORN-approved structural data elements and definitions.)

Although development and validation of the structural elements was part of the original charge of the group working on data elements, it was not submitted to the ANA for recognition as part of the data set. The DECC members decided to limit the

submitted materials to nursing diagnoses, interventions, and outcomes that together formed the PNDS. The rationale for this decision was based largely on the fact that the AACD lexicon is copyrighted by that organization and that clinical testing of this type of terminology would be best conducted from a multidisciplinary perspective.

PERIOPERATIVE PATIENT FOCUSED MODEL

The Perioperative Patient Focused Model (**Figure A-1** and inside front cover) is the conceptual framework for the PNDS and the model for perioperative nursing practice. The patient and his or her family, at the core of the Model, provide the focus of perioperative nursing care. Within the Model, concentric circles expand beyond the patient and family representing the perioperative nursing domains and elements. The Model illustrates the relationship between the patient, family, and care provided by the perioperative professional nurse.

The three patient-centered domains were derived from a survey of experienced perioperative nurses (N=239) who indicated the frequency with which specific patient diagnoses occurred in their daily practice (1=never, 5=all of the time). Following an exploratory principal components factor analysis, three domains of perioperative practice were labeled—patient and family behavioral responses to surgery (26.7% of the variance, Cronbach's alpha = 0.92), perioperative patient safety (10.1% of variance, Cronbach's alpha = 0.89), and perioperative physiological responses to surgery (5.7% of variance, Cronbach's alpha = 0.87).[15] These domains represent concerns, problems, or risks that nurses manage when caring for perioperative patients. The domains constitute the phenomena of concern in the practice of perioperative nursing.

The Model is thus divided into four quadrants, three representing patient-centered domains:
- safety of the patient,
- patient physiologic responses to surgery, and
- patient and family behavioral responses to surgery.

The fourth quadrant represents the health system in which the perioperative care is delivered. The health system domain designates administrative concerns and structure elements (ie, staff, equipment, environmental factors, supplies) essential to successful surgical intervention.

The Model is patient focused. The patient is at the center of the Model, which clearly represents the true focus of perioperative patient care. Regardless of practice setting, geographic location, or nature of the patient population, there is nothing more important to the practicing perioperative nurse than his or her patient. This Model makes this concept of patient care "visible" in and between all other variables in the surgical setting.

Nursing diagnoses, nursing interventions, and patient outcomes comprise the patient safety, physiologic response, and behavioral response domains. These foci represent the phenomena of concern to perioperative nurses and the needs of surgical patients and their families. These components of the Model are in continuous interaction with the health system encircling the focus of perioperative nursing practice—the patient. The fourth domain, the health system, is composed of the structural data elements and focuses on clinical processes and outcomes.

The Model focuses on outcomes. This is important, as nursing theories and models should embrace and represent all elements of the nursing process, including outcomes. AORN's Model represents the outcomes focus of perioperative nurses by placing outcomes immediately adjacent to the patient care domains. The Project Team members believed that perioperative nurses have a unique knowledge base that supports high-quality patient outcomes in surgical settings. An individualized patient assessment guides the identification of nursing diagnoses and selection of nursing interventions for each patient.

Components of the Model, such as safety, physiologic responses, and behavioral responses of patients and families, reflect the nature of the surgical experience for the patient and guiding precepts for providing care by perioperative nurses. The Model is logical, and the concepts and principles are supported in practice environments. Although this Model and the theoretical concepts that underpin it are descriptive in nature and in early stages of development, it holds much promise for research.

The Model represents the "real world" for practicing perioperative nurses and has utility for practicing nurses, educators, and researchers. A simultaneous simplicity and elegance is reflected in this Model. The interrelationships of the domains and concepts provide a picture of the building blocks of perioperative nursing practice in a way that instructs and educates the student, guides nursing practice, and offers infinite opportunities for testing and further validation through research.

The Model as a whole illustrates the dynamic nature of the perioperative patient experience and the nursing presence throughout that process. Working in a collaborative manner with other members of the health care team and the patient, the nurse establishes outcomes, identifies nursing diagnoses, and provides nursing care. The nurse intervenes within the context of the health care system to assist the patient to achieve the highest attainable health outcomes (ie, physiological, behavioral, and safety) throughout the perioperative experience.

References

1. H H Werley, C R Zorn, "The nursing minimum data set and its relationship to classifications for nursing practice," in *Classification Systems for Describing Nursing Practice: Working Papers* (Kansas City, Mo: American Nurses Association, 1989) 50-54.

2. J Clark, N Lang, "Nursing's next advance: An internal [international] classification for nursing practice," *International Nursing Review* 39 (July August 1992) 109-111, 128.

3. International Organisation for Standardisation, *International Standard ISO 1087 Terminology Principles and Coordination* (Geneva: International Organisation for Standardisation, 1990).

4. A R Killen et al, "The prevalence of perioperative nurse clinical judgments," *AORN Journal* 65 (January 1997) 101-108.

5. S V M Kleinbeck, "In search of perioperative nursing data elements," *AORN Journal* 63 (May 1996) 926-931; Killen et al, "The prevalence of perioperative nurse clinical judgments," 101-108.

6. North American Nursing Diagnosis Association, *Nursing Diagnoses: Definitions and Classification 1995-1996* (St Louis: North American Nursing Diagnosis Association, 1994).

7. North American Nursing Diagnosis Association, *Nursing Diagnoses: Definitions and Classification 1999-2000* (Philadelphia: North American Nursing Diagnosis Association, 1999).

8. AORN National Committee on Education, *Preceptor Guide for Perioperative Nursing Practice* (Denver: Association of Operating Room Nurses, Inc, 1998).

9. Association of Operating Room Nurses, Inc, *AORN Standards of Practice* (Denver: Association of Operating Room Nurses, Inc, 1978).

10. Association of Operating Room Nurses, Inc, *AORN Standards and Recommended Practices for Perioperative Nursing* (Denver: Association of Operating Room Nurses, Inc, 1982).

11. Association of Operating Room Nurses, Inc, *Perioperative Nursing Data Elements: Outcomes and Interventions, Version 1* (Denver: Association of Operating Room Nurses, Inc, March 1995).

12. D G Huber et al, "A nursing management minimum data set: Significance and development," *Journal of Nursing Administration* 22 (July/August 1992) 35-40.

13. Association of Anesthesia Clinical Directors, "Procedural times glossary—glossary of times used for scheduling and monitoring of diagnostic and therapeutic procedures," *Surgical Services Management* 3 (September 1997) 11-15.

14. Association of Operating Room Nurses, Inc. *Standards, Recommended Practices, and Guidelines* (Denver: Association of Operating Room Nurses, Inc, 2002).

15. S V M Kleinbeck, "Dimensions of perioperative nursing for a national specialty nomenclature," *Journal of Advanced Nursing* 31 (March 2000) 529-535.

EXHIBIT A-1:
WORKING DEFINITIONS ESTABLISHED BY THE
TASK FORCE ON PERIOPERATIVE DATA ELEMENTS (1993–1995)

Actual Problem: "An existing deviation from health." Source: M Gordon, *Nursing Diagnosis Process and Application* (New York: McGraw-Hill Co, 1982) 3.

Classification System: "The ordering of phenomena in a systematic way for some purpose." (Example: classifying students as freshman, sophomore, junior, senior). "Used to sort and code phenomena of interest." (Example: biology and chemistry). Source: M Gordon, *Nursing Diagnosis Process and Application* (New York: McGraw-Hill Co, 1982) 304.

A process of categorizing clients according to their nursing care requirements. It can be based on single or multiple indicators of care needs. Source: M Gordon, *Nursing Diagnosis Process and Application* (New York: McGraw-Hill Co, 1982) 286.

Data Element: Discrete entities that are described without interruption, information as data that has been interpreted, and knowledge as information that has been synthesized so relationships are identified. Source: S A Kilby, M N McAlendon, "Searching the literature yourself. Why, how, what to search," in *Computer Applications in Nursing Education and Practice*, J M Arnold, G A Pearson, eds (New York: National League for Nursing, publ no 14-2406, 1992) 23.

Data Set: A collection of related data items. Source: N M Lang et al, "Toward a national database for nursing practice," in *An Emerging Framework: Data System Advances for Clinical Nursing Practice* (Washington, DC: American Nurses Association, 1995) 4.

Database: "An organized collection of data or information." Source: K J Hannah, M J Ball, M J A Edwards, *Introduction to Nursing Informatics* (New York: Springer-Verlag, 1994) 288.

"A collection of interrelated files with records organized and stored together in a computer system." Source: N M Lang et al, "Toward a national database for nursing practice," in *An Emerging Framework: Data System Advances for Clinical Nursing Practice* (Washington, DC: American Nurses Association, 1995) 4.

Diagnostic Category(ies): Concept(s) of health problem(s) when specifically defined represent a division in a classification system of named problems. They permit discrimination among different health problems. They represent the typical signs and symptoms of a health problem. They provide a means for ordering and coding clinical data so meaning can be derived. Source: M Gordon, *Nursing Diagnosis Process and Application* (New York: McGraw-Hill Co, 1982) 10-11.

Diagnostic Concept(s): "Nursing diagnoses are abstractions, they summarize a cluster of signs, symptoms and inferences. A mental grasp of a cluster of observations and their interrelationships is called a concept. Important concepts are named and defined to prevent miscommunication." Source: M Gordon, *Nursing Diagnosis Process and Application* (New York: McGraw-Hill Co, 1982) 10.

Diagnostic Process: "A process of determining a client's health state and evaluating the etiological factor influencing that state. It involves four activities: 1) collecting information, 2) interpreting the information, 3) clustering the information, 4) naming the cluster." Source: M Gordon, *Nursing Diagnosis Process and Application* (New York: McGraw-Hill Co, 1982) 12-13.

Guidelines: Guidelines relate to clinical conditions and contain suggestions for interventions for specified outcomes. They describe a process of patient care management that has the potential to improve the quality of clinical and consumer decision making. Source: N M Lang et al, "Toward a national database for nursing practice," in *An Emerging Framework: Data System Advances for Clinical Nursing Practice* (Washington, DC: American Nurses Association, 1995) 9.

Intervention(s): Actions taken to help the client move from a present state to the state described in the projected outcome(s). The type of nursing intervention selected depends on the nursing diagnosis and outcome(s). Source: M Gordon, *Nursing Diagnosis Process and Application* (New York: McGraw-Hill Co, 1982) 242.

Language: "A social collective contract which one must accept in its entirety if one wishes to communicate. It has elements and these each have value in themselves and in relation to other elements. One uses or gives a name to something one wishes to focus upon, learn, define, and count. Consensus about terms, words, signs—a language." Source: P B Kritek, "Conceptual considerations, decision criteria, and guidelines for the nursing minimum data set from a practice perspective," in *Identification of the Nursing Minimum Data Set,* H H Werley, N M Lange, eds (New York: Springer Publishing Co, 1988) 31.

Nomenclature: "A compilation of approved terms for describing phenomena." (Example: airway clearance, ineffective). Source: M Gordon, *Nursing Diagnosis Process and Application* (New York: McGraw-Hill Co, 1982) 304, 325.

Nursing Diagnosis/Clinical Diagnosis: "Made by professional nurses to describe actual or potential health problems which nurses by virtue of their education and experience are capable and licensed to treat." Source: M Gordon, *Nursing Diagnosis Process and Application* (New York: McGraw-Hill Co, 1982) 2.

Nursing Minimum Data Set (NMDS): A minimum set of items of information with uniform definitions and categories concerning the specific dimensions of nursing that meets the information needs of multiple data users in the health care system. There are 16 elements. Source: H H Werley et al, "The nursing minimum data set: An abstraction tool for standardized, comparable, essential data," *American Journal of Public Health* 81 (April 1991) 421-426.

Nursing Outcome: An aspect of patient or client health status that is influenced by nursing intervention and recorded at specific times for an episode or encounter of care. The nursing outcome is linked to the nursing diagnosis and recorded as resolved, not resolved, or referred for continuing care. Source: K Marek, "Classification of outcome measures in nursing care," in *Classification Systems for Describing Nursing Practice* (Kansas City, Mo: American Nurses Association, 1989) 39.

Nursing Process: "A systematic approach used to carry out nursing's independent function." "It provides organization and direction of nursing activities, a means for predicting outcomes and

evaluating results, and a method for establishing standards of nursing care." "It is a five step process:
1. Assessment: collection of patient data of pertinence to nursing.
2. Data Analysis: using the collected data to identify the patient's health care needs that can be influenced by nursing care (nursing diagnosis).
3. Planning: determining priorities, expected patient outcomes, and specific nursing actions.
4. Implementation: carrying out the planned nursing actions necessary to accomplish the defined goals.
5. Evaluation: determining the extent to which the goals have been achieved."
Source: B C Long, W J Phipps, V L Cassmeyer, *Medical-Surgical Nursing: A Nursing Process Approach,* fourth ed (St Louis: C V Mosby, 1993) 8.

Outcome: "Achieving a desired conclusion and/or reducing the probability of undesired outcomes as perceived by the patient and according to a well-defined and properly implemented practice outlined in the *AORN Patient Outcome Standards for Perioperative Nursing.*" Source: J C Rothrock, *Perioperative Nursing Care Planning* (St Louis: C V Mosby, 1990) 497.

Perioperative Outcomes: Outcomes that are observable or measurable physiological, psychosocial, and psychological responses to perioperative nursing interventions. They provide direction for judging patient responses and result from care provided by the health care team members. The perioperative outcomes focus on high-risk areas for patients undergoing surgical, diagnostic, or therapeutic interventions in which the patient's protective reflexes may be compromised. There currently are six outcome standards:
1. The patient demonstrates knowledge of the physiological and psychological responses to surgical intervention;
2. The patient is free from infection;
3. The patient's skin integrity is maintained;
4. The patient is free from injury related to positioning, extraneous objects, or chemical, physical, and electrical hazards;
5. The patient's fluid and electrolyte balance is maintained;
6. The patient participated in the rehabilitation process. Source: Association of Operating Room Nurses, Inc, *Standards and Recommended Practices* (Denver: Association of Operating Room Nurses, Inc, 1993) 89-90.

Potential Problem/High-Risk State: "Presence of a set of risk factors." Source: M Gordon, *Nursing Diagnosis Process and Application* (New York: McGraw-Hill Co, 1982) 3.

Recommended Practice: Practices approved by AORN based on principles of microbiology, research, review of the scientific literature, and opinions of experts knowledgeable in the subject. They are statements of optimum performance criteria on the various aspects of technical and professional perioperative nursing practice. They do not attempt to gain consensus among users. Source: Association of Operating Room Nurses, Inc, *Standards and Recommended Practices* (Denver: Association of Operating Room Nurses, Inc, 1993) 93.

Standard: Authoritative statement that describes the responsibilities for which nursing practitioners are accountable. They reflect the values and priorities of the profession. They are a means to direct and evaluate professional nursing practice. Source: Association of Operating Room Nurses, Inc, *Standards and Recommended Practices* (Denver: Association of Operating Room Nurses, Inc, 1993) 61.

Taxonomy: "The theoretical study of classification and of the classification system that results." Source: M Gordon, *Nursing Diagnosis Process and Application* (New York: McGraw-Hill Co, 1982) 304.

"The science of classification, laws, and principles covering the classifying of objects, the science of grouping things and the resultant grouping is often called a taxonomy." Source: P B Kriteck, "An introduction to the science and art of taxonomy," in *Classification Systems for Describing Nursing Practice* (Kansas City, Mo: American Nurses Association, 1989) 6.

Uniform Language System: A major goal in the use of NMDS. This will be achieved through careful definition of data items, using existing nursing practice language. Where items overlap with existing health care, NMDS items should be defined uniformly. Source: P B Kritek, "Conceptual considerations, decision criteria, and guidelines for the nursing minimum data set from a practice perspective," in *Identification of the Nursing Minimum Data Set,* H H Werley, N M Lange, eds (New York: Springer Publishing Co, 1988) 31.

Uniform Minimum Data Sets (UMDSs): UMDSs provide core minimum sets of items of information with common definitions concerning a specific aspect of the health care system that meet the essential needs of a variety of health care users. Source: C M Freeman, "Annotated bibliography about minimum data sets and computer use by nurses," in *Identification of the Nursing Minimum Data Set,* H H Werley, N M Lang, eds (New York: Springer Publishing Co, 1988) 434.

EXHIBIT A-2:
AORN STRUCTURAL DATA ELEMENTS

A. UTILIZATION AND EFFICIENCY INDICES

Percentage of operating room utilization without turnover time: Total actual utilized hours (patient in the room/patient out of the room) without turnover time divided by total available operating room hours.

Percentage of operating room utilization with turnover time: Total actual utilized hours (patient in the room/patient out of the room) including turnover time divided by total available operating room hours.

Percentage of utilization by hour of day: Total actual utilized hours by hour of day divided by total available hours by hour of day.

Percentage of utilization by shift: Total actual utilized hours by shift divided by total available hours by shift.

Percentage of utilization by day of week: Total actual utilized hours by day of week divided by total available hours by day of week.

Percentage of hours of utilization by surgical specialty: Total hours of utilization by surgical specialty divided by total hours of utilization for all specialties.

Percentage of case utilization by surgical specialty: Total number of cases performed by surgical specialty divided by total number of cases performed by all specialties.

Percentage of hours of utilization by outpatient: Total hours of utilization (patient in the room/ patient out of the room) by outpatient divided by total hours of utilization for all patients.

Percentage of hours of utilization by inpatient: Total hours of utilization (patient in the room/ patient out of the room) by inpatient divided by total hours of utilization for all patients.

Percentage of case utilization by outpatient: Total number of outpatients divided by total number of cases.

Percentage of case utilization by inpatient: Total number of inpatients divided by total number of cases.

Average minutes per case: Total minutes of utilization (patient in the room/patient out of the room) divided by total number of cases.

Average minutes per outpatient case: Total minutes of outpatient utilization (patient in the room/patient out of the room) divided by total number of outpatient cases.

Average minutes per inpatient case: Total minutes of inpatient utilization (patient in the room/ patient out of the room) divided by total number of inpatient cases.

OR turnover time: The time between the exit of one patient from the room until the entrance of the next patient into the room. (Usually only calculated between cases that are scheduled "to follow" each other.)

Surgeon turnover time: The time between the exit of the surgeon from the room until the surgeon enters the room for the following case. (Usually only calculated between cases that are scheduled "to follow" each other.)

Anesthesia turnover time: The time between the exit of the anesthesiologist from the room until the anesthesiologist enters the room for the following case. (Usually only calculated between cases that are scheduled "to follow" each other.)

Percentage of case cancellation: Total number of cases cancelled (cancelled once scheduled) divided by total cases scheduled, excludes urgent and emergent. (May be further delineated by reason for cancellation [eg, physician, patient, OR].)

Percentage of case delays: Total number of cases delayed (starting 15 minutes or more after the scheduled start time) divided by total number of scheduled cases, excluding urgent and emergent cases.

Preoperative length of stay: The total time elapsed from the time the patient enters the health care facility as an outpatient until they are transferred to the operating room.

PACU length of stay: The total time elapsed from the time the patient is admitted to the postanesthesia care unit (PACU) until they are discharged from the PACU.

Postoperative length of stay: The time elapsed from the time the patient is admitted to the postanesthesia care unit until they are discharged from the hospital.

B. PATIENT CATEGORIES*

Elective: A nonemergent, nonurgent procedure that is prescheduled. Elective surgery is performed at the patient's and surgeon's convenience. It can be completed within days or even months of the diagnosis.

Urgent: A non-life-threatening condition which may lead to complications if not performed within 24 hours or a procedure that needs to be done within 24 hours. Urgent cases generally are added to the schedule rather than replacing a procedure already scheduled and generally will follow elective scheduled procedures.

Emergency: A life-threatening or potential life-threatening condition that requires immediate intervention. The procedure must be done immediately because of the threat to vital life and/or limb function. Emergency cases take precedence over other previously scheduled elective or urgent procedures.

Acuity: The categorization of patients according to some assessment of the direct and indirect nursing care requirements over a specified period of time.

*Other structural elements to be included are the ASA classification and wound classification (CDC).

C. STAFFING

Personnel: The various individuals who are included in the staff roster for the operating room. (They may include management, staff, and support personnel.)

Direct care time: The time that staff members are involved in providing direct hands-on care to patients. Direct care in the operating room also includes the time spent in setup and cleanup of rooms as it is directly related to the care of an individual patient.

Indirect care time: The time that staff members are involved in activities indirectly related to patient care. This includes such things as instrument processing, education, breaks, lunch, and housekeeping.

Productive hours: The hours that staff spend in activities related to patient care. This includes regular, overtime, and call hours.

Nonproductive hours: The hours that staff spend in activities not related to patent care. This includes vacation, sick time, and orientation.

Actual operating room hours: Total paid staff hours divided by total actual operating room hours.

Productive hour productivity: Total paid productive staff hours divided by total actual operating room hours.

Productivity per case: Total paid staff hours divided by total cases.

Total productivity for productive hours per case: Total paid productive staff hours divided by total cases.

Percent of overtime: Total overtime staff hours paid divided by total paid hours.

Percent of call: Total call staff hours paid divided by total paid hours.

Percent of regular hours: Total regular staff hours paid divided by total paid hours.

Direct care staff ratio: Total RN FTE in direct care compared to total non-RN FTE in direct care.

Total staffing ratio: Total clinical (RN, technician) FTE in direct care compared to total non-clinical staff in indirect care.

Direct care costs: Total staff paid engaged in direct care activities.

Indirect care costs: Total staff paid engaged in indirect care activities.

D. FINANCIAL

Total cost per OR minute: Total costs (staff, direct billable supplies, and overhead [equipment, nonbillable supplies]) divided by total actual utilized minutes.

Direct staff costs per OR minute: Total paid direct staff divided by total actual utilized minutes.

Indirect staff costs per OR minute: Total paid indirect staff divided by total actual utilized minutes.

Productive staff costs per OR minute: Total paid productive staff divided by total actual utilized minutes.

Nonproductive staff costs per OR minute: Total paid nonproductive staff divided by total actual utilized minutes.

Total cost per case: Total costs (staff, direct billable supplies, and overhead [equipment, non-billable supplies]) divided by total actual cases.

Supply costs per case: Total direct billable supplies divided by total actual cases.

Revenue per case: Total actual revenue divided by total actual cases.

Total expense budget: Total costs including staff, overhead, and supplies.

Percent supply costs of total expenses: Total direct billable supply costs divided by total expenses.

Percent staff costs of total expenses: Total paid staff divided by total expenses.

E. ENVIRONMENTAL MONITORING

Room temperature: Ambient air temperature within the operating room.

Room humidity: Relative humidity within the operating room.

Air exchange: Total air exchange per hour per operating room.

Used by permission. The complete *Glossary of Times Used for Scheduling and Monitoring of Diagnostic and Therapeutic Procedures* is available from the American Association of Clinical Directors, http://www.aacdhq.org. Copyright © 1997. All rights reserved.

The PNDS in Action:
Sample Documentation and Care Planning

The documentation and care planning examples on the following pages are representations of many of the data fields used in the majority of hospital settings. Their purpose is to demonstrate a consistent approach to documenting nursing assessment; identification of clinical problems; and nursing interventions, activities, and outcomes in a paper format. It is expected that clinicians will use these samples as a beginning point to develop population-specific and facility-pertinent clinical records.

Such clinical records should incorporate data fields that best represent the case types, clinical situations, and patient experiences within a particular setting. Such records could build upon these samples, but also should reflect departmental/facility policies and procedures, AORN recommended practices, and any pertinent regulatory requirements. In addition, any clinical record should provide an opportunity for clinicians to document the unique needs of the patient as well as age-specific and cultural needs and interventions. For a paper record, additional (addendum) forms might be required. For example, an orthopedic specialty hospital might have an addendum form for the numerous implants it might use for a single case or an addendum form for blood administration.

Some data fields in the same records have the PNDS unique identifier in parentheses to illustrate how the PNDS terminology can be used in patient records. These identifiers do not need to appear on a facility's paper or electronic record.

Sample documents included in this appendix:

Policies and Procedures: Fire Safety in Perioperative Settings

Clinical Competencies: Perioperative Medication Competency

Sample Care Plan: Intraoperative

Sample Care Plan: Ambulatory Surgery

Sample Care Plan: Perioperative

Perioperative Clinical Pathway: Total Hip Arthroplasty

Job Description: Perioperative Case Manager

Job Description: Perioperative Team Leader

Job Description: Perioperative Registered Nurse

Electronic Perioperative Record

For additional applications, visit the PNDS section of *AORN Online* at http://www.aorn.org/PracticeResources/PNDS/PNDSResources.

Policies & Procedures:
Fire Safety in Perioperative Settings

Copyright © 2006 AORN, Inc. All rights reserved.

Surgical and procedural fires

Domain: Safety—Freedom from acquired physical injury. (D1)

INTRODUCTION

Seventy percent of reported surgical and procedural fires result from electrosurgical equipment use, and an additional 10% involve lasers. The remaining 20% occur from other heat-producing sources found in surgical and procedural settings, such as fiber-optic light sources, high-speed power equipment, electrocautery devices, and electrical shorts in equipment. The oxygen-enriched environment found in perioperative settings and the presence of alcohol-based prepping agents contribute to approximately 79% of all surgical fires.[1]

Events reported to health care regulatory and research agencies identify the prevalence of patient injury as follows:
- 21% involve the airway or oropharyngeal locations;
- 44% involve the head, neck or upper chest;
- 26% are other patient surface fires; and
- 8% of reported fires occur inside the patient.[1,2]

Outcomes
The patient is free from signs and symptoms of injury caused by extraneous objects. (O2)
The patient is free from signs and symptoms of chemical injury. (O3)
The patient is free from signs and symptoms of electrical injury. (O4)
The patient is free from signs and symptoms of laser injury. (O6)
(For associated PNDS interventions, see **Exhibit B-1** at the end of this document.)

POLICY

Fire prevention is the responsibility of every member of the perioperative team. The promotion of a culture of fire safety relies on department leadership (directors, managers, educators, clinical nurse specialists) to maintain safety standards, identify safety protocols, and implement staff education and instruction on fire prevention methodology and strategies. Clinical staff (perioperative nurses, technicians, support personnel, surgeons, residents, anesthesia providers and visiting health care vendors and students) are accountable for participation in department fire safety training and a minimum of one mock evacuation a year.

IMPLEMENTATION PROCEDURE

1. **Education and training** prepare the perioperative clinician to deliver care in a fire-safe environment and includes at a minimum:
   - Knowledge of the elements of the Fire Triangle and perioperative risk assessment;
   - Participation in department fire drills and mock evacuation scenarios;
   - Knowledge of "defend in place" versus when to evacuate environment;
   - Skill demonstration in fire extinguishing techniques, including use of fire-fighting equipment;
   - Knowledge of rescuer methods;
   - Identification of department evacuation routes for each room and fire extinguisher locations;
   - Knowledge of medical gas panel location and operation;
   - Knowledge of ventilation and electrical system locations and operation, including personnel authorized to turn off and when;
   - Initiation of the fire alarm or emergency notification system; and
   - Specific procedures for contacting the local fire department.

2. **Safety strategies** are used to interrupt elements of the Fire Triangle.
   (See associated PNDS Interventions in **Exhibit B-1** at the end of this document.)

Fire occurs when all three elements of the Fire Triangle—oxidizers, fuels sources, and ignition sources—come together. Surgical and procedural settings require clinicians to use these elements in close proximity for perioperative patient care. Perioperative clinicians can prevent the sides of the Fire Triangle from making contact by following the suggested strategies below:

Strategies to Manage Fuel Sources
- Prior to the start of the procedure:
    - Assess the flammability of all materials used on or around the patient.
    - Do not allow skin prep solutions to pool on or around the patient; remove prep soaked linen and disposable prepping drapes before start of the procedure.
    - Allow skin prep agents to dry before draping the patient and the procedure begins; conduct a skin prep "time out" to validate agent is dry.
    - Do not trap volatile chemicals or chemical fumes (eg, alcohol, collodion, tinctures) beneath the drapes; allow chemicals to dry thoroughly and vapors to dissipate before beginning procedure.
    - Configure surgical drapes to allow sufficient venting of oxygen delivered to the patient.
    - Coat facial hair near surgical site with water-soluble surgical lubricant to decrease flammability.
- During the procedure:
    - Do not allow drapes or linens to come in contact with activated ignition sources
    - Moisten drapes, towels, sponges that will be in close proximity to ignition sources.
    - Ensure that oxygen is not accumulating beneath the drapes.
    - Evacuate surgical smoke to prevent accumulation in small or enclosed spaces (eg, back of throat).
    - Exercise caution when using electrosurgery or laser in the presence of intestinal gases; do not use an ignition source to enter the bowel when distended with gas.
    - If drapes ignite, smother small fires with a wet sponge or towel. Remove burning material from patient.
    - Extinguish any burning material with water or saline or an approved fire extinguisher* if appropriate.
    - Do not use fire blankets in surgical or procedural patient care settings.

Strategies to Manage Ignition Sources
- Use the lowest possible power setting for the ESU.
- Place the patient return electrode on a large muscle mass close to the surgical site
- Always use a safety holster for ignition sources when available
- Do not coil the active electrode cords
- Do not use the ESU in the presence of flammable solutions
- Do not use the ESU near oxygen or nitrous oxide; if *not* possible, stop supplemental oxygen or nitrous oxide for one minute before using electrosurgery, electrocautery or laser for head, neck, or upper chest procedures.[1]
- Inspect active electrodes, electrical cords and plugs for integrity
- Do not place fluids on top of the ESU
- Do not bypass ESU safety features (including dimming audible alarms)
- Keep the active electrode tip clean
- Do not use active electrodes or return electrodes that are not manufacturer approved for the type and model of ESU being used
- Use wet sponges/towels to help retard fire potential
- Do not use protective covers created from rubber catheter or packing materials as insulators on the active electrode tip
- Use cut or blend instead of coagulation when possible
- Do not open the circuit to activate the ESU

- Ensure the active electrode is not switched on in close proximity to another metal object that could conduct heat or cause arcing
- Remove active electrode tip from electrosurgical or electrocautery unit before discarding
- After prepping, allow skin prep agent to dry and fumes to dissipate before using an ignition source

Laser: Use only an approved laser-resistant endotracheal tube for upper airway procedures.
- Wet sponges around the tube cuff to provide extra protection and help retard fire potential.
- Do not use liquids or ointments that could be combustible.
- Inflate endotracheal tube cuff with tinted saline (eg, methylene blue) to detect inadvertent rupture.

Fiber-optic light sources: Place the light source in standby mode or turn off when a cable is not in active use (eg, used within 5-10 seconds).
- Ensure light cables are in good working order and do not have broken light bundles.
- Do not allow a light cable that is connected to a light source to contact drapes, sponges or other flammable materials.
- Place operating telescopes in standby mode when not in a body cavity.

Drills, saws: A slow drip of saline on a moving drill/burr/saw blade helps reduce heat buildup.
- Do not place drills, burrs, or saws on the patient when not in use.
- Ensure that all equipment is periodically inspected by biomedical personnel for proper function.
- Check biomedical inspection stickers on equipment for currency.

Defibrillator paddles: Select paddles that are the correct size for the patient.
- Use only manufacturer recommended gel for paddle lubrication.
- Ensure paddle placement is appropriate for patient and optimal contact with skin is made.

Strategies to Manage Oxidizers
- Oxygen supports combustion and should be used with caution in the presence of ignition sources.
- Question the use of 100% oxygen; titrate oxygen to the lowest percentage to support the patient's physiologic needs using a pulse oximeter.
- Check anesthesia circuits for possible leaks.
- When possible, use cuffed endotracheal tubes during LASER or ESU techniques.
- Pack wet sponges around the back of the throat to help retard oxygen leaks.
- Use suction to help evacuate any accumulation of oxygen under the drapes or within a body cavity, such as mouth or chest.
- Do not use the laser or ESU where oxygen is flowing; stop supplemental oxygen or nitrous oxide for one minute before using electrosurgery, electrocautery, or laser for head, neck, or upper chest procedures.[1]
- Use conformable drapes to allow sufficient venting of oxygen when using mask or nasal oxygen.
- Have an emergency tracheostomy tray available for head, neck, and upper airway procedures.
- The same strategies used to manage oxygen also are used to manage the risks associated with nitrous oxide.
- Turn off the flow of oxygen at the end of each procedure.

3. **Emergency procedures** include the following.

    - In the event of *a small fire on the patient*, immediately:
        - Smother or douse the fire, and
        - Remove burning materials from the patient.

    - In the event of a *large fire on the patient*, immediately:
        - Stop the flow of breathing gases to the patient
            - Have another team member extinguish the burning material.
            - If needed, use a fire extinguisher to put out the fire involving the patient.

- ▪ Care for the patient
  - o Resume patient ventilation.
  - o Control bleeding; protect the surgical field.
  - o Activate Fire Safety/Evacuation plan.

- • At the first sign of a *tracheal tube fire*, immediately and rapidly:
  - ▪ Disconnect the breathing circuit form the tracheal tube.
  - ▪ Remove the tracheal tube.
    - o Have another team member extinguish the fire
    - o Remove cuff protective devices and any segments of the burned tube that may remain smoldering in the airway
  - ▪ Care for the patient
    - o Re-establish the airway and resume ventilating with room/medical air until the airway is free from burning materials; switch to 100% oxygen or as appropriate for patient.[3]
    - o Examine the airway to determine the extent of damage, and treat patient accordingly.

> **Save all involved materials and devices for later investigation**

* Contact the local Fire Department for an approved listing of fire extinguishers that may be used in perioperative practice areas.

References

1. ECRI, "Guidance article: Surgical fire safety," *Health Devices* 35 no 2 (February 2006) 45-66.
2. M E Bruley, "Surgical fires: Perioperative communication is essential to prevent this rare but devastating complication," *Quality and Safety in Health Care* 12 (June 2004) 467-471, available http://qhc.bmjjournals.com/cgi/content/full/13/6/467 (accessed 4 January 2006).
3. ECRI, "Surgical fires," *Operating Room Risk Management* (November 2004) 15.

Resources

"AORN guidance statement: Fire prevention in the operating room." In *Standards, Recommended Practices, and Guidelines* (Denver: AORN, Inc, 2006) 251-259.
ECRI. "A clinician's guide to surgical fires: How they occur, how to prevent them, how to put them out." *Health Devices* 32 no 1 (January 2003) 1-24.
ECRI. "Only you can prevent surgical fires: Surgical team communication is essential," in "Guidance article: Surgical fire safety." *Health Devices* 35 no 2 (February 2006) 54.
Inova Fairfax Hospital—Perioperative Services. "Fire safety in the operating room." Department policy (November 2005).

Exhibit B-1: PNDS Interventions

The Perioperative Nursing Data Set (PNDS) is recognized by the American Nurses Association as the standardized language for perioperative nursing practice. The PNDS should be reflected in the documentation of perioperative nursing care and can be linked to department policies in the form of desired patient outcomes. The following are suggested nursing interventions for the PNDS outcomes identified in the preceding document.

The patient is free from signs and symptoms of injury caused by extraneous objects (O2)
- Implements protective measures prior to operative or invasive procedure (I138)
  - The patient equipment and environment are prepared to ensure safety during operative or other invasive procedure
  - Removes environmental hazards (eg, remove malfunctioning equipment)
- Implements protective measures to prevent skin or tissue injury due to thermal sources (I176)
  - Removes body jewelry within the operative field or in direct line of ESU return electrode pathways
  - Monitors active electrode of electrosurgical unit (ESU) or electrocautery device during procedure; holsters ignition sources as appropriate
  - Monitors function of patient return electrode of electrosurgical unit during procedure
  - Protects skin and internal organs from heat transfer by endoscopes or other hot instruments
- Implements protective measures to prevent skin/tissue injury due to mechanical sources (I77)
  - Selects safest method of hair removal (if indicated) that preserves skin integrity
  - Inspects, tests, and uses powered surgical instruments according to manufacturers' documented instructions
- Maintains continuous surveillance (I128)
  - Communicates patient's risk status to appropriate member(s) of the health care team
  - Monitors and controls clinical environment for safety or potential hazards
  - Monitors patient for changes in status that requires immediate nurse attention
  - Troubleshoots surgical equipment and clinical systems

The patient is free from signs and symptoms of chemical injury (O3)
- Implements protective measures to prevent skin and tissue injury due to chemical sources (I75)
  - Removes prep soaked linen and disposable prepping drapes before procedure start
  - Allows for flammable solutions (eg, alcohol, acetone, fat solvents) to dry and fumes to dissipate before draping or activating electrosurgical or laser equipment.

The patient is free from signs and symptoms of electrical injury (O4)
- Implements protective measures to prevent injury due to electrical sources (I72)
  - Implements general electrosurgical and electrocautery safety precautions
  - Implements active electrode safety precautions
  - Implements dispersive patient electrode safety precautions
  - Implements general high powered drill and saw safety precautions
  - Inspects equipment, including laser, for electrical hazard

The patient is free from signs and symptoms of laser injury (O6)
- Implements protective measures to prevent injury due to laser sources (I73)
  - Removes patient makeup, jewelry from surgical site
  - Protects skin and non-targeted tissues from unintended laser beam exposure
  - Implements fire protection measures

Source: Perioperative Nursing Data Set: The Perioperative Nursing Vocabulary, *revised 2nd ed (Denver, AORN, Inc, 2007).*

Perioperative Medication Competency

<table>
<tr><td colspan="3">COMPETENCY STATEMENT:
The perioperative registered nurse demonstrates the ability to safely administer medications.</td></tr>
<tr><th>Patient Outcome</th><th>PNDS Interventions as Measurable Criteria</th><th>Recommendations for Validation of Competency</th></tr>
<tr>
<td>O9 The patient receives appropriate medication(s), safely administered, during the perioperative period.</td>
<td>(I123) Verifies allergies
Identifies allergies, idiosyncrasies, and sensitivities to medications, latex, chemical agents, foods, and/or adhesives.
<ul>
<li>Queries patient about allergies or hypersensitivity reaction to adhesive products, latex or iodine product.</li>
<li>Queries patient about medications and foreign proteins that cause anaphylaxis (eg, antibiotics, opiates, insulin, vasopressin, protamine, allergen extracts, muscle relaxants, vaccines, local anesthetics, whole blood, cryoprecipitate, immune globulin, iodinated contrast media)</li>
<li>Determines type of food, nutritional supplements, or substance and type of reaction experienced, if any, as reported by the patient</li>
<li>Records and communicates to the anesthesia care provider a patient history of anaphylaxis, asthma, or other respiratory difficulties related to the presence of allergens, toxins, or antigens</li>
</ul></td>
<td><ul>
<li>Direct observation of patient assessment</li>
<li>Peer review of patient care documentation</li>
<li>Verification of communications with patient care team members</li>
<li>Other:_____</li>
</ul></td>
</tr>
<tr>
<td></td>
<td>(I141) Prescribes medications within scope of practice (RNFA)
Prescribes medications in accordance with state and federal rules and regulations and facility policies
<ul>
<li>Assesses current prescription, over-the-counter medication, and herbal supplemental use</li>
<li>Collaborates with surgeon to establish medication protocols applicable to specific patient populations (RNFA)</li>
<li>Assess allergies and/or any limitations to medications protocol (RNFA)</li>
<li>Prescribes medications when authorized by state rules and regulations and approved by facility policy (RNFA)</li>
<li>Instructs patients regarding side effects of self-administered medications, herbs, and food supplements</li>
<li>Evaluates response to prescribed medications</li>
</ul></td>
<td><ul>
<li>Peer review of patient care documentation</li>
<li>Verification of communications with attending physician</li>
<li>Verification of current credentialing status</li>
<li>Evidence of continuing education in area of medication expertise</li>
<li>Other:_____</li>
</ul></td>
</tr>
<tr>
<td></td>
<td>(I8) Administers prescribed medication and solutions
The correct prescribed medication or solution is administered to the right patient, at the right time, in the right dose, via the right route.
<ul>
<li>Reviews patient's history and assessment to identify potential allergies, medication interactions and contraindications</li>
<li>Identifies patient's culturally based home health remedies and any influence on medication management</li>
<li>Identifies patient's over-the-counter self-medication use and herbal practices</li>
<li>Reviews medication orders and understands each medication action, indications, contraindications, adverse reactions, and emergency management</li>
<li>Reviews patient's medication record to determine dosaging schedule</li>
<li>Verifies patient identification, medication or solution, dose, route, and time for administration</li>
<li>Verifies the medication name, dose, and route of administration with the physician and scrub person before transferring medication to the sterile field</li>
<li>Verifies the patient's written consent before administration of experimental medications</li>
</ul></td>
<td><ul>
<li>Observation of patient assessment</li>
<li>Demonstration of patient education related to perioperative medication administration</li>
<li>Peer review of patient care documentation</li>
<li>Completion of facility Occurrence Reporting forms as appropriate</li>
<li>Verification of accuracy of drug calculations</li>
<li>Completion of department specific medication administration module</li>
<li>Other:_____</li>
</ul></td>
</tr>
</table>

Perioperative Medication Competency *(continued)*

Patient Outcome	PNDS Interventions as Measurable Criteria	Recommendations for Validation of Competency
	• Verifies verbal orders before administration by performing a read-back process • Identifies patient by using two different patient identifiers prior to medication administration • Questions orders that appear to be erroneous, illegible, or incomplete • Gathers prescribed medications/solutions and necessary supplies and equipment • Prepares and administers medications/solutions according to facility policy, manufacturers' documented instructions, and federal and state regulations • Calculates drug dosages using weight in kilograms • Ensures the five rights of medication administration are followed during medication administration: 　– Right patient　– Right dose　– Right time 　– Right medication　– Right route • Prepares a written label for all medications placed on the sterile field • Injects local anesthesia when within scope of practice *(RNFA)* • Recognizes medication reactions, complications, and contraindications • Documents medication reactions, complications and contraindications on intra-operative record • Identifies potential drug-drug, herb-drug, and over-the-counter drug-prescription drug interactions • Determines specific antidotes and other emergency medications and equipment are available • Uses resources as needed (eg, product literature medication bulletins, hospital formulary, PDR) • Communicates with facility's pharmacist as needed • Offers instruction about medication actions to patient and family as appropriate • Maintains and follows policies, procedures, guidelines, and/or protocols for safe medication administration • Assess the patient's history for chemotherapy treatment plans (ie, chemotherapeutic and cytotoxic agents) 　▪ Reviews facility's chemotherapy protocols 　▪ Reviews facility's protocols in the event of an accidental spill or exposure to chemotherapeutic agents (hazardous/chemical waste) 　▪ Reviews physician's (ie, oncologist) orders for chemotherapeutic medications 　▪ Reviews lab results before administration of chemotherapeutic medications 　▪ Verifies concentration and stability of chemotherapeutic agent with pharmacist 　▪ Follows facility's procedural guidelines for safe handling, administration, and disposal of chemotherapeutic medications in the operating room 　▪ Revaluates patient's response to chemotherapeutic medication administered	• Evidence of continuing education on general principles for medication administration • Evidence of continuing education related to drug-drug, herb-drug, over-the-counter drug-prescription drug interactions • Evidence of individual annual review of facility policies and procedures related to medication administration • Other: _____

Perioperative Medication Competency (*continued*)

Patient Outcome	PNDS Interventions as Measurable Criteria	Recommendations for Validation of Competency

O29 The patient demonstrates and/or reports adequate pain control throughout the perioperative period	**(I54) Evaluates response to pain management interventions**
	Assesses patient's responses to pain management interventions, including physiological parameters and subjective and objective findings
	• Establishes a safe therapeutic environment during moderate sedation/analgesia or local anesthesia
	  ▪ Establishes and maintains IV access as indicated by procedure and physician order
	  ▪ Uses facility-approved pain scale to assess pain control interventions
	  ▪ Administers prescribed medication or solutions to the right patient, at the right time, in the right dose, via the right route
	  ▪ Implements alternate, non-chemical, methods of pain control including, but not limited to
	    o Positioning to augment pain control
	    o Therapeutic touch
	    o Meditation
	    o Breathing techniques
	• Acts as a patient advocate by protecting the patient from incompetent, unethical, or illegal practices
	  ▪ Maintains continuous surveillance/monitoring of patient data to evaluate reactions to medication administration
	  ▪ Determines patient's maximum limitations for prescribed medications and communicates patient's response to surgeon
	  ▪ Intervenes to protect the patient's safety as needed
		• Review of patient care documentation for continuing assessment and interventions of pain management
		• Completion of annual facility competency specific to moderate sedation/analgesia
		• Evidence of continuing education modules on moderate sedation/analgesia and/or local anesthesia
		• Evidence of annual review of facility policies and procedures for moderate sedation/analgesia and local anesthesia
		• Demonstrates alternative techniques to promote pain relief
		• Other: _____

O3 The patient is free from signs and symptoms of chemical injury	**(I7) Administers prescribed antibiotic therapy and immunizing agents as ordered**
	Verifies physician orders for antibiotic therapies and immunizing agents and safely administers
	• Determines if physician orders for antibiotic therapy have been written
	  ▪ Verifies physician orders and determines that orders are appropriate
	    o Consults with physician as needed
	    o Consults with pharmacist as needed
	  ▪ Determines indications, doses, and intended effects of prescribed medications, as well as interactions with other medications that the patient is receiving
	  ▪ Confirms patient compliance with prescribed prophylactic therapies ordered to be self-administered
	  ▪ Assesses patient before administering, delaying, or withholding medication if necessary
	  ▪ Compares physician's order with label on medication container
	  ▪ Confirms correct medication is administered to the right patient, at the right dose, via the right route, at the right time
	  ▪ Notes expiration date
	  ▪ Safely administers antibiotic therapy as prescribed
	  ▪ Recognizes and identifies adverse effects, toxic reactions, and medication allergies
	  ▪ Evaluates the patient's response to medication administered
		• Observation of medication order review and physician interactions
		• Verification of accuracy for drug calculations
		• Review of patient care documentation for correct dosage of medication and desired effects of medication administration
		• Observation of medication administration technique
		• Completion of facility Occurrence Report form for adverse medication effect
		• Other: _____

Perioperative Medication Competency *(continued)*

Patient Outcome	PNDS Interventions as Measurable Criteria	Recommendations for Validation of Competency
	• Assesses the patient's immunization history for recommended immunizations (eg, vaccines, antisera, immune globulins) ▪ Obtains physician's order for any required immunizations as appropriate ▪ Follows above procedure for safely administering immunizing agents ▪ Safely administers immunization agents as prescribed ▪ Recognizes and identifies adverse effects, toxic reactions, and medication allergies ▪ Evaluates patient's response to medications administered	
O19 The patient demonstrates knowledge of medication management	**(I51) Evaluates response to medications** Observes for response and adverse reactions to medications administered • Monitors patient for demonstrated signs of therapeutic effect • Monitors patient for signs of allergic effects • Monitors patient for signs and symptoms of medication toxicity, including nausea or vomiting • Monitors patient who identifies significant home remedies/over-the-counter medications for potential complications and/or drug interactions • Reports signs or symptoms of adverse reactions to the appropriate member of the health care team	• Evidence in patient care documentation of physiologic monitoring and effects of medication administration • Completion of facility Occurrence Report form as appropriate for untoward medication effect • Other: _____
	(I17) Assesses psychosocial issues specific to the patient's medication management Identifies any variances in medication plan related to psychosocial status. • Identifies barriers to communication • Determines knowledge level • Verifies patient's ability to understand information • Approaches patient in a calm and unhurried manner • Obtains interpreter if needed • Identifies influence of health beliefs and folk practices • Provides culturally sensitive nursing care • Reviews current medication regimens in detail with patient and family members • Reviews factors that may prevent the patient from taking medications as prescribed • Identifies effects of medication use on patient's lifestyle • Evaluates psychosocial issues specific to patient's medication administration	• Evidence of patient response to intervention(s) in patient care document • Evidence of cross-disciplinary collaboration for psychosocial interventions for patient (ie, referrals to case management, visiting nurse) • Evidence of continuing education in cultural competence • Other: _____
	(I104) Provides instruction about prescribed medications Provides information about prescribed medications, such as purpose, administration, and desired side and adverse effects. • Verifies any allergies and sensitivity reactions • States names and purpose of medications • Identifies dose, route, and appropriate times of administration • Instructs patient/family member of specific procedures necessary before medication administration (eg, checking pulse) • Provides clear, understandable explanations about procedures • Communicates discharge instructions verbally and in writing	• Review of individualized patient teaching tools • Peer review of performance • Positive comments on patient satisfaction survey • Evidence of patient/family teaching • Other: _____

Perioperative Medication Competency (*continued*)

Patient Outcome	PNDS Interventions as Measurable Criteria	Recommendations for Validation of Competency

	• Assesses patient's/family member's ability to understand information
	• Encourages family member participation in the instructional process
	• Offers teaching methods relevant to the patient's ability to comprehend information
	• Evaluates the patient's ability to safely and correctly self-administer medications
	• Provides instruction about prescribed medications, to include:
	  ▪ How to obtain and store medications
	  ▪ The purpose and action of medications
	  ▪ Differences in name and appearance of generic and brand names of medications
	  ▪ Doses and times
	  ▪ How medications should be given
	  ▪ Side effects/adverse reactions that may occur
	  ▪ Side effects/adverse reactions to be reported immediately
	  ▪ Symptoms indicating a medication is not effective
	  ▪ Any dietary or fluid restrictions that accompany prescribed medications
	  ▪ Activity restrictions when taking medications
	  ▪ Signs and symptoms of over and under dose
	  ▪ Consequences of not taking or abruptly discontinuing medications
	  ▪ Risks of taking expired medications
	  ▪ Proper disposal of needles and syringes and where to dispose of sharps in the community
	  ▪ Action to be taken if a dose is missed
	  ▪ Applicable food/medication interactions
	  ▪ Appropriate storage practices and care of devices required for medication administration
	• Provides written instructions
	• Instructs patient to take a list of all medications to doctor's office appointment
	• Evaluates patient's responses to instruction
		response to teaching documented in patient care record
		• Patient/family's expressed satisfaction of teaching
		• Review of individualized written patient instructions
		• Review of patient/family member return demonstration of appropriate medication administration
		• Patient/family member verbalization of safety concerns related to prescribed medications
		• Other: _____

	(I48) Evaluates response to instruction about prescribed medications Evaluates understanding of medication instruction by listening to explanations and observing return demonstrations of activities related to the administration and management of medications. • Requests patient/family member to verbalize name of medication prescribed and its purpose • Reviews any cultural practices related to medication administration • Requests patient/family member to verbalize dose, route, and frequency of medication administration • Request patient/family member to verbalize action to be taken when a dose is missed • Requests patient/family member to demonstrate specific procedures required before medication administration (eg, check pulse) • Encourages and answers questions	• Review of patient/family member's return demonstration of medication administration • Patient/family member verbalization of safety concerns related to cultural beliefs and prescribed medications • Other: _____

Perioperative Medication Competency (*continued*)

Patient Outcome	PNDS Interventions as Measurable Criteria	Recommendations for Validation of Competency
O20 The patient demonstrates knowledge of pain management	**(I61) Identifies cultural and value components related to pain** Provides pain control considering cultural factors and manifestations of values (eg, stoicism, alternative therapy, verbalization, meditation). • Reviews patient record for type of pain being treated, medical condition, demographics, and cultural cues • Establishes rapport • Evaluates language and cognitive skills relative to age and developmental stage • Identifies barriers to communication • Identifies presence of altered thought processes • Determines educational background • Obtains interpreter if needed • Requests patient to verbalize pain management protocol and its purpose • Identifies patient's preference of pain therapy and coping methods • Asks patient to describe pain and its intensity • Offers assessment tool most appropriate to patient need (ie, numerical scale, color scale, face scale) • Verifies assessment tool is clearly understood • Provides culturally sensitive nursing care • Identifies mutual goals of care that consider different preferences (eg, alert versus pain free)	• Evidence of patient's understanding of cultural belief system and medication safety concerns in the patient care record • Evidence of positive patient/family-nurse interactions (eg, peer report) • Presence of interpreter or evidence of translation line accessed • Review of pain assessment using appropriate pain scale; nursing interventions, and patient response to interventions as documented in patient care record • Other: _____
	(I108) Provides pain management instruction Provides information about the purpose; administration; and desired side and adverse effects of prescribed medications and non-pharmacological techniques for managing pain. • Validates orders for prescribed medication • Verifies patient's ability to understand information • Provides patient with time to process information • Identifies patient's cultural practices • Obtains interpreter if needed • Verifies allergies and any sensitivity reactions • Explains names and purposes of medications • Identifies dose, route, and appropriate times of administration • Instructs patient/family member on specific protocols for medication administration (eg, use of patient controlled analgesia pump) • Reviews actions to be taken if a dose is missed • Encourages notification of health care provider when discomfort is unrelieved by ordered medications or is worsening • Reviews desired side and adverse effects • Reviews applicable food/medication interactions • Reviews appropriate storage practices and care of equipment • Provides written instructions • Encourages family member participation in the instruction process • Evaluates patient's understanding of medication administration, purpose and effects	• Observation of patient education/instruction • Presence of interpreter or evidence of translation line accessed • Identification of patient allergies in patient care record and use of facility allergy alert system (ie, arm band) • Patient/family verbalization of steps taken for missed medication dose and identification of adverse side effects • Evidence of continuing education in cultural competence • Other: _____

Perioperative Medication Competency (*continued*)

Patient Outcome	PNDS Interventions as Measurable Criteria	Recommendations for Validation of Competency
	(I53) Evaluates response to pain management instruction Evaluates understanding of pain management instruction by listening to explanations and observing return demonstrations. • Requests patient/family member to verbalize understanding of pain medication and its purpose • Requests feedback on level of pain management achieved using a recognized pain measurement tool (eg, numbers, faces) • Observes patient for nonverbal cues regarding pain (eg, grimacing with movement, splinting) • Reviews cultural influences on pain assessment and management • Requests patient/family member to verbalize dose, route, and frequency of medication • Requests patient/family member to verbalize action to be taken when a dose is missed • Requests patient/family member to identify where written instructions will be kept for reference • Determines patient's understanding to notify health care provider if pain is not controlled or is worsening • Encourages questions and clarifies information	• Review of patient/family medication instruction sheet • Peer review of patient responses to nursing interventions • Evidence of assessment of patient/family understanding of pain management in patient care documentation • Observation of nurse interventions related to patient's nonverbal responses to pain • Other: _____

Sample Care Plan: Intraoperative

Nursing Diagnosis	Expected Patient Outcome	Nursing	Y ☐	N ☐	N/A ☐	Evaluation of Patient Outcomes	Y ☐	N ☐	N/A ☐
Potential for risk of injury.	The patient is free from signs and symptoms of injury.	1. Verifies patient identity, operative site, operative procedure, and consents.	☐	☐	☐	1. Patient is optimally prepared for surgery. 2. Patient is free from signs and symptoms of injury related to	☐	☐	☐
		2. Verifies NPO status.	☐	☐	☐	• physical injury.	☐	☐	☐
		3. Assesses/verifies known allergies.	☐	☐	☐	• foreign objects (eg, sponges).	☐	☐	☐
		4. Implements protective measures to prevent injury related to electrical, chemical, and laser sources.	☐	☐	☐	• chemical injury (eg, prep solutions).	☐	☐	☐
						• electrical injury (eg, electrocautery).	☐	☐	☐
		5. Implements procedure for sponge and sharps counts.	☐	☐	☐	• laser injury.	☐	☐	☐
		6. Uses supplies and equipment within safe parameters.	☐	☐	☐	• positioning.	☐	☐	☐
		7. Identifies physical alterations that may affect procedure-specific positioning.	☐	☐	☐				
Potential for risk of infection.	The patient is free from signs and symptoms of infection.	1. Implements/ensures that sterile technique is maintained.	☐	☐	☐	Sterile technique is maintained.	☐	☐	☐
		2. Classifies surgical wound.	☐	☐	☐				
		3. Performs skin preparations.	☐	☐	☐				
		4. Minimizes length of procedure by planning care.	☐	☐	☐				
		5. Assists with wound dressing at completion of procedure.	☐	☐	☐				
Potential for risk of altered body temperature.	Body temperature will remain within expected range.	1. Collaborates with anesthesia in maintenance of normothermia.	☐	☐	☐	Patient is at or returning to normothermia at the conclusion of the intraoperative period.	☐	☐	☐
		2. Implements thermoregulation measures.	☐	☐	☐				
		3. Evaluates responses to thermoregulation.	☐	☐	☐				

Sample Care Plan: Intraoperative (continued)

Nursing Diagnosis	Expected Patient Outcome	Nursing Interventions	Y ❏	N ❏	N/A ❏	Evaluation of Patient Outcomes	Y ❏	N ❏	N/A ❏
Potential for risk of impaired skin integrity.	Patient has wound/ tissue perfusion consistent with or improved from baseline levels established preoperatively.	1. Assesses for pre-existing conditions that predispose to inadequate tissue perfusion. 2. Identifies baseline tissue perfusion. 3. Utilizes proper positioning aids. 4. Evaluates postoperative tissue perfusion.	❏ ❏ ❏ ❏	❏ ❏ ❏ ❏	❏ ❏ ❏ ❏	Other than the surgical site, skin remains smooth, intact, non-reddened, non-irritated, and free of bruising.	❏	❏	❏
Potential for compromised cardio-respiratory function.	Patient will maintain optimal cardiopulmonary function.	1. Collaborates with anesthesiologist on cardiorespiratory function and fluid management. 2. Assists with administration of blood product therapy as required.	❏ ❏	❏ ❏	❏ ❏	Patient did not experience cardiopulmonary event related to surgical procedure.	❏	❏	❏

Comments: _____

_____

_____

Signature   Title   Date

Sample Care Plan: Ambulatory Surgery

Nursing Diagnosis	Expected Patient Outcome	Nursing Interventions	Y ❑	N ❑	N/A ❑	Evaluation of Patient Outcomes	Y ❑	N ❑	N/A ❑
PREOPERATIVE PHASE									
Anxiety and fear related to knowledge deficit regarding preoperative sequence of events and perioperative experience.	The patient will be optimally prepared for surgery.	1. Implement protocol for presurgical patient screening.	❑	❑	❑	1. The patient is prepared and ready for surgery.	❑	❑	❑
		2. Implement protocol for perioperative care of the ambulatory surgical patient.	❑	❑	❑	2. The patient is transferred to operating room.	❑	❑	❑
		3. Provide appropriate patient education.	❑	❑	❑				
INTRAOPERATIVE PHASE									
Potential for risk of injury.	The patient is free from signs and symptoms of injury.	1. Verifies patient identity, operative site, operative procedures, and consents.	❑	❑	❑	1. Patient is optimally prepared for surgery. 2. Patient is free from signs and symptoms of injury related to:	❑	❑	❑
		2. Verifies NPO status.				• physical injury.	❑	❑	❑
		3. Assess/verifies known allergies.	❑	❑	❑	• foreign objects (eg, sponges).	❑	❑	❑
			❑	❑	❑				
		4. Implements protective measures to prevent injury related to electrical, chemical, and laser sources.	❑	❑	❑	• chemical injury (eg, prep solutions).	❑	❑	❑
		5. Implements procedure for sponge and sharps counts.	❑	❑	❑	• electrical injury (eg, electrocautery).	❑	❑	❑
		6. Uses supplies and equipment within safe parameters.	❑	❑	❑	• laser injury.	❑	❑	❑
		7. Identifies physical alterations that may affect procedure-specific positioning.	❑	❑	❑	• positioning.	❑	❑	❑
Potential for risk of infection.	The patient is free from signs and symptoms of infection.	1. Implements/ensures that sterile technique is maintained.	❑	❑	❑	Sterile technique is maintained.	❑	❑	❑
		2. Classifies surgical wound.	❑	❑	❑				
		3. Performs skin preps.	❑	❑	❑				
		4. Minimizes length of procedure by planning care.	❑	❑	❑				
		5. Assists with wound dressing at completion of procedure.	❑	❑	❑				

Sample Care Plan: Ambulatory Surgery *(continued)*

Nursing Diagnosis	Expected Patient Outcome	Nursing Interventions	Y ☐	N ☐	N/A ☐	Evaluation of Patient Outcomes	Y ☐	N ☐	N/A ☐
Potential for risk of altered body temperature.	Body temperature will remain within expected range.	1. Collaborates with anesthesia provider to maintain normothermia. 2. Implements thermo-regulation measures. 3. Evaluates responses to thermoregulation.	☐ ☐	☐ ☐	☐ ☐	Patient is at or return-ing to normothermia at the conclusion of the intraoperative period.	☐	☐	☐
Potential for risk of impaired skin integrity.	Patient has wound tissue perfusion consistent with or improved from baseline levels established preoperatively.	1. Assesses for pre-existing conditions that predispose to inadequate tissue perfusion. 2. Identifies baseline tissue perfusion. 3. Utilizes proper positioning aids. 4. Evaluates postopera-tive tissue perfusion.	☐ ☐ ☐	☐ ☐ ☐	☐ ☐ ☐	Other than the surgical site, skin remains smooth, intact, non-reddened, non-irritated, and free of bruising.	☐	☐	☐
Potential for compromised cardio-respiratory function.	Patient will maintain optimal cardiopulmonary function.	Collaborates with anesthesia provider on maintaining cardio-respiratory function and fluid management.	☐	☐	☐	Patient did not experience cardiopul-monary event related to surgical procedure.	☐	☐	☐
POSTOPERATIVE PHASE									
Potential for compromised physical state related to surgery/ anesthesia.	Patient will regain optimal functioning/ homeostasis.	Implement protocol for perioperative care of the ambulatory surgical patient.	☐	☐	☐	1. Vital signs are stable. 2. Patient is alert and oriented. 3. Dressing on surgical site is dry and intact. 4. Minimal or absent signs of nausea or vomiting. 5. Patient is tolerant to fluid intake. 6. Patient is able to void.	☐ ☐ ☐ ☐ ☐ ☐	☐ ☐ ☐ ☐ ☐ ☐	☐ ☐ ☐ ☐ ☐ ☐
Alteration in comfort/pain.	Patient verbalizes a comfort level of 0–5 using a Pain Scale of 0–10.	1. Patient verbalizes adequate pain control. 2. Patient/family verbalizes under-standing of discharge pain management plan.	☐ ☐	☐ ☐	☐ ☐	1. Implement pain management protocol. 2. Administer analgesics per order. 3. Apply cryotherapy (cold therapy) to surgical site.	☐ ☐ ☐	☐ ☐ ☐	☐ ☐ ☐

Sample Care Plan: Ambulatory Surgery *(continued)*

Nursing Diagnosis	Expected Patient Outcome	Nursing Interventions	Y ❏	N ❏	N/A ❏	Evaluation of Patient Outcomes	Y ❏	N ❏	N/A ❏
						4. Teach comfort measures (eg, controlled deep breathing exercises, proper positioning/ elevation of extremity, application and importance of cryotherapy). 5. Provide prescription and instruction regimen for pain medication.	❏	❏	❏
Potential risk for peripheral and neurovascular dysfunction related to surgery/anesthesia.	The patient will not experience peripheral neurovascular dysfunction.	Implement protocol: "Management of the Patient with High Risk for Peripheral Neurovascular Dysfunction."	❏	❏	❏	Neurovascular status intact.	❏	❏	❏
Knowledge deficit related to rehabilitation, discharge experience, and care after discharge.	The patient will understand rehabilitation protocol and demonstrate safe functioning. The patient/family will verbalize understanding of discharge instructions. The patient will be discharged to an environment that is congruent with patient's needs.	1. Reinforce instructions provided in patient education manual. 2. Reinforce rehabilitation regimen and use of equipment. 3. Ensure that patient knows when to return to surgeon's office for postop visit. 4. Teach surgical site care and signs and symptoms of infection. 5. Instruct patient on how to proceed in event of an emergency.	❏ ❏ ❏ ❏ ❏	❏ ❏ ❏ ❏ ❏	❏ ❏ ❏ ❏ ❏	1. Patient/family express understanding of discharge instructions and rehabilitation protocol. 2. Patient discharged to home accompanied by a responsible adult. 3. Patient transferred to inpatient unit for further recovery.	❏ ❏ ❏	❏ ❏ ❏	❏ ❏ ❏

Comments: _____

_____

_____

Signature   *Title*   *Date*

Sample Care Plan: Perioperative

System	Patient Problem	Interventions	Outcomes	Preop			Intraop			Postop		
Coping, psychosocial	Anxiety related to periop experience.	Offers reassurance, emotional/physical support Administers anti-anxiety medications as ordered	Patient exhibits appropriate coping behaviors	Y	N	N/A	Y	N	N/A	Y	N	N/A
Safety	Potential for injury in periop environment	*Refer to standards of care* Allergies verified Fall precautions implemented	Patient is free from physical injury unrelated to the intervention	Y	N	N/A	Y	N	N/A	Y	N	N/A
Comfort	Pain related to diagnosis and or surgery	*Refer to standards of care* Assess verbal and nonverbal signs and symptoms of pain Instruct and use pain scale related to age and need Administer pain medication as ordered Utilize other treatment modalities	Patient reports pain is tolerable	Y	N	N/A	Y	N	N/A	Y	N	N/A
Cultural/ Spiritual	Fear/anxiety related to periop experience	*Refer to standards of care* Interpreter PRN Privacy provided Preserve/protect autonomy/ dignity	Patient expresses satisfaction with delivered care	Y	N	N/A	Y	N	N/A	Y	N	N/A
Cardiovascular	Altered tissue perfusion: cardiac or peripheral	*Refer to standards of care*	VS within +/- 20% of baseline	Y	N	N/A	Y	N	N/A	Y	N	N/A
Neuro	Potential alteration in neuro status	*Refer to standards of care* Assess neurological status	Sensory/motor and cognitive function appropriate to intervention	Y	N	N/A	Y	N	N/A	Y	N	N/A
Respiratory	Potential for impaired gas exchange	*Refer to standards of care*	Airway patent, maintain 02 sat at 92% or +/- 2% of baseline	Y	N	N/A	Y	N	N/A	Y	N	N/A
Nutrition	Potential for inadequate caloric intake Potential for fluid and electrolyte imbalance	Maintain NPO status Functional nutrition screen completed on day of surgery Identify priority status for follow-up by inpatient unit • High—within 24 hrs • Med—within 48 hrs • Low—within 72 hrs	Patient's caloric and hydration needs are met	Y	N	N/A	Y	N	N/A	Y	N	N/A
Skin/Tissue	Potential for skin/tissue injury	*Refer to standards of care*	Skin/tissue integrity unchanged other than surgical incision/IV site	Y	N	N/A	Y	N	N/A	Y	N	N/A
Education	Knowledge deficit	Provide information to patient/family throughout the periop period	Patient/family verbalizes understanding of care	Y	N	N/A	Y	N	N/A	Y	N	N/A

Circle one: Y = Outcomes met; N = Outcomes not met; N/A = Not applicable.

Sample Care Plan: Perioperative *(continued)*

System	Patient Problem	Interventions	Outcomes	Preop	Intraop	Postop
Medical conditions	❑ Malignant hyperthermia (MH)	MH precautions and protocol instituted	Absence of MH symptoms	Y N N/A	Y N N/A	Y N N/A
	❑ Diabetes	Diabetic protocol	Glucose within defined parameters	Y N N/A	Y N N/A	Y N N/A
	❑ Latex allergy	Implement latex precautions	Absence of allergic reaction to latex	Y N N/A	Y N N/A	Y N N/A
	❑ Potential for seizures	Seizure precautions instituted	Absence of injury as a result of seizure	Y N N/A	Y N N/A	Y N N/A

Circle one: Y = Outcomes met; N = Outcomes not met; N/A = Not applicable.

Comments: _____

_____

_____

Signature   *Title*   *Date*

Perioperative Clinical Pathway: Total Hip Arthroplasty

Multidisciplinary Action Plan	Arrival to Holding Avg time = ___ min	Holding Area Time Avg time = ___ min	Arrival to OR to Incision = 40 min	Incision to End of Procedure = 2 hrs	End of Procedure to Arrival in PACU = 15 min
Clinical and Learning Outcomes *(PNDS elements in parentheses)*	Pt free from signs and symptoms of injury from transfer/ transport (O8)	*Nsg Dx: Fear and anxiety related to surgery* Consent signed Right to privacy maintained (O25) Pt is free from signs and symptoms of physical injury (O1) Pt demonstrates knowledge of the physiological and psychological responses to the operative procedure (O31) Pt participates in decisions affecting perioperative plan of care (O23)	*Nsg Dx: Risk for impaired skin integrity, neuro-muscular injury, circulatory compromise* *Nsg Dx:* Risk of infection related to surgical wound Pt care is consistent with perioperative plan (O24)	*Nsg Dx: Risk of injury related to extraneous objects* *Nsg Dx:* Risk of infection related to surgical wound Pt is free from injury related to extraneous objects (O2) Pt is free from signs and symptoms of infection (O10) Pt receives appropri-ate prescribed medications, safely adminis-tered during the periop period (O9) Pt receives consis-tent level of care from all caregivers regardless of the setting (O27) Pt's value system, lifestyle, ethnic-ity, and culture are considered, respected, and incorporated in the plan of care (O28)	*Nsg Dx: Risk of injury related to extraneous objects* *Nsg Dx:* Risk of infection related to surgical wound Pt is free from signs and symp-toms of injury related to positioning (O5) Pt is free from signs and symp-toms of injury related to electrocautery device (O4) Pt free from signs and symptoms of injury related to chemical sources (O3) Pt is free from signs and symptoms of injury related to transfer/transport (O8) Pt is free from signs and symp-toms of infection (O10) Pt returned to normothermia (O12)
Consults		Dept of Anesthesia			
Discharge Planning	Pt's family identified, directed to lounge	Immediate postop disposition identified Family or other support person identified		Status reports given to family	OR record complete Prosthesis docu-mented; implants communicated to Materials Mgmt
Assessment		History & physical, labs, ECG, chest x-ray, hip films to chart Allergies identified and charted	Vital signs per Anesthesia. Confirms identity and operative site prior to incision (I26); charted	Vital signs per Anesthesia. Classifies surgical wound (I22)	Vital signs per Anesthesia. Pt meets criteria for successful emer-gence per anes-thesia protocol

Perioperative Clinical Pathway: Total Hip Arthroplasty *(continued)*

Multidisciplinary Action Plan	Arrival to Holding Avg time = __ min	Holding Area Time Avg time = __ min	Arrival to OR to Incision = 40 min	Incision to End of Procedure = 2 hrs	End of Procedure to Arrival in PACU = 15 min
		Verifies consent; operative site identified and marked; matches consent (I23-I26) Verifies NPO status (I125) Identifies barriers to communication (I65) Identifies baseline tissue perfusion (I60) Assesses readiness to learn (I20) Family contact identified Verifies presence of prosthetic or corrective devices (I27)			Skin assessed for signs and symptoms of injury related to positioning, electrical, chemical, or mechanical sources (I36-43) Assess for pain control (I16)
Interventions	Length of invasive procedure minimized by planning care (I85)	Administers prescribed antibiotic (I7) Administers other prophylactic treatment PRN. (I10)	Positions patient (I96) Applies safety device (I11) Performs skin preparation (I94) Implements protective measures to prevent injury due to electrical sources (I72) Implements thermo-regulatory measures (I78)	Implements aseptic technique (I70) Collaborates in fluid management (I23) Performs required counts (I93) Provides update to family (I10) Records devices implanted (I12)	Administers care to wound site (I3, 31) Transports according to individual needs (I118) Continuity of care provided (I27)
Tests		Missing labs located, performed PRN	ABG per Anesthesia		
Meds		Antibiotics as ordered; IV and sedation per Anesthesia	Per Anesthesia	1 g Ancef/1L NS irrigation; anesthetic per Anesthesia	Per Anesthesia
Treatment & Equipment: Related periop data elements *(data-type in parentheses)*	Holding area time in/out *(date/time)* Mode of transport *(dictionary/table)*	Chart complete *(y/n)* Consent signed/site verified *(y/n)* Pt verbalizes correct procedure *(y/n)*	Pt time in *(date/time)* Surgical team *(dictionary/table)* Positioned per protocol *(y/n)*	OR laminar flow room *(y/n)* Sterile field maintained *(y/n)* Counts correct *(C or NC)*	Sterile dressing type/location *(dictionary/table)* Bovie site intact *(y/n)* Pt safely transferred to cart *(y/n)*

Perioperative Clinical Pathway: Total Hip Arthroplasty *(continued)*

Multidisciplinary Action Plan	Arrival to Holding Avg time = ___ min	Holding Area Time Avg time = ___ min	Arrival to OR to Incision = 40 min	Incision to End of Procedure = 2 hrs	End of Procedure to Arrival in PACU = 15 min
	Siderails up *(y/n)* ID band on and verified *(y/n)*	Warm blanket applied *(check vs null)* Preop checklist complete *(y/n)* Access to pt care area restricted *(y/n)* Access to pt information restricted Antibiotic start/stop *(date/time)* Implants *(y/n)*	Devices documented *(dictionary/table)* Safety strap applied *(y/n)* Surgical prep type *(dictionary/table)* Bovie pad applied/ location *(unit #)* Temperature-regulating blanket applied *(unit #)*	Updates to family *(date/time)* Implants confirmed w/ surgeon prior to delivery to sterile field *(y/n)* Implants documented *(lot #, sterile date/time, date of surgery)* Procedure end *(date/time)* Wound class *(table)*	Siderails up *(y/n)* PACU notified OR record complete Pt time out *(date/time)*
Activity	Pt states name ID band checked	Pt states name ID band checked Pt confirms operative side Pt verifies NPO status	Thermoregulatory measures verified by pt's body temperature		Pt stable for transport per anesthesia protocol Pt's skin remains intact and non-reddened; no bruising Pt remains afebrile
Nutrition		IV per Anesthesia	IV per Anesthesia	IV per Anesthesia	IV per Anesthesia

JOB DESCRIPTION
Position Title: Perioperative Case Manager

JOB SUMMARY

The Perioperative Case Manager is a Registered Professional Nurse who has 24-hour accountability for the intraoperative nursing care provided in his/her designated surgical specialties. In this capacity, the Perioperative Case Manager works with specialty physicians and clinical and administrative leaders to provide quality care at optimal cost. The Perioperative Case Manager will provide direct care and supervise the care given by others. He or she will participate in the development of Critical Pathways pertinent to his/her designated surgical specialty. He or she will orient staff members and evaluate staff performance. The Perioperative Case Manager provides continuing education and is responsible for the development of staff members. In conjunction with the Administrative Director, the Perioperative Case Manager is also responsible for securing and maintaining supplies and equipment necessary to the delivery of care. He or she is also responsible for their participation in the formation of the annual budget and its monthly monitoring. Additionally, the Perioperative Case Manager will perform case cost analysis and work with physician members to improve cost per case ratios.

RESPONSIBILITIES AND DUTIES

1. **Demonstrates knowledge of facility CARE protocol.**

   Considerate
   - Be courteous; introduce yourself and treat each customer as you would a guest in your home.
   - Use good judgment; customers are everywhere, and you are always "on stage."

   Attentive
   - Always acknowledge someone waiting for your attention.
   - Maintain a clean and professional environment.

   Responsive
   - Take initiative; ask how you can help and make a good first impression.
   - Find answers; don't assume someone else will take care of it.

   Empathetic
   - Treat people with dignity; respect the privacy and confidentiality of each patient.
   - Anticipate your customer's needs and freely offer your help.

2. **Demonstrates knowledge and application of facility policies and procedures that apply to job and area of responsibility.**

3. **Assesses the physiological and psychosocial needs of the patient.**
   - Confirms identity, verifies operative site, surgical procedure, NPO status, and any patient allergies. (PNDS I123 through I125)
   - Identifies baseline skin condition, body mobility, sensory impairments, cardiovascular and respiratory status. (PNDS I59, I60)
   - Assesses and reports any deviations from normal in preoperative diagnostic studies. (PNDS I110, I111)
   - Assesses readiness to learn based on pt's perceptions and expectations of care. (PNDS I19, I20, I57, I65–I68)
   - Identifies any spiritual, cultural, and/or philosophical beliefs that may impact care provided.(PNDS I17, I18)

4. **Provides intraoperative nursing care.**
   - Implements aseptic technique by creating and maintaining a sterile field.(PNDS I70)
   - Monitors physical status of patient, to administer drugs, solutions as prescribed. (PNDS I51)
   - Monitors and controls the environment and considers all assessment information for the plan of care and demonstrates individual choice based on identified patient needs. (PNDS I30)
   - Applies safety devices. (PNDS I11)
   - Assesses the timing and need for a sponge, needle, and instrument count and performs required counts accurately. (PNDS I93)
   - Manages culture/specimen collection, handling, and disposition according to facility policy and procedure. (PNDS I83-I84)
   - Classifies surgical wound per policy. (PNDS I22)
   - Collaborates in fluid management. (PNDS I23)
   - Provides status report to family/support person. (PNDS I109)

5. **Performs activities that demonstrate nursing accountability.**
   - Respects patient rights and practices within ethical and legal guidelines. (PNDS I116)
   - Completes required competencies and training in assigned timeframe.
   - Performs QI activities in conjunction with department leadership.
   - Demonstrates the ability to process through to solution a variety of problems.
   - Exercises safe judgment in decision making and demonstrates tact and understanding when dealing with patients, team members, members of other disciplines, and the public. (PNDS I92)
   - Demonstrates flexibility and adaptability to changes in nursing practice and responds in a positive manner to constructive criticism.

6. **Safely and adequately provides and utilizes equipment and supplies based on patient needs.**
   - Minimizes the length of invasive procedure by planning care: anticipates needs for equipment and supplies and selects in an organized and timely manner. (PNDS I85)
   - Uses supplies and equipment within safe parameters by ensuring all equipment is functioning before use and removing malfunctioning equipment from use. (PNDS I122)
   - Implements protective measures to prevent injury due to electrical, laser, radiation, chemical, thermal, or mechanical sources. (PNDS I72 through I77)
   - Uses supplies and equipment in a judicious and cost-effective manner and documents utilization.
   - Records devices implanted during the operative or invasive procedure. (PNDS I112)

7. **Evaluates patient outcomes.**
   - Evaluates for s/s of injury related to chemical, electrical, thermal, or mechanical sources. (PNDS I36-I38, I41, I43)
   - Evaluates for s/s of injury as a result of positioning or pt transfer/transport. (PNDS I38, I42)
   - Evaluates response to pain management interventions. (PNDS I54)

8. **Participates in the professional development of self and team members.**
   - Actively participates in educating and mentoring colleagues and team members to the job or team duties.
   - Participates in professional organization and/or performs educational inservicing for team members.
   - Creates a positive learning environment for new team members.
   - Provides ongoing assessment of professional growth and the level of development of each staff member through observation, evaluation, counseling, problem-solving, and emotional and situational support to increase retention and decrease turnover.
   - Utilizes knowledge and skill to facilitate warranted change.
   - Responsible for the continuing education and development of staff.

9. **Participates in unit management as appropriate.**
   - Performs QI activities in conjunction with the departmental leadership.
   - Acts as a resource person for problem solving in the operating room and facility-wide.
   - Provides supervision for the operating rooms in the absence of the Clinical Director.
   - Maintains 24-hour accountability for services.
   - Interviews, selects, counsels, mentors, and evaluates staff in accordance with facility guidelines.
   - Develops and uses interdepartmental contacts to promote quality patient care.
   - Participates as a member of the Perioperative Case Manager Team in the OR.

10. **Demonstrates problem solving/critical thinking skills.**
   - Demonstrates the ability to process through to solution a variety of problems.
   - Displays a clear understanding of the organizational structure of the operating room and facility.
   - Must be able to maintain his or her problem-solving skills under very stressful conditions.
   - Demonstrates flexibility and adaptability to changes in nursing or administrative practice and responds in a positive manner to constructive criticism.
   - Exercises safe judgment in decision making and demonstrates tact and understanding when dealing with patients, team members, members of other disciplines, and the public.

11. **Demonstrates knowledge of case management and analysis.**
   - Responsible for inventory of equipment, special supplies, and their maintenance.
   - Performs case cost analysis and works with physician members to reduce cost per case ratios.
   - Participates in the negotiation for and evaluation of surgical supplies and equipment.
   - Participates in the preparation and monthly monitoring of annual budget.
   - Works with Administrative Director to maintain appropriate level of inventory.
   - Participates on assigned committees to improve performance of operating room.
   - Periodically meets with service specific physicians to coordinate activities and identify needs.
   - Monitors block utilization for service specific physicians and suggests reallocation based on activity.

JOB DESCRIPTION
Position Title: Perioperative Team Leader

JOB SUMMARY

The Perioperative Team Leader is a clinically competent RN who assumes accountability for the quality of nursing care delivered on specified surgical services. In this capacity, the Team Leader gives direct care and oversees the care given by other nursing personnel on the services. The Team Leader orients staff members, participates in evaluating their performance, and provides continuing education. In conjunction with the Case Manager, the Team Leader is responsible for securing and maintaining the supplies and equipment necessary for the delivery of care. The Team Leader reports to the Case Manager responsible for his or her service in the operating room.

RESPONSIBILITIES AND DUTIES

1. **Demonstrates knowledge of facility CARE protocol.**

   Considerate
   - Be courteous; introduce yourself and treat each customer as you would a guest in your home.
   - Use good judgment; customers are everywhere, and you are always "on stage."

   Attentive
   - Always acknowledge someone waiting for your attention.
   - Maintain a clean and professional environment.

   Responsive
   - Take initiative; ask how you can help and make a good first impression.
   - Find answers; don't assume someone else will take care of it.

   Empathetic
   - Treat people with dignity; respect the privacy and confidentiality of each patient.
   - Anticipate your customer's needs and freely offer your help.

2. **Demonstrates knowledge and application of policies and procedures that apply to your job and area of responsibility.**

3. **Assesses the physiological and psychosocial needs of the patient.**
   - Confirms identity, verifies operative site, surgical procedure, NPO status, and any patient allergies. (PNDS I123 through I125)
   - Identifies baseline skin condition, body mobility, sensory impairments, cardiovascular, and respiratory status. (PNDS I59, I60)
   - Assesses and reports any deviations from normal in preoperative diagnostic studies. (PNDS I110, I111)
   - Assesses readiness to learn based on pt's perceptions and expectations of care.(PNDS I19, I20, I57, I65-I68)
   - Identifies any spiritual, cultural, and/or philosophical beliefs that may impact care provided.(PNDS I17, I18)

4. **Provides intraoperative nursing care.**
   - Implements aseptic technique by creating and maintaining a sterile field. (PNDS I70)
   - Monitors physical status of patient, to administer drugs, solutions as prescribed. (PNDS I51)
   - Monitors and controls the environment and considers all assessment information for the plan of care and demonstrates individual choice based on identified patient needs. (PNDS I30)
   - Applies safety devices. (PNDS I11)
   - Assesses the timing and need for a sponge, needle, and instrument count and performs required counts accurately. (PNDS I93)
   - Manages culture/specimen collection, handling, and disposition according to facility policy and procedure. (PNDS I83-I84)
   - Classifies surgical wound per policy. (PNDS I22)

- Collaborates in fluid management. (PNDS I23)
- Provides status report to family/support person. (PNDS I109)

5. **Performs activities that demonstrate nursing accountability.**
   - Respects patient rights and practices within ethical and legal guidelines. (PNDS I116)
   - Completes required competencies and training in assigned timeframe.
   - Performs QI activities in conjunction with department leadership.
   - Demonstrates the ability to process through to solution a variety of problems.
   - Exercises safe judgment in decision making and demonstrates tact and understanding when dealing with patients, team members, members of other disciplines, and the public. (PNDS I92)
   - Demonstrates flexibility and adaptability to changes in nursing practice and responds in a positive manner to constructive criticism.

6. **Safely and adequately provides and utilizes equipment and supplies based on patient needs.**
   - Minimizes the length of invasive procedure by planning care: anticipates needs for equipment and supplies and selects in an organized and timely manner. (PNDS I85)
   - Uses supplies and equipment within safe parameters by ensuring all equipment is functioning before use and removing malfunctioning equipment from use. (PNDS I122)
   - Implements protective measures to prevent injury due to electrical, laser, radiation, chemical, thermal, or mechanical sources. (PNDS I72 through I77)
   - Uses supplies and equipment in a judicious and cost-effective manner and documents utilization.
   - Records devices implanted during the operative or invasive procedure. (PNDS I112)

7. **Evaluates patient outcomes.**
   - Evaluates for s/s of injury related to chemical, electrical, thermal, or mechanical sources. (PNDS I36-I38, I41, I43)
   - Evaluates for s/s of injury as a result of positioning or pt transfer/transport. (PNDS I38, I42)
   - Evaluates response to pain management interventions. (PNDS I54)

8. **Participates in the professional development of self and team members.**
   - Actively participates in educating and mentoring colleagues and team members to the job or team duties.
   - Participates in professional organization and/or performs educational inservicing for team members.
   - Creates a positive learning environment for new team members.
   - Utilizes knowledge and skill to facilitate warranted change.

9. **Demonstrates leadership.**
   - Performs QI activities in conjunction with the departmental leadership.
   - Acts as a resource person for problem solving in the operating room and facility-wide.
   - Provides supervision for the operating rooms in the absence of the control desk manager or on off-shifts.
   - Develops and uses interdepartmental contacts to promote quality patient care.
   - Functions on a daily basis as an expert in his or her specialty in both the scrubbing and circulating role.

10. **Demonstrates problem solving/critical thinking skills.**
    - Demonstrates the ability to process through to solution a variety of problems.
    - Displays a clear understanding of the organizational structure of the operating room and facility.
    - Must be able to maintain his or her problem solving skills under very stressful conditions.
    - Demonstrates flexibility and adaptability to changes in nursing or administrative practice and responds in a positive manner to constructive criticism.
    - Exercises safe judgment in decision making and demonstrates tact and understanding when dealing with patients, team members, members of other disciplines, and the public.

JOB DESCRIPTION
Position Title: Perioperative Registered Nurse

JOB SUMMARY
Provide preoperative, intraoperative, and postoperative nursing care of the surgical patient.

RESPONSIBILITIES AND DUTIES
1. **Demonstrates knowledge of facility CARE protocol.**

   Considerate
   - Be courteous; introduce yourself and treat each customer as you would a guest in your home.
   - Use good judgment; customers are everywhere, and you are always "on stage."

   Attentive
   - Always acknowledge someone waiting for your attention.
   - Maintain a clean and professional environment.

   Responsive
   - Take initiative; ask how you can help and make a good first impression.
   - Find answers; don't assume someone else will take care of it.

   Empathetic
   - Treat people with dignity; respect the privacy and confidentiality of each patient.
   - Anticipate your customer's needs and freely offer your help.

2. **Demonstrates knowledge and application of facility policies and procedures that apply to your job and area of responsibility.**

3. **Assesses the physiological and psychosocial needs of the patient.**
   - Confirms identity, verifies operative site, surgical procedure, NPO status, and any patient allergies. (PNDS I123 through I125)
   - Identifies baseline skin condition, body mobility, sensory impairments, cardiovascular, and respiratory status. (PNDS I59, I60)
   - Assesses and reports any deviations from normal in preoperative diagnostic studies. (PNDS I110, I111)
   - Assesses readiness to learn based on patient's perceptions and expectations of care. (PNDS I19, I20, I57, I65-I68)
   - Identifies any spiritual, cultural and/or philosophical beliefs that may impact care provided. (PNDS I17, I18)

4. **Provides intraoperative nursing care.**
   - Implements aseptic technique by creating and maintaining a sterile field. (PNDS I70)
   - Monitors physical status of patient, to administer drugs, solutions as prescribed. (PNDS I51)
   - Monitors and controls the environment and considers all assessment information for the plan of care and demonstrates individual choice based on identified patient needs. (PNDS I30)
   - Applies safety devices. (PNDS I11)
   - Assesses the timing and need for a sponge, needle, and instrument count and performs required counts accurately. (PNDS I93)
   - Manages culture/specimen collection, handling, and disposition according to facility policy and procedure. (PNDS I83-I84)
   - Classifies surgical wounds per policy. (PNDS I22)

- Collaborates in fluid management. (PNDS I23)
- Provides status report to family/support person. (PNDS I109)

5. **Performs activities that demonstrate nursing accountability.**
   - Respects patient rights and practices within ethical and legal guidelines. (PNDS I116)
   - Completes required competencies and training in assigned timeframe.
   - Performs QI activities in conjunction with department leadership.
   - Demonstrates the ability to process through to solution a variety of problems.
   - Exercises safe judgment in decision making and demonstrates tact and understanding when dealing with patients, team members, members of other disciplines, and the public. (PNDS I92)
   - Demonstrates flexibility and adaptability to changes in nursing practice and responds in a positive manner to constructive criticism.

6. **Safely and adequately provides and utilizes equipment and supplies based on patient needs.**
   - Minimizes the length of invasive procedure by planning care; anticipates needs for equipment and supplies and selects in an organized and timely manner. (PNDS I85)
   - Uses supplies and equipment within safe parameters by ensuring all equipment is functioning before use and removing malfunctioning equipment from use. (PNDS I122)
   - Implements protective measures to prevent injury due to electrical, laser, radiation, chemical, thermal, or mechanical sources. (PNDS I72 through I77)
   - Uses supplies and equipment in a judicious and cost-effective manner and documents utilization.
   - Records devices implanted during the operative or invasive procedure. (PNDS I112)

7. **Evaluates patient outcomes.**
   - Evaluates for s/s of injury related to chemical, electrical, thermal, or mechanical sources. (PNDS I36-I38, I41, I43)
   - Evaluates for s/s of injury as a result of positioning or pt transfer/transport. (PNDS I38, I42)
   - Evaluates response to pain management interventions. (PNDS I54)

8. **Participates in the professional development of self and team members.**
   - Actively participates in educating and mentoring colleagues and team members to the job or team duties.
   - Participates in professional organization and/or performs educational inservicing for team members.
   - Creates a positive learning environment for new team members.
   - Utilizes knowledge and skill to facilitate warranted change.

ELECTRONIC PERIOPERATIVE RECORD

Below are two sample screens from an electronic perioperative record using PNDS. The appearance of an electronic record is significantly different from the traditional paper record. The structural design of individual software systems and facility preference further enhances the look of the electronic perioperative record. The example below demonstrates the application and documentation of the nursing process using PNDS. Referring to Outcome O5, "The patient is free from signs and symptoms of injury related to positioning" (pages 41-42), note that intervention I127, "Verifies presence of prosthetics or corrective devices," was completed in the preoperative phase (**Figure B-1**) and the correlating intraoperative interventions are documented in **Figure B-2** with the following PNDS interventions:

- I96 Positions the patient.
- I11 Applies safety devices.
- I38 Evaluates for signs and symptoms of injury as a result of positioning.

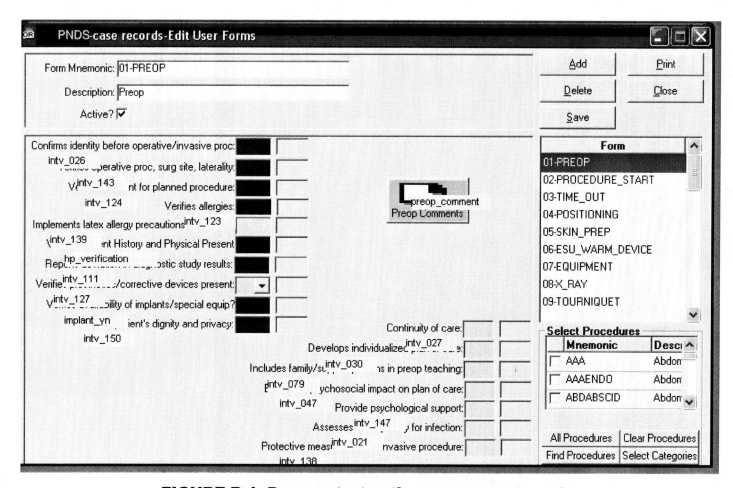

FIGURE B-1. Demonstrates the assessments and verifications completed preoperatively.

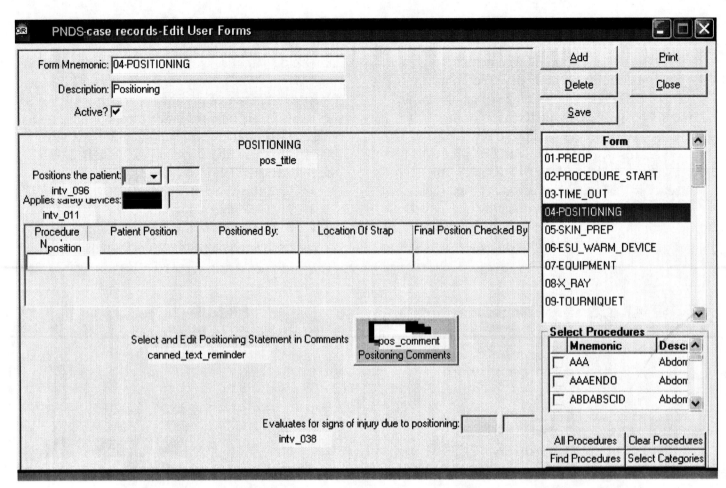

FIGURE B-2. Demonstrates the intraoperative application.

Screen samples reprinted with permission from Sisters of Charity, Leavenworth Health System.

Index to PNDS Revised Second Edition

Outcome Topics in Alphabetical Order

NOTE: **For the complete coding document containing the PNDS Domains, Outcomes, Nursing Diagnoses, and Interventions in numerical order, see Chapter 3, "The Conceptual Framework of the PNDS."**